Critical Thinking in Nursing

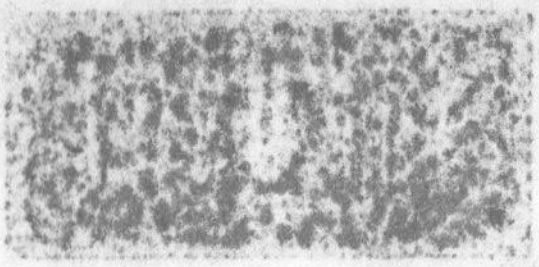

Critical Thinking in Nursing

Elsie L. Bandman, R.N., Ed.D., FAAN
Professor of Nursing
Hunter-Bellevue School of Nursing
Hunter College of the City University of New York
New York, New York

Bertram Bandman, Ph.D.
Professor of Philosophy
Brooklyn Campus, Long Island University
Brooklyn, New York

APPLETON & LANGE
Norwalk, Connecticut/San Mateo, California

0-8385-1330-1

Notice: The author(s) and publisher of this volume have taken care that the information and recommendations contained herein are accurate and compatible with the standards generally accepted at the time of publication.

88 89 90 91 92 / 10 9 8 7 6 5 4 3 2 1

Prentice-Hall International (UK) Limited, *London*
Prentice-Hall of Australia Pty. Limited, *Sydney*
Prentice-Hall Canada, Inc., *Toronto*
Prentice-Hall Hispanoamericana, S.A., *Mexico*
Prentice-Hall of India Private Limited, *New Delhi*
Prentice-Hall of Japan, Inc., *Tokyo*
Simon & Schuster Asia Pte. Ltd., *Singapore*
Editora Prentice-Hall do Brasil Ltda., *Rio de Janeiro*
Prentice Hall, *Englewood Cliffs, New Jersey*

Library of Congress Cataloging-in-Publication Data
Bandman, Elsie L.
Critical thinking in nursing / Elsie L. Bandman, Bertram Bandman.
p. cm.
Includes index.
ISBN 0-8385-1330-1
1. Nursing—Philosophy. 2. Critical thinking. 3. Reasoning.
I. Bandman, Bertram. II. Title.
[DNLM: 1. Cognition. 2. Nursing. 3. Philosophy, Nursing.
4. Thinking. WY 86 B214c]
RT84.5.B36 1988
610.73—dc19
DNLM/DLC
for Library of Congress 88–11625
CIP

Production Editor: Tim Condon
Designer: Steve M. Byrum

PRINTED IN THE UNITED STATES OF AMERICA

TO

ERNA BANDMANN,
A bright, vital, caring person who shall be greatly missed (1908–1988).

NANCY BANDMAN, Our daughter,
For her loving, good-humored, continuing support.

Contents

Part III: Structures of Argument in Nursing

Preface

Purpose

The purpose of this book is to identify and strengthen the critical thinking skills of nurses by demonstrating the role of scientific reasoning, logic, and philosophy in increasing the effectiveness of the nursing process, and everyday nursing decisions. Included in this work are aspects of deductive and inductive arguments, informal and formal reasoning relevant to nursing process, practice, and theory. Its use enhances the critical, analytical skills of the learner in thinking through problems perceived as unsolvable, fearful, detestable or obvious. The reader will see how critical thinking applies the use of systematic reasoning to the clarification of problems. Students, nurse practitioners, educators, managers, and researchers who practice critical thinking and use logic will enhance their conceptual acuity.

Nursing practice, education, research and administration are significant to the health and well being of all people. Therefore, nurses who create and generate these activities will benefit from the critical examination of the basic assumptions and presuppositions of their work. The arguments on which decisions of allocation of personal, material, and financial resources are made calls for critical scrutiny.

Organization and Content

Part I, The Uses of Argument in Nursing, is the first of three major themes around which the book is organized. This part includes chapters on critical thinking in nursing, the functions of nursing arguments and fallacies in reasoning. Part II, The Dynamics of Practical Arguments, includes chapters on the role of critical thinking in scientific reasoning, in the use of the nursing process, in decision making, and in resolving controversial moral issues. Part III, The Structures of Argument, includes three chapters on deductive reasoning and three chapters on inductive reasoning. The deductive reasoning chapters introduce patterns of deduction and apply classical syllogistic and modern symbolic reasoning to nursing problems. The three inductive chapters are concerned with induction and analogies, cause–effect relations, and the role of evidence and probability judgments in nursing. The work concludes with a summary of the values of critical thinking in science and in nursing. There are nearly 300 exercises with answers interspersed throughout, and a glossary of key terms to facilitate the student's engagement with the content. Graduate students will benefit by critically examining the arguments on which they base their life's work.

The book has been organized for use as the basis of a single course on critical thinking or as a supplementary text in major clinical courses. It can be used at the undergraduate level to teach beginning scientific reasoning and nursing process or at the graduate level to teach beginning logic and scientific reasoning to students in all clinical specialties. The contents are practical and immediately applicable to problems of a professional and personal nature. The process of critical thinking is specific, universal, and timeless in its application.

Acknowledgments

To produce a text on critical thinking applied to nursing—the first we believe—has been an arduous task. Without Marion Kalstein-Welch's unflagging editorial support, enthusiasm, and encouragement, the work would not have been possible. We are deeply appreciative to Tim Condon and Danielle Ponsolle for their splendid editorial assistance. The support of our respective institutions was also significant. The Trustee Awards Committee on Research and Released Time of the Brooklyn Campus of Long Island University enabled Bert to pursue research on this topic for a part of each semester for three years. Robert D. Spector, Director of the Humanities Division gave support and encouragement for Bert's research, as did Kenneth Bernard of the English Department of Long Island University's Brooklyn Campus. Dean Evelyn C. Gioiella of the Hunter-Bellevue School of Nursing of Hunter College of the City University of New York granted release time for part of two semesters to Elsie to attend a Faculty Development Course on Critical Thinking at the Graduate Center. The teacher of this course Professor Lewis M. Schwartz and Professor Richard L. Mendelsohn, co-author of the book *Basic Logic,* had an important effect on our work. To each, our dean, our director, and our teachers, we are profoundly grateful for their assistance. To our early reviewers, we say "Many thanks. Your reviews were instrumental to developing this book." Because this is the first critical thinking book for nurses, your comments are appreciated. We hope it will encourage others to think critically about nursing.

Reviewers

Anna Marie Brock, Ph.D., R.N.
Villa Marie College
Erie, Pennsylvania

Leah Gorman, Ed.D., R.N.
Emory University
Atlanta, Georgia

Hesook Suzie Kim, Ph.D., R.N.
University of Rhode Island
Providence, Rhode Island

Dee Putzier, Ph.D., R.N.
University of Oregon
Portland, Oregon

Nell Hodgson Wodruff, SON
Emory University
Atlanta, Georgia

Part I
USES OF ARGUMENT IN NURSING

Chapter 1

Use of Critical Thinking in Nursing

Study of this chapter enables the learner to:

1. Define the goals, processes, methods, and significance of critical thinking.
2. Identify important uses of language in nursing.
3. Use criteria of critical thinking to evaluate the uses of language in nursing.
4. Distinguish between vagueness and ambiguity in the use of language.
5. Analyze the difference between factual and verbal disputes.
6. Differentiate between lexical, stipulative, theoretical, and persuasive definitions.
7. Distinguish definitions from value judgments and slogans.
8. Apply methods of evaluation to uses of language in nursing.

INTRODUCTION

Why think critically? To think critically is to show that we are aware and reflective of our place in the world, in relation to things, events, and other people. To think critically is to examine assumptions, beliefs, propositions, and the meaning and uses of words, statements, and arguments. By clarifying both the means and ends of living, critical thinking helps to focus and sharpen awareness.

Critical thinking is of practical assistance in nursing. By defining the conditions under which sound and valid conclusions are drawn, critical thinking facilitates the use of the nursing process. Critical thinking is a liberating force in all human thoughtful activity, but especially to nurses for whom this book is intended. The habitual use of criteria and procedures of critical thinking helps us reason more effectively in all aspects of life and work.

Nursing is in a state of change; active in defining its theory, practice, and social mandate and critical toward its current status. Some nursing texts present knowledge from a singular, monolithic, concrete point of view. Such an approach eliminates the possibility of doubt, questioning, inquiry, curiosity, examination, or consideration of alternatives.[1] Critical thinking offers methods to transform students into "active participants in their own intellectual growth."[2] On an open-ended view, "education is training in how to think rather than in what to think; it is a confrontation, a dialogue between ways of assessing evidence and supporting conclusions."[3]

According to Thomas Kuhn, change occurs only when a field is in turmoil.[4] The nursing profession is experiencing distress and pressure from within and without regarding its purposes, educational preparation, practice, roles, theory, research, and in its relation to medicine. This is, therefore, an auspicious time in which to use canons of critical thinking and logic to inquire openly into the assumptions, beliefs, goals, and values that characterize nursing. The aim of this text is to facilitate conscious, systematic reasoning based on logical, philosophical principles and modes of inquiry. Critical thinking helps us to decide what really matters, what is important.

CRITICAL THINKING—THE CURRENT STATE OF THE ART

Definitions of critical thinking variously emphasize its goals, its process, its methodology, its essential characteristics, or its scope. R. Ennis emphasizes the focus of critical thinking as "deciding what to believe or . . . do" based on "reasonable, reflective thinking . . . ."[5] Harvey Siegel defines critical thinking as being "appropriately moved by reasons and . . . to generate and seek out good reasons."[6] For Ennis, belief and action are connected, but are preceded by thinking through reflectively about what to do and what to believe. According to Ennis, critical thinking must fit or relate to the context. In contrast, Trudy Govier defines critical thinking in a narrow, technical way as "thinking about another product of thought (an argument, claim, theory, definition, question, problem (hypothesis), a comparison, synthesis, simplification, and much else, in a special, skeptically deliberative, evaluative way."[7] This definition implies that critical thinking is a process of evaluating cognitive products and processes. J. Anthony Blair identifies critical thinking as "an activity, whereas informal logic has a subject matter . . . critical thinking applies to a lot more than arguments, . . . the central focus of informal logic is argument."[8] Blair views the usefulness of critical thinking as threefold:

> First, there are certain concepts, tools or mechanisms that can be, and indeed must be, employed everywhere, regardless of the subject matter or content. . . . Second, the vocabulary of criticism contains terms which have general application, even if the specifics of their application vary from field to field. . . . Third, certain habits of mind or disposition, and various habits of critical reaction, can transfer from one subject to another.[9]

According to Blair, "argumentation belongs at the center of critical thinking, as a *sine qua non* of the enterprise."[10]

Richard Paul makes a distinction between a narrow, weak sense and a broad, strong sense of critical thinking. He regards the conception of critical thinking in the narrow, weak sense as skills that can be tacked onto other learning, but remain extrinsic or external to the character of the person. In the broad, strong sense of critical thinking, Paul views critical thinking skills as integrated within the individual with insight into the thinking and feeling processes and further emphasizes critical thinking skills as essential to the "free, rational, autonomous mind."[11] He sees the narrow aspect of critical thinking as consisting of formal, inductive, and informal logic. His broad interpretation consists of the extension of logic to the rational examination of controversial social, ethical, political, economic, and religious issues, such as abortion, euthanasia, and terrorism.

Paul divides all issues into monological issues (having one logic or a single structure of rationality) or multilogical issues (having more than one logic, or alternative structures of rationality). The monological system prevails when one set of rules defines the system, such as in a game of chess, contract bridge, international lawn tennis, or Olympic foot races. Nurses who practice in a health care system that operates only on a medical model, with medical rules of evidence and diagnosis are in a monological system. Nurses who practice in a system that recognizes and supports two competing and also complementary frames of reference, the medical model and the nursing model of using evidence and diagnosing, are in a multilogical system. Almost every important issue and system is multilogical. Yet, nurses, physicians, and most people are trained for a monological world and thrown into one that is multilogical. Nurses and physicians, in particular, need to be trained to identify and analyze health care issues from the perspective of more than one point of view, to reconstruct those points of view and to argue for those issues that they actively oppose as an example of critical thinking.

A nurse, for example, assigned to care for a client with acquired immune deficiency syndrome (AIDS) may be actively and intensely repelled by all that this illness implies. This nurse may be fearful of catching the infection through nursing contact with bodily fluids. This nurse may sense that this person may be facing imminent death; the nurse is forced to confront issues of human fragility and the powerlessness of science to cure this dreaded disease. The nurse may be ethnocentric, identifying only with her own culture in agreeing with traditional religious beliefs that are biased against homosexuality. Some religious believers regard disease as punishment for evil deeds. The critical thinker will view this situation from the point of multilogical issues. One issue is that of AIDS as a contagion based on scientific evidence of disease etiology and communicability. A second issue is that of sexual preference from the perspective of psychosocial theories of human development. A third issue is that of the nursing code of ethics respecting persons irrespective of the nature of the health problem. Using a multilogical system, the nurse reflects and analyzes the reasons underlying each issue from a different frame of reference. The critical thinker views AIDS as a communicable disease that can be contained by specific precautions related to sexual practices, body fluids, transfusions, the use of needles, and pregnancy. The nurse assesses the situation from multiple points of view.

Nurses operating under a monological frame are not able to examine the implications and evidence of their view, able to argue against it, or able to construct a different point of view based on the use of critical thinking; they are unable to make a fundamental change requiring a new frame of reference. These nurses see the world from only one perspective and are unaware of the variety of existing differences and possibilities.

CRITICAL THINKING IN EDUCATION

Siegel discusses the role of critical thinking in education and sees critical thinking to be an educational ideal. He views the important issue not to be the question of whether or not there is a generalized skill of critical thinking but rather inquiry surrounding the ways critical thinking manifests itself. Siegel takes the position that critical thinking is "both subject specific . . . and general."[12] We concur with his view and argue for it here.

Siegel identifies three imperatives for teaching critical thinking. First, to teach critical thinking is to facilitate students' self-sufficiency and autonomy, to help students "to act and judge . . . on the basis of . . . a reasoned appraisal of the matter at hand."[13] This is incompatible with any educational program that aims to prepare students for a preconceived slot or role without active participation in those arrangements.[14] To treat students with respect means to recognize their rights to use independent judgment and evaluation on the basis of honest reasons and explanations that are questioned, challenged, and justified.[15]

Siegel's second imperative for teaching critical thinking is to "empower the student to control his or her own destiny . . . to encourage them to ask questions, to look for evidence, to seek and scrutinize alternatives, to be critical of their own ideas as well as those of others."[16] Such persons are liberated because they are free of the control of unjustified beliefs and attitudes that cannot be supported.[17] Such persons are able to take charge of their own lives.[18]

Siegel's third imperative for supporting critical thinking as an ideal is to promote rationality as the use of reasons.[19] A scientific researcher identifies and selects "what counts as a good reason for or against some hypothesis, theory, or procedure,"[20] how much weight to give it and how to appraise it in terms of other reasons that seem relevant. The researcher works within the tradition of science that holds to standards and principles that are evolving, but that are impartial and universal in application, for the appraisal of reasons.[21]

DEFINITION OF CRITICAL THINKING FOR NURSING

Critical thinking is defined in this text as the rational examination of ideas, inferences, assumptions, principles, arguments, conclusions, issues, statements, beliefs, and actions. This examination covers scientific reasoning, includes the nursing process, decision making, and reasoning in controversial issues. The four types of reasoning that comprise critical thinking are deductive, inductive, informal or everyday, and practical. To elaborate on this initial definition, critical thinking is reasoning in which we analyze the use of language, formulate problems, clarify and explicate assumptions, weigh evidence, evaluate conclusions, discriminate between good and bad arguments, and seek to justify those facts and values that result in credible beliefs and actions. We may further particularize this definition by providing the following checklist of critical thinking functions in nursing.

1. Use the processes of critical thinking in all of daily living.
2. Discriminate among the uses and misuses of language in nursing.
3. Identify and formulate nursing problems.[22]
4. Analyze meanings of terms in relation to their indication, their cause or purpose, and their significance.
5. Analyze arguments and issues into premises and conclusions.
6. Examine nursing assumptions.
7. Report data and clues accurately.
8. Make and check inferences based on data, making sure that the inferences are, at least, plausible.
9. Formulate and clarify beliefs.
10. Verify, corroborate, and justify claims, beliefs, conclusions, decisions, and actions.

11. Give relevant reasons for beliefs and conclusions.
12. Formulate and clarify value judgments.
13. Seek reasons, criteria, and principles that effectively justify value judgments.
14. Evaluate the soundness of conclusions.

THREE MODELS OF TEACHING AND LEARNING CRITICAL THINKING IN NURSING

By way of an overview, three models help orient the teaching and learning of critical thinking in nursing.[23] Adapted from the context of teaching, they are the Feeling model, the Vision model, and the Examination model.

The Feeling model emphasizes feelings, impressions, and data, the given. Feelings call for observation, sensitivity, care, concern, alertness for vital signs, symptoms, and clues, and attention to a patient's state of mind. The Feeling model includes "hands on" nursing. But feelings are not enough. We also need ideas, vision, and insight into those feelings, impressions, and data.

The Vision model is used to generate a pattern of thought, to organize and interpret feelings, to assemble a patient's data, and to formulate a hypothesis, an inference, a guess, an idea about the patient's health care problem. To engage in critical thinking is to search for insightful principles and rules that may guide appropriate responses to the expressions of both the nurse's and the patient's feelings.

But even the best hypotheses can be wrong. There is a need to test the ideas and hypotheses a nurse formulates. Consequently, the Examination model is used to reflect on the ideas, insights, and visions. Nurses examine their ideas with the help of relevant criteria, referred to by philosopher L. Wittgenstein (1891–1952) as "outer criteria." According to Wittgenstein, "an inner process is in need of outer criteria."[24] Nurses use the Examination model to search for appropriate rules of inference, investigation, testing, inspecting, verification, confirmation, corroboration, and justification. These models provide a framework for teaching students how to think critically. Skills, habits, ability, and attitudes are all involved in critical thinking, and in the appropriate use of these models.

The role of critical thinking in nursing means movement from freedom of expression to an enriched freedom of reasoned restraints. The rules of inference say in effect, "If you want to think critically and reason correctly, then follow these rules and guideposts." Critical thinking in nursing consists in sharpening the distinctions between certainty, near certainty, and degrees of uncertainty. A nurse learns to discriminate by understanding and observing appropriate criteria.

USES OF LANGUAGE IN NURSING

To think is to use language. Nurses use language to make inferences, to corroborate inferences, and to communicate ideas, thoughts, information, facts, feelings, beliefs, and attitudes. To think critically is to use language reflectively. Nurses think critically by reflecting on their ideas, beliefs, and feelings. Nurses think critically by asking challenging questions, questioning assumptions, assessing, investigating, inquiring, and solving complex health care problems.

To impose organization out of the various uses of language in nursing, we can identify five main types of language use. The first type seeks to inform and consists of true or false propositions that can be verified. A second use of language is expression of feelings and attitudes, and is neither true nor false. A third use of language is its directive function; it is used for implementing a nursing plan or initiating a nursing action. A fourth use consists in asking questions. Questions have various functions: to collect or request information; to express doubts, wonder, or bewilderment, as in "Oh, how can that really be true?;" to probe, investigate, examine, inaugurate research; to formulate a problem to be solved; or to seek reassurance. A fifth use of language consists of conditionals or subjunctives, such as the expression of regret or recrimination. For example, "If I hadn't smoked all these years, I would not need to have a lung removed." Conditional judgments are also used as indicatives, as in the statement "If I do X for my patient, then my patient will have effect Y, which we both desire."

There are overlaps between these uses of language; however, we can single out five—directive, informative, expressive, interrogative, and conditional—as major uses of language in nursing.

Directive Use of Language

In the directive use of language we consider whether giving an order is useful for the goal intended. For example:

> Teach the client foods to avoid while taking anticoagulants.[25] Lanoxin 0.125 mg qd is prescribed along with the directive to count apical pulse before every medication. Give Lanoxin 0.125 mg at 8 AM qd if pulse above 60 beats per minute.[26]

This or any other medical prescription may be evaluated by considering its appropriateness and accuracy.

Informative Use of Language

In contrast, the informative function of language in nursing is fairly easy to evaluate. The criteria of truth and falsity, validity and invalidity are used by appealing to relevant evidence or to formal rules of logic or mathematics. An example of appeal to relevant evidence follows.

> Digibind . . . draws digoxin molecules away from receptor sites and binds with them to reverse digoxin toxicity. The drug . . . is for use against severe, otherwise intractable cases of digoxin toxicity. In trials with more than 150 patients, toxicity often was reversed completely within four hours and arrhythmias were abolished in some cases in as little as 30 minutes.[27]

Expressive Use of Language

A more complicated issue is in the use of standards of critical thinking to evaluate the expressive and directive uses of language in nursing. If linguistic expressions achieve the intended goal, then such expressions are effective. For example, announcing "Fire" over the hospital loudspeaker system is effective if measures are taken to evacuate the patients and visitors, and to control the fire and safeguard lives. Judging a language use in relation to its intended goal is called the *pragmatic test.*

In connection with the expressive use of language, problems arise because of people's diverging interests and values. People disagree about whether the quality of life is more important than its length; criteria for judging quality of life; and who is most suited to judge the quality of life.

Interrogative and Conditional Uses of Language

One also uses interrogatives, as in "Why did Jones, in Room 304, expire suddenly?" and conditionals, as in, "If I give Ms. Smith digitalis as prescribed, then her cardiac symptoms will be relieved."

Exercises

1. How many uses of language are there?
   Answer: Multiple uses, as many as there are activities of life.
2. Identify the different uses of language in these passages:
   a. "First, I would like to know what medications he was on."
      Answer: Indirect command, stating, "Tell me the medication he is on."
   b. "The patient is on digoxin 0.25 mg qd, HCTZ 50 mg bid, KCl 20 mEq bid, prednisone 40 mg qd, Theodor 300 mg qid."
      Answer: Informative use.
   c. What's his blood pressure?
      Answer: Question and indirect command: "Tell me his blood pressure."
   d. 140/90.
      Answer: Informative.[28]

Mixed Uses of Language

Words, phrases, sentences, and paragraphs may have mixed meanings. Language communicates information, expresses attitudes, directs behavior, and calls for action. To say "The ice is thin" is both descriptive and warns a skater about the ice. This use of language prescribes as well. A nurse's statement over the loudspeaker, "Visiting hours are over" both informs visitors and directs them to leave. The language of nursing has informative, directive, and expressive functions (Table 1–1).

If nurses communicate directly with patients in an effort to coerce them to comply with a regimen, they might use this approach. In general, nurses do not transmit information in such a blunt fashion with any expectation that it will be accepted. For our purposes, however, effective communication may consist of combining functions of language, as illustrated in this example.

Emotive Use of Words

We may use different words to convey pro, con, or neutral attitudes. Bertrand Russell, quoted by I. Copi, cites this amusing example to illustrate how one can use words to reflect feelings or attitudes toward others.

> I am firm; you are obstinate; he is a pig-headed fool.
> I have reconsidered it; you have changed your mind; he has gone back on his word.[29]

A nursing example is:

> I give individualized care; you are inefficient; she is slow and disorganized.

Some other examples are:

> I am a nursing practitioner; you are a bedside nurse; she is a physician's handmaiden.
> I am a sanitation technician; you are a refuse collector; he is a garbage man.

TABLE 1-1. FIVE FUNCTIONS OF LANGUAGE

Directive and interrogative	Nurse: "Wouldn't you like to take your insulin, follow your diet, and test your urine as I've taught you?"
Informative and conditional	Because, if you don't, you may develop diabetic coma or complications such as stroke, heart and kidney failure, blindness, or gangrene of your extremities.
Expressive and conditional	I assume that you want to avoid these conditions, since you enjoy your life and want to go on living.

The point to recognize is that we can use emotionally charged words to suit our purpose. Critical thinking is necessary to recognize that words can be used to express different attitudes; and that language can be emotive and not provide a way to decide what is rational or irrational.

Exercises

1. Give three conjugations of verbs of your own in and outside nursing: (a) Use the first person, *I,* in conjugation to make yourself look good; use a second person pronoun, *you,* to characterize another person neutrally; and use a third person pronoun to characterize a derogatory situation or person.
2. Take a passage from a poem and translate it into ordinary literal language.
3. Take an editorial from *Nursing Research,* the *American Journal of Nursing, Nursing Management,* or *Nursing Outlook* and identify three emotionally charged words in each editorial; then re-express them.

If–Then Use of Language

The *if–then* use of language is worthy of special attention. Medical directives and nursing actions, including the use of the phases of the nursing process, are examples of a critical thinking model identified as an if–then model. Here, the *if* states the antecedent, assumptions, premises. The if can be used to state the health care goals, priorities, problems, obstacles, and resources. The *then* or *therefore* can be used to state the nursing action, intervention, drug treatment, or policy intended to solve the problem. We can also use if to state the intervention, the means, in a means–ends analysis, where the if cites the indicated treatment and the then states the hoped for or expected outcome, such as restoration of a patient's health.

The if–then model is also used in nursing diagnosis, as in "If the patient is immobile and elderly, and has poor nutrition, then the probability of decubitus is 95 percent."[30] The if–then form of reasoning, when applied to practical problems, is called the use of hypothetical imperatives. A nursing example of a hypothetical imperative is: If you want to prevent decubitus in an elderly, immobile, malnourished patient, then improve his or her nutrition and regularly change his or her position to avoid pressure areas.

Even after using the if–then reasoning, there may be ifs or assumptions that have to be decided before taking the needed nursing action. For example, if a staff nurse meets all of the nursing needs of her first patient of the day, she may never have sufficient time to give needed care to other patients. There are all sorts of open-ended value aspects and complications, involving competing demands and limited resources. There are, consequently, difficulties in adequately assessing hypothetical forms of if–then uses of language.

Use of If–Then to Make First- and Second-Order Changes

One form of if–then thinking is illustrated by Watzlawick's distinction between first- and second-order changes.

One interpretation of Watzlawick's first-order change is as follows: A medical prescription of Lanoxin 0.125 mg qd for a cardiovascular action is a first-order change. Changes that fit within the if–then reasoning, where the goals of change are acceptable, are first-order changes.[31] First-order changes use conventional means to achieve prior, agreed upon goals. Such if–then or means–ends changes are successful if they achieve the goals they are designed to achieve. Such changes occur "within a specific frame . . . which excludes undesirable outcomes."[32] Traditional nursing was based on strict compliance with physicians' orders and institutional policy on the assumption that if the nurse obeyed the commands of expert physicians and administrators, then nursing care would be accurate and appropriate. The language of nursing was likewise used to achieve traditional medical goals. The language of orders and obedience was judged within this first-order frame. As the first-order change frame showed that the command–obedience model of physician–nurse relations did not work as effectively as shared decision making, the traditional model gave way to newer forms of authority relationships. But the newer model was nevertheless oriented by the first-order change model. Within this model, it even worked best to have more decision making placed in the hands of patients than the previous command–obedience model provided for.

Within first-order changes, there is sometimes the illusion of choice. For example, a nurse may ask a patient, "Would you like your enema or your injection first?" or "Do you want your dressing changed now or later?" These questions offer an illusion of choice because the patient is not expected to refuse any nursing measure. Health professionals commonly assume that because the patient voluntarily entered the hospital, this implies the voluntary agreement to each and every procedure.

Watzlawick points to the commonality in these interventions. Unwanted alternatives are excluded in this first-order frame; options are ruled out. If the issue is that of helping the patient to rise and walk either in the morning or afternoon, the first-order frame restricts options.

In contrast, second-order changes require reframing. An everyday example of reframing is that of a bottle that is half-filled. The optimist sees the bottle as half full. The pessimist sees the same bottle as half empty. These are the same first-order realities, but viewed as "two very different world images, creating two very different (second-order) 'realities.' "[33] This example of reframing supports Watzlawick's contention that "we never deal with reality per se, but with images of reality—that is, with interpretations. While the number of potentially possible interpretations is very large, our world image usually permits us to see only one—and this one therefore appears to be the only possible, reasonable, and permitted view . . . (and) suggests only one possible, reasonable, and permitted solution, and if we don't succeed at first we try and try again . . . we resort to the recipe of doing more of the same."[34] There is a resistance to second-order change, even though reframing a situation with a new way of seeing relationships may help resolve a difficulty.

If critical thinking in the form of reframing is successful, it gives the situation a new meaning that is more convincing and appropriate than the previous form of thinking about a situation. A nursing example is the nurse explaining the importance of, and the discomfort associated with, a particular diagnostic procedure. The patient only sees the possibility of refusing it, because it is painful, or the patient accepts the procedure and the pain that goes with it. The nurse reframes the situation by explaining that the patient is under no obligation to like the procedure or the care provider, and should complain loudly in response to all pain and demand alleviation of the pain.

The nurse who uses language to think critically about nursing judgments, activities, and human rights, tends to be an advocate of patients' and nurses' rights to question, refuse, or terminate the continuation of existing activities or policies. The introduction of patients' and nurses' rights reframes a situation and provides an example of a second-order change in nursing.

In a second-order change, major assumptions in the first-order frame are questioned. Economic constraints in health care, for example, may require that nursing providers make sweeping second-order changes in practice and education. One example is for nurses to develop and manage independent, home health services and long-term care facilities.

In the language of means–ends relationships used earlier, examples of first-order changes are to determine how soon to discharge the patient after uncomplicated surgery, such as an appendectomy or a herniorraphy. A second-order change is to question the ends and purposes of any action. A second-order change includes deciding whether to resuscitate or treat a patient with a hopeless prognosis; or to do all routine surgery on an ambulatory basis, or to make all long-term care facilities nonprofit. First-order change presents a means–ends question and second-order change involves the justification of ends. In the rational order of things, second-order change comes first or has priority. But in dealing with the language of second-order change, we again meet open-ended values without rationally acceptable criteria for settling disagreements about ends.

The Manifest–Latent Distinction

To apply critical thinking to the use of nursing language is to make relevant distinctions in the use of language. Watzlawick's distinction between first- and second-order changes implies that the way we send a message is also important. His distinction is similar to the one developed by Robert Merton.[35] He distinguishes between the manifest functions of a hospital or nurse, such as care of the sick, and the latent or hidden functions of a hospital or nurse, such as self-maintenance activities.

On the manifest level, a nurse who is asked by a patient why a preoperative saline enema is given has only to answer that it was ordered or that the colon needs to be clean before the operation. But a nurse, who is intellectually trained, skillful and sensitive, caring and thoughtful, is aware of the possibility of the latent function of the question, namely deep anxiety about the immediate and long-term consequences of the surgery.

The nurse who engages in critical thinking will be aware of the manifest and latent functions of nurse–patient relationships. To fulfill the latent functions of patient care calls for more knowledge, training, skills, and the formation of beliefs and attitudes other than the manifest functions call for. The manifest–latent distinction along with the first-order and second-order distinction give added perspectives to the multiple uses of language.

Summary of Uses of Language

Appropriate uses of language are vital to effective thought and action in nursing. The use of critical thinking is essential to evaluate the uses of language in problem solving. Language and thought are inseparable. One cannot function without the other.

Various uses of language are the primary means for the communication of ideas, thoughts, beliefs, feelings, and attitudes. Critical reflection about the uses of language in nursing helps the nurse to evaluate the content of communication apart from its emotive, directive and informative, interrogative and conditional aspects.

MEANING AND DEFINITION IN NURSING

A major use of language in nursing is the specification of meaning and definition. It is essential to know the meaning of the terms used as a condition of effective communication.

The term *meaning* itself may have several meanings. It is an indication or an implication of a state of affairs. Lots of rainfall may mean that a farmer will reap a bumper crop. If the rain falls at the wrong time, however, it may mean disaster to the farmer's crop. Similarly, cues or clues, such as the pitting edema of a patient's ankles, may indicate or mean worsening of a heart condition.

A second meaning is in asking for the cause or effect, as in "What do the footprints in the sand mean?"[36] Or one may ask, "What do those red, raised spots on this patient's body mean?"

A third meaning refers to intention or purpose. For example, one nurse may ask another, "What was the meaning of your telling the patient to ignore the physician's prescription?"

A fourth meaning refers to implication or significance,[37] as when a nurse asks, "What is the meaning of my involvement with dying patients?" or "What is the meaning of keeping these irreversibly and terminally ill, comatose patients alive on a respirator in an intensive care unit?"

Nurses are not alone in looking for the meaning of life, the meaning of significant relationships, and the meaning of events in patients' health histories. We seek meanings of all kinds. We seek meanings in work and love relations, in the scheme of things, such as the meaning of life, in tragedy and in happiness. To engage in critical thinking is to pursue meaning. We find and form meanings by using and by reflecting on uses of language.

Definitions to Help Search for Meaning

Instruction is helpful to function effectively in the uses of language. To explain the meaning of a word is to understand precise rules for using the word. The rules governing the use of a word are the rules that define the word. A definition limits the meaning of a word; it includes some meanings and excludes others. For example, an ambulance is a vehicle designed to carry a patient in a prone position on a stretcher. By distinguishing an ambulance from an ambulette or bus for wheelchair or ambulatory patients, we achieve a more precise use of language. A nursing student learns precision in distinguishing various medication essential to the proper treatment of patients. Likewise definitions offer sharpened discriminations between various terms. Meaning is clarified by defining terms or by sharpening their usages. Definitions delineate boundaries around concepts, including some things while excluding others. For example, a human female is defined as one with specific reproductive organs, hormones, and processes that exclude male humans in that definition.

Vagueness and Ambiguity

One distinction made in the use of language is between vagueness and ambiguity. A term is *vague* if we have no way of knowing exactly its reference. Words or expressions, such as life, ability, competence, young, old, game, working too slowly, having too many patients, having a troublesome patient, or being burnt out, are vague. In some contexts, vagueness may not matter. But in other contexts, vagueness may prevent the achievement of one's purpose. A term is vague if we have no way of knowing the "cutoff point" between the application and nonapplication of that term or expression. For example, a patient may be "alive," but comatose and completely dependent on a respirator, or be nearly well. A physician or a nurse may have "ability," but the term lacks a clear cutoff point for judging among those with ability. The patient in the next room may be "old," but old may cover a 50-year span from 45 to 95. A nurse may work "too fast," "too slowly," or have "too many patients." But this can only be known if the context makes it clear what it means to work too fast, too slowly, or have too many patients. In contrast, no such question arises for deciding when a woman is pregnant.

A term is *ambiguous* if one is not sure which of several possible meanings applies to that term. For example, one nurse says abortion is murder, whereas another nurse says abortion is the right to decide what to do about one's own body. Similarly, two nurses may disagree about the *definition of death,* whether death means circulatory and respiratory failure or brain death. The term *brain death* may be defined as the loss of all those functions that characterize humanness or complete cessation of all brain activity. Dilemmas as to whether to save a given patient or perform a particular procedure may rest on resolving just such an ambiguity, in which we are unsure which of two meanings to apply to a term. Whether or not to call an RN without a baccalaureate degree a professional nurse, may be based on an ambiguous meaning of professional nursing.

An advantage of ambiguities over vagueness is that in vagueness, we have to decide which of several meanings applies. In ambiguity, we have to decide which of two meanings to apply. The use of both vague and ambiguous terms may lead to a dispute. One way to resolve a dispute is to clarify which of two or more meanings best clarifies the point at issue. Suppose that a nurse says, "This is the same patient I saw last week." There are two senses of "the same." One sense is that a person is essentially the same person she or he was last week. Another sense of a person is that she or he changed within the week, even though such a change may have been imperceptible. But on this second interpretation, the person in question is not the same person she or he was last week. We have to decide which of two meanings prevails in a given case. Similarly, a nurse may say, "I did everything I could to save Mrs. Jones, but she died anyway." Another nurse may respond, "You didn't try everything, since you didn't call for the resuscitation team." Each nurse is using "everything" in a different sense. Deciding which of two disputed senses is appropriate depends on which sense of the term best clarifies the meaning of the term within the context in dispute. For some uses of terms, an ambiguity remains unresolved, a stalemate.

A function of critical thinking is to distinguish vague from ambiguous terms, clarify their senses and determine which meaning is involved. If nurses are not getting a fair salary, that vagueness may be resolved into an ambiguity. The dispute may be about an institutional salary scale or fringe benefits package, or about the conditions of work, which are demanding and unpleasant, such as shift rotation. Once the meanings of terms are made clear, reducing the scope of vagueness may diminish the factors of the dispute and help make it resolvable.

Verbal and Factual Disputes

Another function of definitions is to help distinguish between verbal and factual disputes. If two nurses, A and B, argue over whether a certain medication is appropriate for a particular patient with a specific medical diagnosis, the specifications of that medication make that dispute a *factual* matter. If, however, two nurses, C and D, have a dispute as to whether a specific staff member is "creative" their dispute may well be *verbal.* If two other nurses, E and F, argue about their patient's level of wellness and functions, their dispute may be verbal unless they resort to specific tools of assessment and evaluation upon which they agree. Two nurses, G and H, may disagree as to whether a third nurse, J, is a good nurse. To resolve this dispute, they have to move the dispute from a vague to an ambiguous one. One nurse, G, may define a good nurse as one who makes nursing judgments independently of physicians. Nurse H, on the other hand, may define a good nurse as one who acts in cooperation with physicians' directives. Nurses G and H may then appeal to their preferred nursing theory. Nurse G may prefer M. Rogers' theory of nursing, whereas Nurse H may prefer an institutional assumption of the supremacy of the medical model. According to Rogers, "Nursing has no dependent functions, but, like all other professions, it has many collaborative ones."[38] Nurse H may disagree with this view.

Barbara Stevens cites several examples of terms defined differently by nursing theorists. Stevens refers to these as "commonplaces." These terms include *health, nursing acts,* and *patient.* According to Stevens:

> For one theory a patient may have to be a discrete person. Another theory may grant that the patient may be a group, community or organizational entity . . .[39] Similarly, 'nursing acts' may have different meanings for different theories. These may refer to cognitive acts, behavioral tasks, hands-on care only, or to nursing acts mediated through others (e.g., teaching and administration). 'Health,' similarly, has different meanings for different theorists. For some it represents a full continuum of states of being, ranging from illness to wellness. For other theorists, health only refers to ill health, arising only in a state of deficiency . . .[40]

Other terms that are either vague or ambiguous include *nursing theory, nursing process, problem-solving method, leadership, autonomy,* and *decision making.* Disputes between theorists regarding these important terms are not factual, but verbal. They are not easily resolved or perhaps even resolvable.

If two nurses disagree about their observations of blood in a patient's stool, careful testing for the presence of blood can settle their disagreement. But if two nurses disagree about the meaning of *nursing act,* one insisting that it requires knowledge, cognitive skills, appropriate values, and attitudes, and the other nurse arguing that a nursing act requires hands-on care, this is a verbal dispute. As such, it is not easily resolvable.

One may help clarify such disputes by distinguishing several senses to which a given term applies. Then these nurses will, at least, be clearer about what they are in dispute about. However, some "essentially contestable concepts" or intractable disputes remain, such as whether a ten-week-old fetus is an unborn person or primarily living tissue. Such differences result in either stalemate or some practical compromise.

One reason why some verbal disputes in nursing are more resistant to resolution than others is that some nursing concepts are based on tacit or latent political, ideological, metaphysical, religious, epistemological, and moral views or assumptions of broad human, societal, and cosmic proportions. These disputes need to be made explicit so that the verbal and factual assumptions embedded in them can be disentangled and discussed.

> Two nurses may disagree about abortion as follows:
> Abortion$_1$: The removal of a parasitic tissue from the uterine wall of a human female.
> Abortion$_2$: The murder of an innocent child for the selfish convenience of her/his mother.[41]

We cannot appeal to facts alone to resolve the abortion issue.

Although nursing theories do not exhibit a similar type of divergence, they, too, cannot be rationally resolved as easily as straightforward factual disputes. Nevertheless, a function of critical thinking is to attempt to resolve rationally or to dissolve verbal and factual disputes. One way is to make the meanings of disputed terms clearer. Another is to appeal to relevant evidence. Some issues, however, spill over into attitudinal and value disputes, such as the issue of abortion. Serious psychological or ideological difficulties may stand in the way of overcoming such differences.

Types of Definitions in Nursing

One way to reduce the vagueness and ambiguity of nursing terms is to define the terms used, to distinguish the different definitions, and to note their functions. Four major types of definitions are: *lexical or reportive, stipulative, theoretical,* and *persuasive* (Table 1–2).

TABLE 1-2. TYPES OF DEFINITIONS

Type	Function	Example
Lexical or reportive	Explicates accepted usage/true or false	Dictionary definitions Hole—a depression
Stipulative	Announces speaker's decision	STAT—immediately
Theoretical	Connects definition to a theory	Nursing is holistic
Persuasive	A new usage intended to achieve acceptance	Nursing is the nursing process.[42]

Lexical Definitions. A *lexical* or *reportive definition* is an explication of accepted usage. Lexical definitions are readily found in dictionaries or reference works, nursing and medical dictionaries, and encyclopedias. Acquaintance with lexical definitions is part of a person's socialization and induction into any field. We use lexical definitions to announce the way words, such as *gangrene* and *nursing,* are used. These standard usages are not arguable. They are the reference points people use or assume in any form of dialogue, discussion, or discourse. A lexical definition is an agreement conventionally arrived at for the use of a term. For example, after a gram or a cubic centimeter is distinguished as a unit of measurement, there is no argument whether it is less or more than precisely what it is. Lexical definitions do not comprise *training in uncertainty.* Rather, they are the stock and trade, the essentials of training in certainty. They help us to recognize and appreciate the difference between certainty and uncertainty. If all nursing and all knowledge was uncertain, there could be no distinction between certainty and uncertainty, and no sense of sureness about what could be taken as foundational or basic.

Lexical definitions are free of doubt. A reason they are immune to doubt is that there is little, if anything, to which anyone using lexical definitions commits oneself. Lexical definitions are equations, explications, translations, alternatively equivalent renderings, or substitutions of how we commonly agree to use terms. These equations, nevertheless, enrich our store and stock of available meanings.

Much is at stake in the agreements by members of the human race to use selected terms for certain purposes without argument. If we could not agree on the common meanings of terms, we could not communicate. In nursing, whatever else defines the nursing process, it involves or logically implies assessment, planning, implementation, and evaluation. Diagnosis was at one time a debatable aspect of the nursing process, but not assessment. The nursing process, as it is currently defined, necessarily involves assessment. Assessment leads to planning. Planning, in turn, leads to implementation. At least one nursing scholar notes that "if planning is not put into action, it is useless."[43] Later in the same work, this author writes that "implementation is the actual giving of nursing care."[44] We may correctly say, then, that there is no nursing process without implementation; and there is no implementation without planning; and there is no planning without assessment. To the extent that the nursing profession recognizes the necessity of the phases of the nursing process, such as assessment followed by planning, implementation, and evaluation, we may correctly say that these phases are necessary to the nursing process. If someone argues that the previous sentence is obviously true or redundant, that is precisely the objective of lexical definitions or tautologies, or expressions that mean the *same.* They state whatever has to be. This definition asserts not only true, but necessarily true propositions. These have the highest cognitive status and serve as standards of judgment.

Lexical definitions or tautologies, sometimes known as analytic or a priori statements, are necessarily true, in part, because they depend on no further experience. We need not observe the nursing process over and over to confirm or disconfirm whether the nursing process makes use of planning and implementation.

Stipulative Definitions. In contrast with lexical definitions, there are also stipulations as to how an individual prefers to use a term in a given context. In 1976, Marjory Gordon gave a *stipulative definition* of nursing diagnosis:

> Nursing diagnosis or clinical diagnosis made by professional nurses, describe actual or potential health problems which nurses by virtue of their education and experience are capable and licensed to treat.[45]

In this article, Gordon stipulates or announces how she will use the expression *nursing diagnosis.* Another example of a stipulative term in nursing is *holistic nursing,* meaning concern for the whole human being in contrast with a focus on pathology. A notable example of the use of a stipulative definition is Freud's use of the Greek words, id, ego, and superego, to characterize imaginary psychological structures within a person. Another example is Spearman's *g factor,* connoting general intelligence as the dominant measure of academic grades. Another example, cited by B. Stevens, is Martha Rogers' use of terms, such as *reciprocy,* which means "the assimilation of human and environmental fields."[46]

Other common examples of stipulative definitions are the uses of abbreviations, such as POSDCORB, the acronym for planning, organizing, staffing, directing, coordinating, reporting, and budgeting.[47] Another example is "Code," which is given a specific meaning in a hospital, and not to be confused with the Morse code. A significant difference between lexical and stipulative definitions is that whereas lexical definitions are true or false, stipulative definitions are not true or false; they are used to announce a speaker's use of terms in a given context.

Theoretical Definitions. A *theoretical definition* attempts to make or succeeds in making a theoretical connection between a term and certain cause–effect or explanatory relations.

Examples of theorectical definitions in nursing are Lydia Hall's definition of a nurse, cited by Stevens, as a "body expert,"[48] B. Harmer and V. Henderson's definitions that a nurse provides for a patient's health care deficits;[49] Orem's definition that a nurse helps a patient achieve self-care;[50] that nursing uses a systems' approach; and that nursing is treating the whole patient.[51] Theoretical definitions in nursing make or attempt to make illuminating contributions to nursing by connecting certain terms to cause–effect or explanatory relationships.

Persuasive Definitions. We come now to the most controversial use of definitions. These are called persuasive definitions. A speaker or writer appears to use a term as if it were either lexical or stipulative. Instead, that person uses the term to recommend or try to persuade others to adopt a new usage. If a person defines "holistic nursing" as "caring for the whole patient," such a definition is persuasive because it is impossible to meet all the nursing health care or human needs of the total patient. Or, if a speaker says, "Abortion is murder,"[52] one will not find a definition in a standard dictionary or specialized reference work. This speaker is not using a term in a commonly understood way. Nor is the speaker merely announcing the way she or he wishes to use a term in a given context. Rather, the speaker is using a term, such as holistic nursing, to recommend that nursing be conceptually, legally, and morally identified with taking care of a person's total well being.[53] The speaker who says "abortion is murder" is recommending that abortion be conceptually, legally, and morally identified with murder. Conversely, a speaker may recommend that abortion be identified with a woman's free choice, or with her right to her own body. In these examples, a speaker is presenting her or his preferred usages and attempting to persuade others of its value.

Gordon's definition of nursing diagnosis was not simply an announcement of how she intended to use that expression. She was also recommending a term along with a new usage; the same is true with other nursing theorists who use persuasive definitions. Whether one speaks of Roy's adaptation model, Rogers' systems model, Orem's self-care model, Johnson's behavioral stability model, Levine's model of social integrity, or Peplau's interpersonal model,[54] each nursing theory provides a persuasive definition of the functions of nursing.[55]

A persuasive definition has four functions. First, it expresses the speaker's feelings toward the use of a word, such as nursing or abortion. Second, a persuasive definition, such as "Health is total well being," "Nursing employs the nursing process," or "This theory uses a systems approach to nursing,"[56] attempts to arouse or persuade the hearer(s) to agree with the speaker about the use of that term.

A persuasive definition has a third function. On occasion, a persuasive definition makes an illuminating distinction about the use of a term that had not been considered before, such as the idea that nursing makes use of nursing diagnosis,[57] or that nursing is caring for the whole patient, in contrast to medicine's purported focus on disease.

A fourth function of a persuasive definition is to redefine a term with a shocking and at times misleading and exaggerated set of terms. Some nursing theories and terms, such as nursing diagnosis, seem to have succeeded in performing all four functions of a persuasive definition, especially the third, that of drawing an illuminating distinction between the use of terms, which had previously not occurred to people. A persuasive definition, however, is not true or false. It is a disguised value judgment. A function of critical thinking is to distinguish between these definitions.

Exercises

Explain what kinds of definitions these are and why.

1. The nursing process includes assessment, planning, implementation, and evaluation.
2. Nursing is a form of interaction between a nurse and a patient.[58]
3. Nursing is a form of communication.[59]
4. Morphine is a narcotic designed to relieve pain.[60]
5. Gangrene is local death of soft tissue due to loss of blood supply.[61]
6. A nurse is a person who is skilled or trained in caring for the sick or infirm, especially under the supervision of a physician.[62]
7. All humans are mortal.
8. A triangle has three sides enclosing a common area.
9. An island is a body of land surrounded by water.
10. A widow is a woman who has lost her husband by death.[63]
    Answer: These are all lexical definitions. To deny the predicate is a contradiction of what has been asserted in the subject. These definitions are analytically true in the sense that they could not be false without contradiction.
11. Nursing is the nursing process.
    Answer: Persuasive definition.
12. Nursing is being a body expert who treats a body, a disease, and a person.
    Answer: Lydia Hall's theoretical definition of nursing.[64]

Rules for Definitions in Nursing

A definition consists of a term to be defined and some defining properties. For example, a puppy is a young dog; a kitten is a young cat; a baby is a young human. A good definition states the essential attributes such that the defining characteristics are equivalent to the term to be defined. Using this type of definition, professional nursing is defined as "diagnosing and treating human responses to actual or potential health problems, through such services as case finding, health teaching, health counseling, and provision of care supportive to or restorative of life and well being . . . ."[65] The first rule of a good definition is that it has all three components, a term to be defined, a general category, and a differentiation. The above definition differentiates nursing diagnosis from medical diagnosis.

A second rule of a good definition is that it is not *circular*. This means that the definition does not repeat the term to be defined in the defining expression. To say "Nursing is whatever nurses do" or that nursing diagnosis is diagnosis done by nurses, repeats the term to be defined in the definition. Such a definition fails to distinguish what nurses actually do from what physicians do in diagnosis. A circular definition begs the question at issue.

A third rule of a good definition is that it is neither too broad nor too narrow. To define a nurse as a health professional is too broad; and to define a nurse as a female health professional who works in a hospital in a supervisory position is too narrow. Some nurses are men and not all nurses occupy supervisory positions.

A fourth rule of an effective definition is that it is not ambiguous, obscure, or uses figurative language. To define negentropy as signifying "increasing complexity and heterogeneity" obscures more than it clarifies.[66] This definition is excessively figurative and obscure.

A fifth rule is that a definition be expressed in the positive, not the negative. We do not define a nurse by what she does not do, but by what she does. To define illness as the absence of health violates the rule.

A sixth rule is that an effective definition states the *connotation* or general characteristics, rather than the *denotation* or particular examples that fall under the definition. The term *nurse,* for example, connotes or characterizes general features that apply to all nurses, such as caring for patients. The term *health* characterizes the features that all human beings may possess, such as being well or functioning optimally. The denotation of nurse refers to points to a particular nurse, like Ms. Jones or Mr. Smith. The term health may denote or point to Mr. R's present condition, that of feeling or being well, of being free of medical requirements, or of being capable of self-care. Connotation is general, whereas denotation is particular.

Pictorial, Artistic, Emotive, and Metaphorical Meaning

Definitions are not the only expressions of meaning in nursing. There are other forms of meaning such as the *objective* and *subjective connotations* of a term. In giving an objective connotation, we cite the features of a term that are real. A hospital is a place where the sick are cared for and treated. Subjective connotation, however, consists of the feelings a speaker may communicate in using a word. The word *patient* is objectively a person in need of health care. Subjectively, the word patient may connote an elderly person with many physiological and psychological deficits. Both kinds of connotations may be present in thinking about a particular word. These forms of connotation are not always neatly separable.

Pictorial Meaning. We all have mental pictures of situations. We sometimes communicate using picture language.[67] Writers convey their meaning by providing a word picture of what they have to say.

A mental picture is an emotive and visual effect on a person. A healthy person may be pictured as a lean, muscular, sexy person doing aerobic exercises. Nurses are apt to form mental pictures of their patients, as "cardiacs, diabetics, or cerebral palsy or AIDS victims" and to form judgments partly on this basis. Picture thinking is an important way in which we form our thoughts.

Artistic Meaning. Artists, including novelists, painters, musicians, sculptors, and architects, give meaning to their creations; and do so by attributing to them lifelike proportions. An opera, play, or poem may seem to have a life of its own. Nursing, too, is an art. Nurses try to reshape their patient's conditions from ill health to health. Forms of artistic meaning are largely but not exclusively subjective.

Emotive Meaning. We experience pictorial and artistic images. Dramatizations may make creations seem real. That is one form of meaning. There is another form of meaning that we experience. We are apt to feel sensations of good or bad, pain or pleasure, beauty or ugliness, as we communicate with one another. Words may evoke feelings and attitudes.[68] The words "vacation" and "well-being" evoke feelings of happiness in almost everyone. Words such as "cancer," "mental illness," "mental retardation," "acquired immune deficiency syndrome," "myelomingocele," "sexism," "racism," and "violence" connote negative feelings in the listener or reader.

Slogans. One form of emotive expressions is that of slogans. A *slogan* is a pithy saying easy to remember, a rallying cry that symbolizes the feelings and aspirations of a group of people. A slogan expresses pictorial and emotive meaning in a short statement. This enables a slogan, if it is emotively and pragmatically effective, to be easily remembered and repeated. "Angels of mercy" for nurses, and "Health care is a right" are typical slogans. In nursing and health care, there are slogans that overlap in meaning with persuasive definitions, such as "Optimum health is a state of well being" or "Nursing care is treating the whole person."

The slogan *holistic nursing* emphasizes the belief in the whole patient or the whole nurse as *emergent entities.* The belief in holism attempts to secure moral and political standing, status, and significance for the role of the bedside nurse. In a holistic view, or theory, a nurse is pictured as treating the whole patient, not as a disease entity. The physician, on the other hand, is viewed as primarily treating the disease entity. Holism accordingly gives rise to the resulting widely championed slogan that "The nurse treats the whole patient, not the disease."[69]

Barbara Stevens evaluates the meaning of slogans quite directly:

> Many theorists fall into the trap of nursing slogans, particularly those in vogue at the time the material is written. For example, one sees many theorists who start out by claiming that the patient is a full-fledged par-

> ticipant in determining his plan of nursing care. Yet one often finds that this concept has no place in the theory that follows. Sloganism, then, is a claim, put forth by the theorist that is not substantiated. . . . Indeed, the reader may be suspicious of . . . the following claims: (1) the nurse is a problem solver, (2) the patient participates in his care determination, (3) health is a state of total well-being, (4) nursing employs the nursing process, or (5) this theory uses a systems approach to nursing.[70]

Two kinds of critical thinking questions arise in a review of extant nursing theories: (1) Are slogans out of place in a nursing theory? and (2) Is holism, in particular, "Nurses treat the whole patient, not the disease," as one example of a slogan, indefensible?

We may object to all nursing slogans. That is one option. Or we may find all slogans to be at least emotively meaningful. A third approach is to examine the slogans to determine which ones, if any, are worth taking seriously. We propose to follow the third option as the most rewarding for enriching the prospects of critical thinking in nursing.

A slogan, we recall, is a pithy saying, easy to remember, a rallying cry that symbolizes the feelings and aspirations of a group of people. We propose now to give an analysis of the nursing slogan that the nurse treats the whole patient, noting its strengths and difficulties.

We note first an analogy of this slogan to two educational slogans that gained prominence in the first half of this century. One was "We teach the child, not the subject matter." A second related slogan was "There is no teaching without learning."[71] The first of these educational slogans has a parallel to the nursing slogan, "We treat the whole patient, not the disease." The second educational slogan has a parallel to one in nursing "There is no nursing without a nursing plan." As with any comparison, a strength or weakness of the educational analogy may help us identify the strengths or weaknesses of our nursing example. An analysis of the educational slogan shows that we cannot teach a child without also teaching something. Similarly, the notion that the nurse takes care of the whole patient, whereas the physician treats the disease is not a clearly defensible distinction. A view of a person as a unity fails to account for the existence of disease and its adverse effects on a person's well-being. Even though nursing is responsible for coordinating the care and safety of each patient for 24 hours a day, the nurse no more takes care of the "whole patient" than does the physician. The nurse can only meet some of the psychological, physiological, cultural, and social needs of the patient. Even in primary care nursing, nurses can only partially satisfy the patient's requirements for physical, emotional, social, economic, religious, nurturant, and curative assistance. In doing so the nurse treats part of the patient. The nurse does not treat solely for health, whereas the physician treats the disease. In caring for the patient, with the goal of raising "levels of wellness" the nurse also treats disease or illness and a physician, in treating illness or disease, treats to restore health.

Exercises

1. How are persuasive definitions similar to slogans? What place, if any, do slogans have in nursing theory? Compare Stevens's treatment of "sloganism" with one that endorses that uses of slogans in practice fields.
2. Is holism, in particular, as one example of a nursing slogan, rationally defensible?
3. Distinguish the following kinds of definitions:
   a. Morphine is a pain reliever.
   b. Euthanasia is murder.
   Answer: The first is a lexical definition, the second is a persuasive definition.

Nursing Metaphors. Pictorial, artistic, or emotive meanings are sometimes associated with or imply analogies, comparisons, or metaphors. A *metaphor* is a word picture used to help draw a comparison and thereby clarify an unknown state. If, for example, microorganisms are perceived as threatening to a patient's life, the patient's body is compared to a fortress or to a nation's defense system. The struggle between the body and its invader is regarded as a battle or war, such as the statements, "He is fighting for his life," "She lost her last fight," or "This treatment will kill the cancer cells;" or a nurse refers to "the invading pathogens," again implying a military metaphor. Some health care metaphors, such as these examples, may be identified as military metaphors.

Other metaphors in health care, such as the notion of a *team,* suggest comparisons between health care providers and athletic players, a game, opposing sides, winners and losers, and a referee or umpire. The team analogy implies players, a coach, and a captain. The use of such a metaphor, then, raises questions, such as "Who is the captain or coach?" Nurses, in certain contexts, may find the implication arguable that physicians are the captains in all respects. At any rate, a characteristic of critical thinking is to be aware of the implications and questions that a metaphor or analogy raises.

METHODS OF EVALUATION AND REFUTATION

Fortunately, there are methods of evaluating whether a definition, slogan, or metaphor helps clarify the meaning of a term.

Reductio Ad Absurdum

One method of evaluating a definition is to trace the consequences or implications of the definition. We do this to note if there are absurd results. The definition of nursing that says "the preservation of, the fostering of, the maintenance of, and the facilitation of the integrity of all the human needs of the person(s) is the territory of nursing,"[72] is absurd in its implications for and demands on nursing.

Inconsistencies

To achieve clarity calls for the exposure of inconsistencies in reasoning.[73] An example of an *inconsistency* is for a nurse to say, "We treat the whole patient, not the disease," while treating the patient's infection, tumor, electrolyte imbalance, knowledge deficit, or other health problems related to the disease.

Category Mistakes

Another method of evaluation and refutation consists in showing that a statement commits a category mistake. A *category mistake* consists of using the terms of a sentence that belong to one category or type and treating them as if they belonged to a category or kind to which they logically cannot belong. For example, we may say logically that people go to bed; but logically we cannot put a nursing unit to bed. Likewise, it may be said of a patient who just died, that he or she "passed away" and is now "resting in peace." However, only living persons rest peacefully or fitfully.

Serious consequences may ride on a category mistake. To call an embryo or fetus "an unborn child" or a comatose person a "vegetable," strictly speaking, commits a category mistake. A fetus is growing within the maternal uterine cavity and is not a child. The comatose person is unresponsive to stimuli, but is not thereby a cabbage or a carrot.

A defender of odd usages may respond that this is merely a metaphorical way of speaking. But the point in exposing category mistakes is to demonstrate the misuse of language that is identified in critical thinking. According to G. Ryle, who developed this notion, a category mistake is the "presentation of facts belonging to one category in the idiom appropriate to another."[74]

Testing Nursing Language

There are criteria for evaluating nursing arguments, definitions, analogies, metaphors, and related uses of language. According to I. Scheffler, a metaphor may break down in application.[75] In connection with analogies, the distinction between nursing diagnosis and medical diagnosis may break down if the nursing diagnosis is not clearly differentiated from the medical diagnosis.

A second criterion for testing a nursing metaphor, according to Scheffler, is to note whether the metaphor or definition is trivial in context. Some nursing arguments, metaphors, and definitions are illuminating; others less so. Lydia Hall's notion of the nurse as a "body expert," seems illuminating and interesting.[76] Some preferred definitions of nursing, however, may be trivial in the context of their application.

A third consideration of a persuasive definition or metaphor in nursing is its plausability. An example of an implausible definition of nursing is that "the preservation of, the fostering of, the maintenance of, and the facilitation of the integrity of all the human needs of the person(s) is the territory of nursing."[77]

In nursing dialogue there are no indisputable, mathematical, or airtight logical proofs for showing whether nursing theories, definitions, arguments, or analogies and metaphors are significant or farfetched, or trivial in the context of their application. Instead we examine reasons that purport to justify nursing decisions, conclusions, claims, beliefs, definitions, and metaphors. In nursing dialogue, refutation, rebuttal, and examination of meanings take place, which are analogous to the role of true and false judgments in factual discourse. The criteria for assessing nursing concepts are admittedly fuzzier and less exact. Nevertheless, there are criteria for judging the role of nursing theories, metaphors, slogans, and persuasive definitions. Such criteria include these "how-to-do-it" procedures: We examine nursing theories to note (1) if they are trivial or significant in the context of their application, (2) if they break down in application, and (3) if they are farfetched or plausible. We may suggest further criteria for judging persuasive definitions, models, metaphors, and nursing theories. We may test a nursing theory for (4) consistency, (5) adequacy, (6) coherence (7) openness to refutation, and (8) freedom from category mistakes.

Exercises

1. In dialogue with another student, argue for the conclusion that "Nursing is a learned profession and an independent discipline." Summarize your arguments in the form of premises in support of a conclusion.
2. Exercise in reciprocity. After five minutes, with your partner, reflect, question, and reconstruct an alternative point of view on the conclusion that "Nursing is an occupation subject to the market forces of labor supply and demand."
3. Exercise in critical inquiry, critical dialogue, and critical reflection. Question the assumptions, reasons, evidence, conclusions, and implications of the following nursing arguments:
   a. Entry into practice and licensure as a professional nurse should be based on a Baccalaureate degree educational program with the Associate Nurse title reserved for the graduates of associate degree programs.
   b. The current situation of three levels of educational preparation leading to license as a professional nurse should be maintained.
   c. A Master's degree level of preparation should be the first professional degree leading to licensing as a professional nurse.
4. Exercise in critical thinking. The evidence is that an intelligent, well-educated male patient of 40 years of age with severe essen-

tial hypertension is noncompliant with his medication and diet regimen. Formulate alternative inferences and data required to support or refute these.

5. Exercises in egocentrism and sociocentric thought.
   a. Either orally or in writing, individually or as a class, list associations with the concept of nurse and physician.
   b. Discuss actual persons and examples that conflict with these associations.
   c. Discuss the associations that youth, middle-aged, or elders might make with the concepts of nurse and physician.
6. Identify inconsistency and double standards in the way patients are treated in public and nonpublic health care institutions on the basis of age, sex, race, socioeconomic standards, education, and diagnosis.

CONCLUSION

This chapter shows that a function of definitions is to clarify language uses and meanings. Definitions range from logically "airtight" lexical definitions—which are true or false—to forms of persuasion that, in some instances, may be more subjective than objective. An analysis of definitions shows that not all definitions are purely objective or subjective. Some persuasive definitions may, for example, have cognitive as well as emotive meaning.

Meanings are not confined only to definitions. There are also expressions of pictorial, artistic, and emotive meaning. These may sometimes be expressed as slogans or metaphors. There are reasoned ways to evaluate these forms of meaning and definition in nursing.

Definitions and forms of meaning range from the almost purely cognitive to the almost purely emotive. The greater the latitude of meaning, the more debatable or vague the meaning or definition is apt to be. The more airtight the definition is, as with a lexical definition, the less interesting and significant it seems to be. That is the final paradox in the search for meaning, including the search for the meaning of life. Exactness and significance seem to be inversely proportional to one another. Nevertheless, on the basis of secure definitions and the conceptual distinctions provided, the propositional planks of arguments, on which so much reasoning in nursing depends, can be constructed.

REFERENCES

1. Ennis, R.H. Critical Thinking Soon: A Status Report of the Illinois Critical Thinking Project, Critical Thinking and Problem Solving 1985; 7(5): 1, May.

2. Paul, R.W. The Critical Thinking Movement. National Forum LXV(1) 1985; 32, Winter.
3. Ibid.
4. Kuhn, T. The Structure of Scientific Revolution (2nd ed.). Chicago: University of Chicago Press, 1970, pp. 174–210.
5. Ennis, R. Goals for Critical Thinking and Reasoning in the Curriculum. Presentation at the Conference on Critical Thinking. California State University at Sonoma, July 20, 1985.
6. Siegel, H. Critical Thinking as an Educational Ideal, The Educational Forum 1980; 7, November.
7. Govier, T. Critical Thinking in the Armchair, the Classroom and the Lab. Unpublished paper quoted by J.A. Blair: Some Challenges for Critical Thinking: Christopher Newport College. Newport News, Va.: Christopher Newport College Press, 1985, p. 70.
8. Blair, J.A. Some Challenges for Critical Thinking, in Hoaglund, J. (Ed.), Conference on Critical Thinking: Christopher Newport College. Newport News, Va.: Christopher Newport College Press, 1985, p. 70.
9. Ibid, p. 73.
10. Ibid, p. 75.
11. Paul, R.W. Critical Thinking Fundamental to Education for a Free Society, Educational Leadership 1984; 5:11, September.
12. Siegel, H. Educating Reason: Critical Thinking, Informal Logic and The Philosophy of Education, Part Two. Philosophical Questions Underlying Education for Critical Thinking, Informal Logic 1985; 7(2&3):69–81, Spring, Fall.
13. Ibid.
14. Ibid.
15. Ibid.
16. Ibid.
17. Ibid.
18. Ibid.
19. Ibid.
20. Ibid.
21. Ibid.
22. Paul, R.W. Critical Thinking, Fundamental to Education for a Free Society.
23. Scheffler, I. Reason and Teaching. Indianapolis: Bobbs Merrill, 1973, pp. 67–82.
24. Wittgenstein, L.W. Philosophical Investigations. Oxford: Oxford University Press, 1952, p. 153.
25. Iyer, P., Taptich, B., & Bermochey-Losey, D. Nursing Process and Nursing Diagnosis. Philadelphia: Saunders, 1986, p. 147.
26. Atkinson, L., and Murray, M. Understanding the Nursing Process (3rd ed.). New York: Macmillan, 1986, pp. 65–66.
27. Drug Capsules. *American Journal of Nursing* 1986; 86(10):1098, October.
28. Tanner, C. Diagnostic Problem Solving Strategies, in Carnevali, D., et al. (Eds.), Diagnostic Reasoning in Nursing. Philadelphia: J.B. Lippincott, 1984, p. 96.
29. Copi, I. Introduction to Logic (7th ed.). New York: Macmillan, 1986, p. 77.
30. Tanner, C. Factors Influencing the Diagnostic Process, in Carnevali, D., et al (Eds.), Diagnostic Reasoning in Nursing, p. 63.
31. Watzlawick, P. The Language of Change, New York: Basic Books, 1978, pp. 74–109.

32. Watzlawick, P. The Language of Change, p. 119.
33. Ibid.
34. Ibid.
35. Merton, R. Societal Theory and Social Structure. Glencoe, Ill.: Free Press, 1949, pp. 21–81.
36. Hospers, J. An Introduction to Philosophical Analysis (2nd ed.). Englewood Cliffs, N.J.: Prentice-Hall, 1967, pp. 11–12.
37. Ibid.
38. Rogers, M. An Introduction to the Theoretical Basis of Nursing. Philadelphia: F.A. Davis, 1970, p. 122.
39. Stevens, B.J. Nursing Theory (2nd ed.). Boston: Little, Brown, 1984, p. 11.
40. Ibid, p. 13.
41. Miller, R.W. Study Guide for Introduction to Logic (6th ed.). New York: Macmillan, 1982, p. 44.
42. Stevens, B. Nursing Theory, p. 15.
43. Marriner, A. The Nursing Process (3rd ed.). St. Louis: C.V. Mosby, 1983, p. 3.
44. Ibid, p. 170.
45. Gordon, M. Nursing Diagnosis and the Diagnostic Process. *American Journal of Nursing* 1976; 76(8):1299, August.
46. Stevens, B. Nursing Theory, p. 46.
47. Ibid, p. 134.
48. Ibid, p. 22.
49. Harmer, B., & Henderson, V. Textbook of the Principles and Practices of Nursing. New York: Macmillan, 1955, p. 4.
50. Orem, D. Nursing: Concepts of Practice (3rd ed.). New York: McGraw-Hill, 1985, p. 105.
51. Stevens, B. Nursing Theory, pp. 241–243.
52. Fogelin, R.J. Understanding Arguments (3rd ed.). New York: Harcourt Brace, 1987, p. 46.
53. Stevens, B. Nursing Theory, pp. 15, 241–243.
54. Brill, E.L., & Kilts, D.F. Foundations for Nursing. New York: Appleton-Century-Crofts, 1980, p. 18.
55. Stevens, B. Nursing Theory, pp. 1–27, 33–35.
56. Ibid, p. 15.
57. Gordon, M. Nursing Diagnosis: Process and Application. New York: McGraw-Hill, 1982, pp. 1–30.
58. Stevens, B. Nursing Theory, pp. 11, 62.
59. La Monica, E. The Humanistic Nursing Process. Monterey, Calif.: Wadsworth, 1985, p. 51.
60. Stevens, B. Nursing Theory, p. 63.
61. Webster's New Collegiate Dictionary. Springfield, Mass.: G. & C. Merriam Co., 1974, pp. 472–473.
62. Ibid, p. 789.
63. Ibid, p. 1340.
64. Stevens, B. Nursing Theory, pp. 22–25.
65. Nurse Practice Act, Title 38, Article 139, New York State Education Law, 1972.
66. Rogers, M. An Introduction to the Theoretical Basis of Nursing, p. 51.
67. Hospers, J. An Introduction to Philosophical Analysis, pp. 49–54.
68. Ibid, pp. 51–52.

69. Gadow, S. Nursing and the Humanities: An Approach to Humanistic Issues in Health Care, in Bandman, E.L., and Bandman, B. (Eds.), Bioethics and Human Rights: A Reader for Health Professionals. Lanham, Md.: University Press of America, 1986, p. 310.
70. Stevens, B. Nursing Theory, p. 15.
71. Scheffler, I. The Language of Education. Springfield, Ill.: Charles Thomas, 1960, pp. 37–46.
72. Yura, H., & Walsh, M.B. The Nursing Process (4th ed.). Norwalk, Conn.: Appleton-Century-Crofts, 1983, p. 79.
73. Stevens, B. Nursing Theory, pp. 54–55.
74. Ryle, G. The Concept of Mind. London: Hutchinson's University Library, 1949, p. 8.
75. Scheffler, I. The Language of Education, pp. 56–58.
76. Stevens, B. Nursing Theory, p. 22.
77. Yura, H., & Walsh, M.B. The Nursing Process, p. 79.

Chapter 2

Structures and Functions of Arguments

The purpose of this chapter is to enable the learner to:

1. Use the structures and functions of nursing arguments.
2. Identify the relations between the different components of arguments, particularly the premises and the conclusion.
3. Evaluate nursing arguments.
4. Construct nursing arguments.

INTRODUCTION

A special function of critical thinking is to present, consider, and evaluate arguments in the field of nursing. This chapter is designed to show the student how to recognize, evaluate, and construct arguments.

WHY ARGUE?

We argue to win or settle a debate or a dispute; to discover or explain new truths; to clarify an issue; to marshal a rational defense for a claim or contention; or to urge a general or particular course of action through a proposal, treatment, plan, or prescription.

WHAT IS AN ARGUMENT?

The word *argument* has several distinct uses. An argument may refer to a quarrel or shouting match. This is a prevalent use of argument in ordinary language; and even textbooks in logic or critical thinking cannot undo this strong association with quarrels.

An argument may also refer to a debate or dispute over an issue, as when politicians or administrators debate cutting appropriations to nursing service, education, or research.

A third use of the word argument is the attempt to persuade individuals or groups to engage in specified action, such as in the advertising and sales language to persuade people to buy a specific product or service.

An argument may also refer to an explanation or demonstration as to why one event or phenomena occurred rather than another. An argument can be presented to explain why people have "slips of the tongue," how AIDS is transmitted, or why a given patient developed side effects to a medication.

An argument may also be used to refer to a logical demonstration of the relation between premises and conclusion. Finally, the word "argument" may also refer to a form of rational persuasion in which an appropriate set of reasons favors one belief, plan, decision, or action over another.

Example:
Doing what helps to avoid harm is good.
Wearing seat belts helps avoid harm.
Therefore (∴), wearing seat belts is good.

An argument is commonly thought of as a dispute or a debate. In the context of critical thinking and logic, an argument is regarded as a connected set of propositions or premises designed to reach another proposition, a conclusion.

A statement or proposition is verifiable as either true or false. Part of an argument, however, may be a command or a value statement that may not be verifiable as being true or false. It may not even be right or wrong. A command, however, may still be part of an argument as the following shows:

Physician: Give all these pneumonia patients antibiotics.
Jones is a pneumonia patient.
∴ Give Jones an antibiotic.

An argument may be perceived as having a goal or a conclusion. Nurse Jones says, "I want Mr. Smith, age 28, the pneumonia patient, to recover."

That is her conclusion. She makes a mental connection, which she states as: "By giving him an antibiotic and skilled nursing care, he should recover soon."

Arguments are not always explicit, they may not be announced. They come in various forms and guises. In the public media, for example, arguments may be hidden or unstated in the effort to persuade us to buy a particular product or service, or to accept some government proposal. One health care ad says "A pain reliever should solve problems, not cause them."[1] It recommends Tylenol. The unstated assumption is that other pain relievers cause problematic side effects.

Arguments delivered in a deep, masculine, authoritative voice persuade us to comply, despite reasons to the contrary. Some ads say, "If you want pleasure, try brand X cigarettes." We then find in a corner of the package the Surgeon General's warning. Arguments may be hidden or implicit in literature, prose, poetry, and opera. Arguments may also be implicit in hypotheses. A nurse may urge the physician to alter the treatment plan for a patient by giving reasons for one treatment plan over another.

INFERENCES

One aspect of an argument is an inference, because to argue is to make inferences. Inferences have a common sense, a psychological and a logical aspect. We make inferences in almost every waking moment of our conscious lives in both practical, theoretical, professional, and personal pursuits. An inference is "the act of passing from one proposition, statement or judgment considered as true to another whose truth is bound to follow from that of the former."[2] If I see a woman with a white coat and a stethoscope walking down a hospital corridor, I infer that this person is a nurse or a physician and not a movie actor, a disguised spy, or a terrorist. We infer that if we have a job and work, we will be paid. A nurse who cares for patients postoperatively after tonsillectomies infers that patients have sore throats. When we hear a siren from a red truck with hoses, we infer that the truck is a fire engine. And when we see smoke we infer that there is a fire. Students infer that if they study hard, they will pass college courses. We make inferences when driving a car, in estimating the width of the road, the distance to be traveled, and the speed of other cars in relation to ours. We make inferences about persons of the opposite sex: their attactiveness, age, social status, occupations, intelligence, and whether they are pleasant or unpleasant to be with in intimate relations. In inferring, we guess about the significance of data and about the consequences of courses of action. Our inferences may be right or wrong, valid or invalid, sound or unsound, relevant or irrelevant, significant or trivial. Trivial references restate the obvious as in the proverbial question, "What color is an orange?" or Groucho Marx's question, "Who is buried in Grant's tomb?" or "There are patients waiting in the emergency room" when all the units and the waiting rooms are filled with people. In the common sense view, we value some people's inferences, which we interchange with *judgments.* When we say, "Nurse Jones used good judgment in taking Mr. Smith's vital signs every 15 minutes," we could interchange "good judgment" with "good inference."

We may study inferences as processes and as products or results. In psychology, the emphasis is on the process of forming inferences. For example, "What role do memory and motivation play in the process of inferring?" In logic and critical thinking, the emphasis is on the finished product of an inference, namely the relation between a set of premises and a conclusion. We judge the inference by noting whether the premises or reasons justify the conclusion.

One way to analyze the logical aspect of an inference is to regard it as an implication. Although inferences occur within, by, and for people, implications are between statements or propositions. Nurse Jones may infer that Mr. Smith, a vastly overweight diabetic, should lose a minimum of 100 pounds. If we recast what Nurse Jones infers about Mr. Smith as a relation between statements or propositions, a statement about an overweight, diabetic patient implies another statement about that patient's need to lose 100 pounds. We could formalize the relation between the premises and conclusion as follows:

- *Premise 1.* Grossly overweight patients who value life should lose weight.
- *Premise 2.* Mr. Smith is a grossly overweight, diabetic patient who values life.
- *Premise 3.* Overweight intensifies a diabetic's problems.
- *Conclusion.* Therefore, Mr. Smith should lose weight.

The relation between the premises or reasons and the conclusion of an implication constitute the terms of an argument. These relations include judgments of validity, soundness, relevance, and significance, as well as invalidity, unsoundness, irrelevance, and triviality.

IF–THEN REASONING

Inferences take an if–then form, in which one reasons from antecedent data to a conclusion. If Mr. Monroe, 56 years old, a known diabetic for many years, has an elevated blood glucose level, sugar in his urine, fruity breath, and drowsiness, then (a consequent, such as the nursing diagnosis), Mr. Monroe has a compliance problem with his diet, activity, and medication regimen, and is in danger of lapsing into a coma.

Critical thinking provides an evaluation of the inferential process.

Critical thinking has rules and procedures to evaluate rationally the completed result of an inference, the upshot, the relation between the premises, and conclusion of an argument.

An inference is analyzed as the relation between premises and conclusions, as a form of if–then reasoning. The premises of an argument belong to the antecedent or *if* part; and the conclusion belongs to the *then* or *therefore* part. All forms of reasoning, including diagnostic reasoning, proceed in this way, by consideration of the relation between the antecedent and the consequent. Using if–then reasoning, there is implication that the premises purportedly justify the conclusion. For example, if a patient is immobile, elderly, and malnourished, then "the probability of decubitus is 95%"[3] Or "if A is present, then B follows."[4] The antecedent contains clues or data and the question is whether these imply the conclusion.

Another way to perceive the relation between the elements of an argument is to note the relationship between reasons, guesses, or estimates and beliefs, claims, decisions, or judgments. The latter refer to end products; the former to data, grounds, supports, and mental processes. Elements, sometimes identified as premises and conclusions, are necessary conditions of arguments.

PREMISES AND CONCLUSIONS

A useful set of clues for determining whether there is an argument is to look at premise and conclusion indicators. These clues include *if* and *then* in passages containing arguments. The clues may be tacit as well as explicit. These clues may not, however, be present at all, as in this example, "Without Ms. Kelly's excellent daily nursing care, Mr. Jones could not have survived. A week after Ms. Kelly retired, Mr. Jones died." Arguments generally have premise and conclusion indicators, but not necessarily.

Some premise indicators are *whereas, since, inasmuch as, in view of, because, for, for the reason that,* and *otherwise.* Some logicians deny that *because* is a premise indicator as they distinguish arguments from explanations, and claim that *because* belongs to a casual explanation rather than to an argument. But an argument against that view is that some casual explanations can also present arguments. For example, "Ms. W is a very good nurse because all her patient interactions are therapeutic."

The following are examples of conclusion indicators: *then, consequently, therefore, so, hence, thus, it follows, this proves that, this confirms that, this shows that, one may infer, this means that, who can deny, how else, the implication is clear,* and *it is inescapable that.* One of the early skills of critical thinking in nursing is to be able to infer from the context and construct arguments, when few, if any of the clues are present. We could reformulate the above examples as follows: "Because Ms. Kelly's excellent nursing care was vital to Mr. Jones' survival, it was not surprising that a week after she retired, he died." I. Copi supplies this example of an argument with an implicit if–then:

> Untreated chronic glaucoma is a leading cause of painless, progressive blindness. Methods of early detection and effective treatment are available. For this reason, blindness from glaucoma is especially tragic.[5]

One could restate this with a premise and conclusion as follows: Because there are (1) methods of early detection and (2) effective treatment for glaucoma, (3) (therefore) blindness from glaucoma is especially tragic.[6] The question is: Do the premises give adequate support to imply the conclusion?

A useful rule of thumb for some critical thinking skills is first to aim for the claim or conclusion and to do so by asking: What is the speaker trying to show? Then look for the support or basis, warrants, reasons, or grounds for the conclusion, which is found in the premises. A second question is: How effectively does the speaker or writer show or substantiate his or her claim? Numbering the premises and conclusion of the argument and diagramming it helps to focus on the relevant issues, and avoids being sidetracked by extraneous or parenthetical materials that may be present within the argument.

A good strategy after numbering premises and conclusion is to focus on the conclusion, and then work your way to the premises. This means that you ascertain what is being claimed or concluded. Then proceed to show that the premises imply or give rational support to the conclusion.

Logic, a feature of critical thinking, is the study of how well the premises of an argument imply conclusions. Previously, we referred to connecting links between premises and conclusions. These links, expressed through some form of if–then, are guided by rules for weighing, estimating, calculating, and evaluating how effectively the premises imply the conclusion. The premises provide reasons for the claim or conclusion.

To analyze an argument, aim first for the conclusion. Ask such questions as "What is being claimed here?" "What is at stake?" "What is the assertion being made?" or "What is the author driving at?" Look for word clues or indicators showing that the author has reached a conclusion and is offering supports for that conclusion. The conclusion may be presented first or last with supporting reasons coming at the beginning, the middle,

TABLE 2-1. FREQUENT ARGUMENT INDICATORS

Because:	Leads to conclusion and to supports
Hence:	Announces conclusion based on premises
Since:	Leads to or implies conclusion
So:	Announces conclusion based on premises
Therefore:	Announces conclusion based on premises or reasons
Thus:	Announces conclusion based on premises or reasons

or the end of the passage. Look for relationships between and among premises and conclusions in the passage rather than the order in which the premises and conclusion are presented. An argument presents a chain of reasoning or links of passage from premises or supporting reasons to a conclusion. Any claim in the form of a conclusion or in the form of supports or grounds for a conclusion is open to question. Premises that are offered in support of an argument may not support the conclusion adequately.

The simplest form of argument includes a premise or premises and a conclusion that follows. A premise is a proposition that generally comes before a conclusion and is either assumed or proved to be true. A simple nursing example is this:

> Anyone who cares for critically ill patients needs scientific knowledge.
> Nurses care for critically ill patients, who receive complex treatment, requiring fast and accurate clinical judgment.
>
> ∴ Nurses need scientific knowledge.

Another example is:

> Anyone making independent judgments of crucial importance to patients' lives needs to know how to think critically.
> Nurses make independent judgments of crucial importance to patients' lives.
>
> ∴ Nurses need to know how to think critically.

Each of these examples makes a claim in the conclusion, and one tries to support it by what is said in the premises.[7]

A useful critical-thinking and problem-solving skill in nursing is to take a sentence, such as the following, and convert it into an argument with a premise and a conclusion. "Radical mastectomy in women is an instance of the general phenomenon of changes in body image." Analysis of this sentence leads to the following if–then sentences: If a woman experiences mastectomy, she will experience changes in her body image." Another example of an if–then sentence is:

> A mother remains with the (hospitalized) child 24 hours a day during the first two days and at least several hours daily thereafter until discharged.[8] The child then displays more mature behavior than a child whose mother stays away during a child's hospitalization.

This applies to children between 14 and 49 months old. The nursing researcher then notices the child's behavior and the effect based on the mother's answers to a questionnaire.[9] We may refer to this analysis of an argument as the setting up of the problem or the laying out of the argument. A function of an argument is to show that one proposition or state of affairs is implied by or logically follows another. We may try to put this argument or problem into if–then terms. We might then compare our interpretation with the author's.

> (If) the mother rooms in with her child during hospitalization for minor surgery, (then) the child will manifest increased maturity in selected . . . behavior compared with the child whose mother does not room in.[10]

One might take this same argument and diagram it by numbering the premises first and then the conclusions as follows: If (1) the mother rooms in with her child during hospitalization, (2) especially for the first 24 hours, then (3) the child will manifest increased maturity. We could display this in the form of an argument tree (shown below) where there is more than one premise, with the premises (1) and (2) shown as roots, implying the conclusion (3), shown as the bark or branches.[11,12]

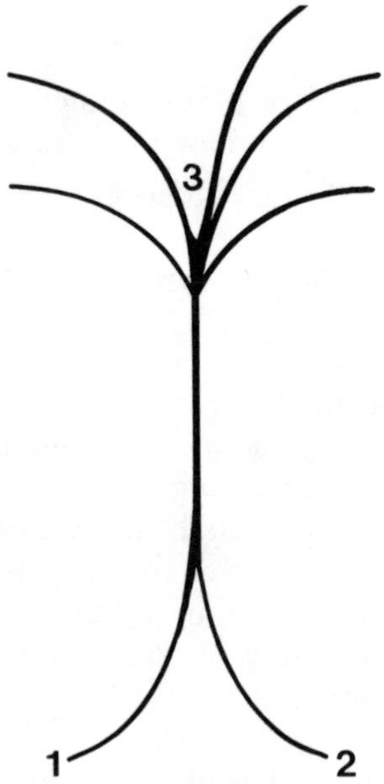

Some other examples of overt if–then's in nursing research are: If (1) an instrument is not valid, then (2) the researcher should delay the proposal until an instrument of demonstrated validity is found.[13] "If (1) patients are the subjects of research, then (2) the task (of finding volunteers) may be more difficult.[14] If (1) appendices are used, then (2) these should be concise, complete, and well organized.[15]

Three points will be made about if–then statements in the language of nursing. First, some if–then statements are descriptive or cast in the indicative mood. For example, if a patient with diabetes takes insulin regularly, then that patient's blood glucose level is likely to be controlled. Some if–then statements are prescriptive, telling someone what to do. For example, persons with hypertension must comply with their medication regimen. Both descriptive and prescriptive if–then statements either assume or claim that if the antecedent is true, the consequent follows as true or justified. In the case of prescriptive if–then statements, the consequent is presumed to be justified because the underlying descriptive if–then is assumed to be true.

A second point is that although imperatives are distinct from indicatives in their logic and critical thinking role, there are no imperatives independent of or isolated from indicatives or descriptions. Imperatives rest on descriptions, as illustrated in the diabetes example. Nursing orders and research protocols or rules are based on descriptions, which are open to empirical or factual challenge or investigation. If, for example, a physician prescribes a beta-blocker to an assumed heart patient who has a hiatus hernia and no heart disease, the nurse may logically question or challenge the basis of such a prescription.

A third point in analyzing arguments is that if–then statements do not come out and announce themselves. We may need to take several steps in analyzing sentences and passages to determine if the sentence or passage is intended to be an argument in which the claim is made or implied that a proposition logically follows from or is derived from another.

Arguments are defined as statement sets in which one part is followed by another. But the word *follow* needs to be explained. In an ordinary language sense follow means that one thing comes before another, the way a locomotive comes before the cars. If that is so, then the thing that comes after follows the thing that comes before. In this language sense, we may use the idea of following another, as in a game of *follow the leader.* But in critical thinking, we define follow not as a geographical or social hierarchical adjacency, but that one statement, claim, or conclusion may be implied by another, the premise or premises; and that the premises give support to the conclusion, claim, or contention. In critical thinking and logic, the latter use of follow is most helpful. The question in critical thinking is: Does the conclusion or claim follow logically from the premises?

Exercises

1. Supply the conclusion.
Premise: If a patient's fluid intake is low or if a patient is dehydrated, force fluids or administer intravenous fluids.
Premise: This patient's fluid intake is extremely low.

Premise: This patient is dehydrated.
Answer: Conclusion: Force fluids or administer intravenous solution.

2. Supply the conclusion.
Premise: Nurses assist patient by supplying self-care deficits.
Premise: This patient is unable to bathe or move himself or herself.
Answer: Conclusion: Nursing agencies will supply self-care deficits for this patient.
3. Rearrange the following statements into a coherent argument with premises and a conclusion.
   a. Diarrhea is one of the most common illnesses in children.
   b. The proper management of this condition and the prevention of dehydration is crucial.
   c. Anything that can be done to prevent diarrhea and dehydration should be done.
   d. In the United States, diarrhea followed by dehydration ranks among the ten leading causes of mortality in children.
   e. In some underdeveloped countries diarrhea followed by dehydration is the most common cause of mortality and morbidity.
   f. Diarrhea, dehydration, a factor in metabolic derangements, is a cause of significant mortality and morbidity.
   One answer: Premises c, d, e, a. Conclusion is b.
4. Arrange these statements into a coherent argument with these premises and a conclusion.
   a. If there is dehydration in a patient, it should be offset by rehydration.
   b. Dehydrated patients have a demonstrable fluid deficit.
   c. Body fluid deficits can be estimated by acute weight losses of 5, 10, and 15 percent over a period of 24 hours, and are termed mild, moderate, and severe dehydration, respectively.
   d. The clinical signs of dehydration include tachycardia, dry skin, and dry mucous membrane.
   e. The most important aspect of treatment for mild to moderate dehydration is maintaining normal fluid and electrolyte balance.
   f. An effective, simple, and inexpensive therapy is rehydration with oral fluids and electrolytes. Fluid and electroylyte replacement should begin quickly. The fluid deficit should be replaced within the first 6 to 12 hours of therapy.
   One answer: Premises a, b, c, d, e. Conclusion: f
5. By appropriate premises, defend the following conclusion: A need then exists for two types of oral electrolyte solutions: one for rehydration of dehydrated patients, and another for maintenance of fluid and electrolyte balance and prevention of dehydration in nondehydrated patients.[16]

One answer: The conclusion is that there is a need for two types of oral electrolyte solutions—one for rehydration and a second for maintenance of fluid and electrolyte balance and the prevention of dehydration. The conclusion is supported in a number of ways: (1) The crucial necessity for proper management of dehydration to prevent child mortality and morbidity all over the world from diarrhea; (2) Specific clinical signs and loss of body weight demonstrate the evidence for a nursing judgment of mild, moderate, or severe dehydration; (3) The most important treatment for mild to moderate dehydration is maintaining normal fluid and electrolyte balance; (4) The goal of therapy is either replacement of fluid deficit or provision for continuing stool losses and normal fluid maintenance requirements.

6. Arrange these nursing statements into premises and conclusion.
a. Dehydration will occur with fluid and electrolyte loss.
b. Death of children is to be prevented whenever possible.
c. Death of children with diarrhea will occur if dehydration is not corrected.
d. Rehydration and maintenance of fluid and electrolyte balance will prevent death of children from dehydration as a result of diarrhea.
e. Whenever there is dehydration, provide for rehydration.
One answer: Premises b, c, a, d. Conclusion: e

ASSUMPTIONS AND IMPLICATIONS IN ARGUMENTS

A supervisor's question to Nurse Kelly, "Why didn't you prevent Mr. Jones's falling out of bed at 7 PM yesterday?" assumes that (1) Ms. Kelly was on duty, (2) that Ms. Kelly was responsible for Mr. Jones, and (3) that Ms. Kelly could have prevented Mr. Jones's fall.

Ms. Kelly could reply, "You're assuming I was on duty at 7 PM, but I wasn't. My shift ended at 6 PM." For the premises to imply a conclusion then, the assumptions must be true. In the case of Ms. Kelly, at least one assumption is false, that she was on duty at 7 PM. If a premise of an argument is false, the conclusion cannot be true. The conclusion that Ms. Kelly was responsible for Mr. Jones's falling, therefore, is not true.

Assumptions are statements that we either take for granted, suppose, or state tentatively. Assumptions may be made explicit or they may be ignored. We can afford to ignore some assumptions, but not others; and it takes an alert, thoughtful, and well-trained person to know the difference. A well-trained and alert practitioner can convert hidden assumptions into explicit assumptions. A health professional may assume that the cause of Ms. S's being pale is that she has anemia, without making this into an explicit assumption. When patients go to a physician or nurse, they may assume that what the physician or nurse says is true. Patients have neither the training, experience, nor knowledge to test all the assumptions that occur or are presupposed in treatment decisions. But to assume that the physician is correct takes it for granted without questioning. A function of critical thinking, however, is to examine assumptions.

Assumptions are beliefs that are regarded as true even though they may not be true. A presumption is an unquestioned assumption. The nurse who assumes that nursing is a learned profession believes educational credentials to be the critical factor in the qualification of a nurse. The physician who assumes nursing to be an occupation ancillary to the practice of medicine, the "handmaiden" concept, believes practical experience to be the critical factor in the qualifications of a nurse. As these examples illustrate, differences in assumptions may become major barriers to understanding.

Arguments in nursing also have implications. Every argument contains an implication relation between the premises and conclusion. For example, "If the guard rails were up, Patient Jones would not have fallen out of bed." Here the premise of the argument is: Had the guard rails been up, the conclusion or implication follows that Patient Jones would not have fallen out of bed.

A second sense of implication is that an entire argument has consequences. An implication or consequence of a nurse on duty at 7 PM who failed to put Patient Jones's guard rails up is that the nurse is legally and morally accountable for this omission.

HIDDEN, MISSING, AND UNSTATED PREMISES

An argument may have a hidden, missing, or unstated premise. For example, Nurse A says to Patient B, a young, severe diabetic "You must lose 50 pounds." The unstated premises are: An obese person requires larger doses of insulin. Larger doses of insulin make blood sugar harder to control. Further unstated assumptions are that the diet must be carefully regulated to control the caloric, fat, carbohydrate, and protein intake. A further assumption is that the client must carefully follow the daily exercise and activity program to help control blood glucose levels. There are further fact–value assumptions as well, such as the desirable consequences of controlling blood sugar.

What do we do with hidden, missing, or unstated premises? We look for them, find them, present them, and evaluate them as being either true or false. What do we do with untested, hidden, or missing conclusions? We supply the conclusions by drawing out the implications within the premises of an argument.

Example:
Nurse Green has a headache.
Nurse Green takes aspirin as an analgesic.
Unstated conclusion: Aspirin is a recommended analgesic and remedy for common headaches.

In ordinary life we recognize that a headache implies an analgesic, and a heartburn indicates an antacid. Physicians and nurses know that certain signs and symptoms imply, indicate, or point to certain remedies. The process of associating a problem with a remedy becomes so habitual that one is apt to leave the conclusion unstated, even though it is not hidden or deliberately missing. It just seems redundant to mention it. If a conclusion is missing, we try to fill in the appropriate conclusion by looking for supporting and opposing evidence. For example, if Nurse Smith wishes to reduce the possibility of death or injury from a car accident, an unstated conclusion, then she abides by the premises that support that conclusion. One such premise is that riding or driving in a car with a seat belt increases safety. We may reformulate this by saying, "Wearing seat belts reduces death and injuries from car accidents. I'll drive now. So I'll wear my seat belt."

We call arguments that have either a hidden, missing, unstated, or suppressed premise or conclusion, an *enthymeme.* To deal with an enthymeme, we explicate what is left implicit. We then determine if the premises validly imply the conclusion, and if the conclusion is true or right.

Exercises

Complete or explicate the following arguments by stating the missing premises or conclusions.

1. Ms. Kay, RN, arrived at 4 PM before Mr. Jones arrested. So, she arrived on time, thank goodness.
   Answer: Missing premise: Ms. Kay arrived in time to be helpful.
2. Give Mr. R. his injection of morphine immediately.
   Answer: Missing premise: Mr. R is in extreme pain. Second premise: Give Mr. R. an effective pain reliever.
3. Nurse Jane is a scrub nurse. So she must work long hours.
   Answer: Missing premise: Scrub nurses work long hours.
4. The nurse in Pavilion 4 is not a geriatric nurse. So the nurse must be a "med–surg" nurse.
   Answer: Missing premise: The nurse must either be a geriatric or a "med–surg" nurse to work in Pavilion 4.
5. Cite the missing conclusion.
   If Jones has a headache, then he is in pain. If Jones has a stomach ache, then he is in pain. Jones is in pain.

Answer: Therefore, either Jones has a headache or Jones has a stomach ache.

6. Cite the missing premise.
Mr. Deeborn, a two-pack-a-day smoker, has heart disease. Therefore, Mr. Deeborn should quit smoking.
Answer: Missing premise: Smoking is harmful for anyone with heart disease or cancer.

7. Cite the missing premise:
Mr. Scott has been sexually promiscuous. Mr. Scott did not use any form of protection in sexual activities. Mr. Scott is diagnosed as infected with AIDS.
Answer: Missing premise: Persons who are sexually promiscuous and who do not use protection are at risk for AIDS.

DEDUCTIVE AND INDUCTIVE ARGUMENTS

Arguments are of two kinds, either deductive or inductive. A deductive argument is one in which the claim is made that the premises supply complete evidence for the conclusion. For such arguments, the conclusion necessarily follows from the premises. If, for example, Nurse A is sitting in front of Nurse B and if Nurse B is sitting in front of Nurse C, then we may conclude that Nurse A is sitting in front of Nurse C. Or if Nurse R works at Montefiore Hospital and if Montefiore Hospital is in the Bronx, then Nurse R works in the Bronx.

An inductive argument is one in which the premises give some evidence, but not conclusive evidence for the truth of the conclusion. For example, Ms. W, a nurse, currently unmarried, has an Italian sounding name. She is, therefore, (probably) of Italian heritage. Or, Mr. E, a lung cancer patient, smoked two packs of cigarettes a day for 40 years. This most likely explains how he got lung cancer. For an inductive argument, the premises probably, rather than necessarily, imply the conclusion. For example, if we claim that in the 1984 election, all nurses voted either for Reagan or for Mondale and Ms. A is a nurse and a voter, then she either voted for Reagan or Mondale. This is a deductive argument, for there is no way the premises could be true and imply anything but that conclusion. On the other hand, if one claims that in the last election 65 percent of nurses voted for Reagan and Ms. A. is a nurse and a voter, then Ms. A most likely voted for Reagan. The argument is inductive, as the premises could be true and still imply a false conclusion, namely that Ms. A voted for Mondale. An inductive argument is one for which the claim is made that the premises provide the probability rather than the certainty that the conclusion is true.

For both kinds of arguments, however, there is still the question: Does the antecedent or premise set imply the conclusion? For even though we have to proceed in health care and nursing largely by depending on induction, our aim is to be able to count on premises implying conclusions. In the sciences we work cumulatively to narrow the gap. For example, the greater the number of infected patients cured by antibiotics, the more confidently one can count on antibiotics working effectively against pathogenic bacteria. To return to our voting example, if the data showed that 85 percent of eligible nurses voted for Mondale instead of 64 percent, that would strengthen the conclusion that Ms. A voted for Mondale. Marjory Gordon cites another example:

> 93 percent of a random sample of American newborns weigh more than 5.5 pounds.
> Baby Jones is a (full-term) newborn American.
> ∴ Jones weighs more than 5.5 pounds.[17]

As Gordon's context makes it clear, her conclusion is intended to be interpreted as a probable judgment.

In nursing research, Seaman and Verhonick point out that "testing hypotheses requires a judgment: Does the data warrant the support of the hypotheses?"[18] The data and criteria for evaluating nursing research are designed to provide a trustworthy guide for choosing a reliable hypotheses. Seaman and Verhonick illustrate this:

> To derive hypotheses from assumptions, the researcher first states the assumption and then predicts what will be found in research. For example, Robischon . . . became interested in pica, the habitual ingestion of nonedible substances, because she was concerned over the poisoning of children from eating lead paint. She believed hand to mouth behavior associated with eating in general was related to development . . . Based on these assumptions, Robischon's hypothesis was children who practice pica have a lower developmental level than children who do not.[19]

An important point to notice is that Robischon "believed hand to mouth behavior associated with eating in general was related to development."[20] Robischon derived an hypothesis from an assumption: Children with a lower developmental level practice pica more than children with a higher developmental level.

ARGUMENT SCHEMES APPLIED TO NURSING

As nursing is a practical field that applies art and science to health care, the nursing arguments are not primarily mathematical or formal. To accommodate the need for practical arguments, several writers, especially Stephen Toulmin, have provided a design or layout of a practical argument. According to Toulmin, in doing practical logic, a "hypothetical bridge" is needed to authorize an inference from a set of premises to a conclusion. To express this, Toulmin suggests a special formula or model in which D stands for data and C stands for claim or conclusion. The conceptual bridge to authorize the inference from D to C is W, or a warrant, a canon, or a criterion of an argument.[21]

For example, Jane earned a baccalaureate degree in an accredited collegiate nursing program and she passed her state board examinations. These are the data (D). The warrant (W) consists in the principle that anyone who graduates from a fully accredited collegiate nursing program and who has passed state boards, is licensed or entitled to practice professional nursing. The claim or conclusion (C) follows: Jane is licensed to practice professional nursing.

Toulmin adds modal terms, such as *necessarily, probably,* or *tentatively,* to qualify the claim. He calls this Q, which indicates the strength of the argument. The relationship between the data, the warrant, and the claim is qualified as either necessarily, probably, presumably, or tentatively justified. Toulmin then adds a rebuttal condition that may set aside the otherwise acceptable justification for the claim or conclusion. To return to our example of Jane, the argument layout is:

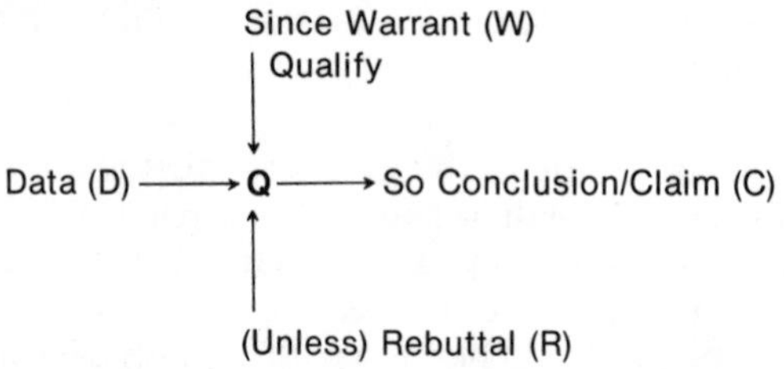

Data (D) Jane graduated from an accredited baccalaureate nursing program and she passed the state board licensing examinations.

Warrant (W): Whoever graduates from an accredited baccalaureate nursing program and passes state board licensing examinations is entitled to become a licensed professional nurse.

Claim or conclusion (C): Therefore, Jane is entitled or licensed to practice professional nursing.

Qualifier of the relationship between data (D), warrant (W), and claim or conclusion (C) is: Presumably or probably.

Unless Jane has committed a serious crime.

Rebuttal or absence of rebuttal condition: Jane has not committed a felony.

Therefore Jane necessarily is entitled or licensed to practice professional nursing.

Qualifier (Q): Unless Jane has been convicted of a felony, Jane necessarily becomes a licensed and professional nurse.

Rebuttal (R): Jane has not been convicted of a felony.

Therefore, the argument stands, without rebuttal, the qualifier supports the conclusion.

Normally, we would use a qualifier modal term such as *presumably* or *probably* in front of the conclusion, as several conditions could defeat the conclusion that Jane is entitled or licensed to practice nursing. One rebuttal or *unless* clause could be that Jane has been convicted of a felony or of professional misconduct with revocation or suspension of her license. But if there is no evidence of a rebuttal, then the claim that Jane is licensed to practice professional nursing would appear justified.

The following qualifiers help identify a conclusion:

- Necessarily
- Certainly
- Presumably
- In all probability
- So far as the evidence goes
- For all we can tell
- Possibly
- Apparently
- Plausibly
- Or so it seems[22]

Some key concepts of critical thinking in nursing include claims or conclusions. These claims take the form of nursing judgments, decisions, or actions. Other key concepts in critical thinking include data, reasons, rules, grounds, backing, or warrants that support nursing judgments. The nursing judgment is qualified by a modality term such as *necessarily* or *probably*. The modality indicates the degree of security with which the nursing judgment is made. Last, there are rebuttals or refuting conditions that, if true, could cancel the conclusion.

The layout of the argument presents several tacit criteria for judging an argument. For example, an argument that lacks a conclusion or premise set is defective; as is an argument without a modality indicative of how strongly the argument is being presented. An argument may be judged by the presence or absence of conditions that refute an argument. An argument without defeating or refuting conditions is weakened by appearing as a dogma. Rebuttal conditions accordingly strengthen the plausibility of an argument. If Supervisor A says give penicillin and Nurse B says it is contraindicated for Patient C, it is important for the sake of rational argument to have a basis for deciding between Supervisor A and Nurse B. The layout of an argument is illustrated with these medical examples (Figs. 2–1 to 2–3).[23]

An argument consists of a conclusion; and a set of premises that, together with modalities and qualifiers, entitles one to draw a conclusion. Figure 2–3 adapts Toulmin's "Layout of Argument" to nursing.[24] In terms of the nursing process, the data, together with assessment and qualifiers and rebuttal provisions, call for an appropriate nursing judgment in the form of a nursing diagnosis.

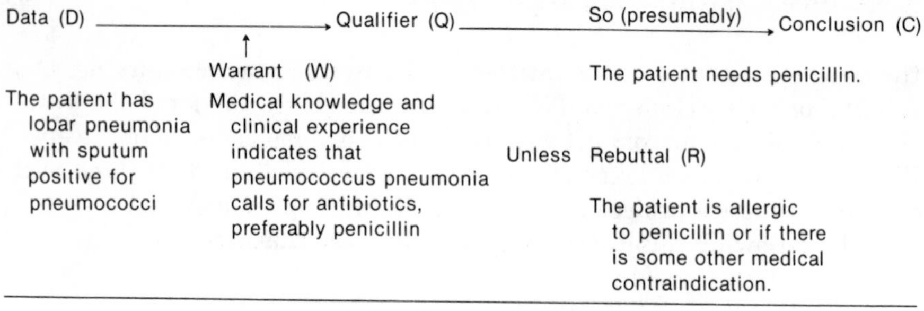

Figure 2-1. The Layout of an Argument

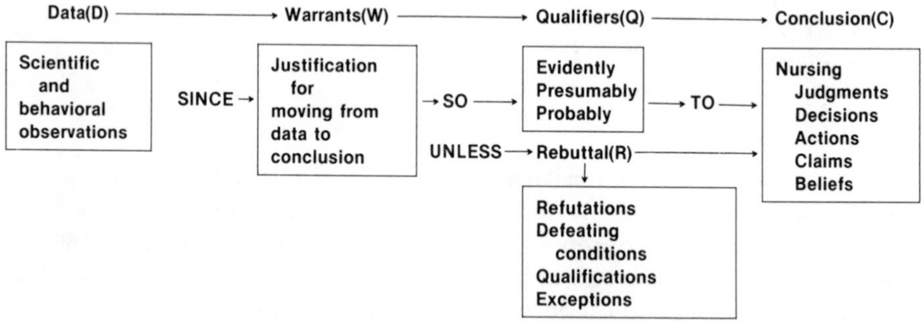

Figure 2-2: The Design of an Argument[25]

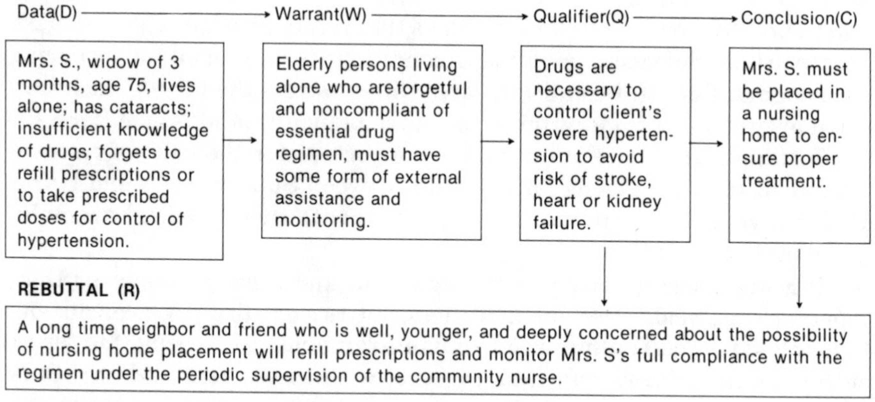

Figure 2-3. A Nursing Argument

Exercises.
Identify the claim, warrants, and backing, and evaluate the following arguments.

1. Mrs. G lives in a trailer. Therefore, she has a low income.
Answer: Poor inference. Patient could have a high income and live in a luxurious trailer.
2. Mrs. G, recovering from coronary bypass surgery, is reluctant to go home after 13 days because she has become dependent.
Answer: Poor inference. Patient could be fearful of postoperative complication. Patient may live alone without any source of help.
3. If Mr. J eats fried foods, he will not reduce weight or lessen the edema.
Answer: Inference by an expert nurse based on data related to the high fat, high cholesterol, high sodium, and high caloric composition of fried foods. Sodium tends to retain fluids.

EXPLANATIONS AS FORMS OF ARGUMENT

In a schematizing explanation, the same if–then form of reasoning can be used as in deductive and inductive inferences. An *explanation* has several major senses that may be distinguished. An explanation may be an effort to prove or demonstrate a theory, a law, or an event. An explanation may be an effort to show why one event is connected to another. An explanation may be an effort to help us understand, learn, or know a relation between two or more events, processes, or occurrences. Or an explanation may be an effort to provide rational accountability for our behavior.

To answer the questions, "Why do objects fall to the ground?," "Why is the earth round?," "Why does the earth move around the sun?," or "Why are we evolved from other animals?" we may attempt to prove or demonstrate which of several alternatives best explains or accounts as an acceptable answer. Or the purpose of explaining an event may be to link cause–effect aspects. Or the purpose of explaining an event may be to understand it. A common pedagogical reason for giving explanations to students is to help them gain an understanding. According to one writer, "the purpose of . . . explanation is to provide understanding . . . Arguments offer justifications; explanations offer understanding."[26] Or an explanation may be demanded from an office boy as to why he is late. In this case, a rational accountability is sought for his lateness.[27] Another view of explanation is, as in to account for an event, "to have found a set of premises from which it can logically be inferred."[28] In scientific explanation, the pattern generally used is a hypotheticodeductive scheme that, although oversimplified, looks like this:

1. General theoretical or lawlike statement predicting and explaining a future event, a principle or guideline, connecting an antecedent to a consequent.
2. Definitions of key terms.
3. Initial conditions, or specifications of conditions.
4. Conclusion predicting that a given event will occur.

Steps 1, 2, and 3 give reasons for the conclusion. For example:

1. If nurses use techniques X in emergencies, then patients' pain will be alleviated.
2. Definitions of pain and alleviation.
3. Jean Brown used techniques X to alleviate Mr. Jones's pain.
4. ∴ Jean Brown alleviated Mr. Jones's pain.

A nursing explanation could be schematized using Toulmin's layout of argument. There are warrants for drawing conclusions, sometimes called *inference tickets* or *inference licenses.*[29]

EVALUATING ARGUMENTS

There are several methods useful to assess rationally the qualities of arguments. One way to evaluate deductive and inductive arguments is to require certainty in deduction while accepting probabilities and uncertainty in inductive arguments. Further specifications for evaluating arguments as either valid, sound, relevant, or significant are developed in subsequent chapters.

Another way to evaluate arguments is to use the features of an argument as a checklist for judging completeness. Arguments contain assumptions, reasons, conclusions or beliefs, implications, or consequences. For a first approximation see Table 2–2.

Let us imagine that Nurse Lee is considering a major career change such as relocating, changing clinical fields, securing advanced educational preparation, or starting independent practice. A nurse using a checklist will ask of each option: (1) What assumptions or presumptions are being made in this situation?, (2) What reasons, premises, warrants, grounds,

TABLE 2–2. STRUCTURE OF AN ARGUMENT

1. Assumptions. Presumptions.
2. Reasons. Premises. Warrants. Grounds. Backing.
3. Conclusions/Beliefs. Claims. Decisions. Judgments.
4. Implications. Consequences.

and backing are there for the course of action I am considering?, (3) What conclusions, beliefs, claims, decisions, or judgments do I act on in this situation?, and (4) What are the likely implications or consequences of my decision, claim, or conclusion? Table 2–3 enlarges our checklist:

A third method of evaluating arguments is suggested by some ancient Greek thinkers such as Socrates. From them we learn that if we cannot prove a conclusion, if we can disprove it or undermine it, its opposite conclusion is thereby strengthened. An effective method of rationally evaluating arguments and explanation includes methods of refutation. It is not enough to confirm a theory continuously. The question is: What would count to refute a given theory or argument, such as holistic nursing and medicine? If there is no method for showing what would count to refute it, that is a methodological weakness of the theory and not a strength. Moreover, as renowned thinkers from Socrates on have shown, the claim that one's beliefs, theories, or arguments are irrefutable has not always withstood the searching scrutiny against these arguments.

The Reductio Ad Absurdum Method

Socrates (470–399 BC) lived in Athens over two thousand years ago. Although he was regarded as a renowned teacher, he was never part of any formal, institutionalized, or salaried school. Instead, he walked the streets of Athens with his followers and opponents, engrossed in arguments about the meaning of such concepts as justice, love, wisdom, courage, and truth. Socrates would not accept any belief or conclusion without good reasons. His probing was continuous with the objections raised to the solutions put forth by his followers. He then asked others to object to his objections. This process of analysis and rigorous examination of the key features of an argument, designed to probe the meaning and truth or falsity of the assertions of an argument, is called the Socratic method.

The Socratic method is identified in technical terms as the *Reductio ad absurdum.* In oversimplified terms, if we generalize, we look for a counter-example to refute the generalization. If, for example, we argue that human rights are unnecessary, we have only to examine the role of women or of nurses without rights to appreciate the need for rights. Or if we argue

TABLE 2-3. STRUCTURE OF AN ARGUMENT APPLICABLE TO NURSING

1. Formulation of the problem
2. Assumptions, presuppositions, presumptions
3. Data, the given
4. Inferences, reasons, hypotheses, activation of hypotheses
5. Conclusions, beliefs, claims, judgments, decisions
6. Tests, implications, consequences
7. Resulting warrants to make further inferences

that informed consent is unnecessary or unjustified, we have only to point to the Tuskeegee racist experiment to challenge the claim that informed consent is unnecessary.

An application of the Reductio method of refutation consists in presenting a counter-analogy to an argument. If, for example, an antiabortionist argues that a fetus has the status of an unborn child and that for a woman to abort at will is murder, we may offer the counter-analogy that a woman is a landlady who may at will evict her tenant. The counter-anology may be no more conclusive than the initial analogy. But the method of offering counter-analogies shows that we can use critical thinking to refute an analogy. The method of refuting analogy with a counter-analogy is also a way to construct and create arguments.

CONSTRUCTING ARGUMENTS

The need for constructing arguments arises in the context of daily involvements with nursing practice and theory. For example, Ms. Brown, a staff nurse is told, "Treat all patients alike," she then asks "What about Mr. Hodges, the comatose patient in Room 407, Ms. Larmoor, the 24-year-old budding actress with AIDS, the 14-year-old appendectomy patient, and Ms. Torrest, age 56, recovering from a stroke: Are they all alike?"

A way to construct arguments is to question claims and commands. Another way to construct arguments is to create counter-arguments. We can do this quite easily by thinking of exceptions. If a supervisor or nursing teacher says, "Always put the client first," ask whether a nurse should put all of an AIDS client's interests ahead of the nurse's interests in surviving. If someone argues that autonomy and self-determination over one's life and body are vitally important values and that coercion and paternalistic interference is bad, we can offer the counter-argument "Is being searched before boarding an airplane a bad idea?" Asking the right question can redirect an inquiry into the construction of new and fresh arguments. Another method is to draw an alternative argument that comes to the opposite conclusion to the one initially presented. Occasionally, bumper stickers and T-shirts express such counter-arguments. For example, the view that "A woman's place is in the house" was refuted by the counter-argument that "A woman's place is in the House of Representatives."

VALUE ARGUMENTS AND THEIR BREAKDOWN

Some deductive or inductive arguments have practical or imperative conclusions, such as people with heart trouble or cancer should not smoke. Mr. Lee has heart trouble. Therefore, Mr. Lee should not smoke, Or, if there is a cardiac arrest, call the Code for CPR. The patient in Room 303 is in cardiac arrest. So, call the Code for CPR.

Arguments with practical or imperative conclusions are sometimes identified as value arguments, even though they fit into a deductive or inductive form. In a valid, deductive argument, the conclusion is certain. In an inductive argument, the conclusion is likely or probable. In some value arguments, however, the values that one person or one group favors may collide with the values held by other persons or groups. In such an event, there may be a moral stalemate. This is illustrated in the value of conserving all human life in collision with the Jehovah's Witness's principle to refuse life-saving blood transfusion.

There are unresolvable moral dilemmas, some of which result in human tragedy. One illustration is the scarcity of health care resources. Thousands of eligible patients apply for the artificial heart to save their lives. Only a few persons, like Barney Clark, have been chosen to receive it, as only a few artificial hearts are available. This example shows that in applying critical reasoning to practical ethical problems, there is a feature that is not always rationally resolvable, namely tragedy. A further elaboration of value arguments occurs in Chapter 7.

TASK AND ACHIEVEMENT SENSES OF AN ARGUMENT

One way to perceive both the structure and dynamics of arguments is to distinguish between an argument as a finished product, an achievement, and an argument as a task or a process.[30] If a nurse, Ms. K, says of another nurse that he used critical thinking, that is an achievement sense of an argument. Critical thinking, in one sense of that expression, is an achievement.

A second sense of use of critical thinking to evaluate an argument refers to a process we go through to arrive at a valid or sound conclusion. This is the *task, try,* or *intentional* sense. This seems to be the main use of critical thinking in nursing. *Treating* rather than *curing* is a task verb. In treating patients, nurses try to raise levels of well-being for their patients rather than achieving absolute health objectives.

To use critical thinking in evaluating arguments is to recognize that arguments have task and success senses; and that arguments generally do not have certain conclusion. The task sense of an argument means that evidence for the conclusions is to be collected rather than assumed. In the prevalent try or task sense, arguments have a tentative, not a conclusive sense. It may seem ironic, even paradoxical to say that for a nurse to be successful at teaching the uses of argument, that success consists largely in teaching students to accept uncertain conclusions; but that is precisely the prevalent use of nursing arguments.

The task sense of arguments also explains the dynamic use of arguments. The process of trying to improve on thinking practices is continuous and challenging. Critical thinking, unlike certain systems of logic, is not a closed or completed system. Critical thinking is open, dynamic, continuous; and to engage in critical thinking is to be receptive to rebuttals, alterations, new insights, ideas, and techniques. Critical thinking is not only a science, but an art of thinking or of trying to think in increasingly rational ways.

CONCLUSION

This chapter demonstrates how nursing arguments have several uses. For certain nursing situations, some uses of argument are more helpful to consider than others. The prevalent uses of argument involve if–then reasoning from data and assumptions to nursing conclusions, beliefs, decisions, and actions. Conclusions in nursing are uncertain, as in other expanding fields. We use the task sense of an argument to achieve a conclusion of an argument, such as cigarette smoking is a cause of cancer. If an argument achieves a degree of credibility, through the marshaling of reasoned evidence, we then have an inference ticket, inference license, or warrant for that conclusion. By citing methods of refutation, we can distinguish between good and bad arguments that apply to nursing.

REFERENCES

1. McNeil Consumer Products Co. Back Cover RN, October, 1986.
2. Webster's New Collegiate Dictionary. Springfield, Mass. G. and C. Merriam and Co., 1974, p. 590.
3. Tanner, C. Factors Influencing the Diagnostic Process, in D. Carnevali, et al (Eds.), Diagnostic Reasoning in Nursing. Philadelphia: J.B. Lippincott, 1984, p. 63.
4. Ibid, p. 63.
5. Copi, I. Introduction to Logic (7th ed.). New York: Macmillan, 1986, p. 11.
6. Harvard Medical School Health Letter, April 1979, p. 2.
7. Weddle, P. Argument: A Guide to Critical Thinking. New York: McGraw-Hill, 1978, p. 2.
8. Seaman, C.C.H., & Verhonick, P.J. Research Methods (2nd ed.). New York: Appleton-Century-Crofts, 1982, p. 65.
9. Ibid.
10. Ibid.
11. Copi, I. Introduction to Logic, pp. 18–20.
12. Beardsley, M. Practical Logic, Englewood Cliffs, N.J.: Prentice-Hall, 1950.
13. Seaman, C.C.H., & Verhonick, P.J. Research Methods, p. 67.
14. Ibid, p. 82.
15. Ibid, p. 99.

16. Fischer, R.G., Morgan, R.S., & Parks, B. Pediatric Drug Information. *Pediatric Nursing* 1985; 11(3):315, May/June.
17. Gordon, M. Nursing Diagnosis. New York: McGraw-Hill, 1982, p. 14.
18. Seaman, C.C.H., & Verhonick, P.J. Research Methods, p. 27.
19. Ibid.
20. Ibid.
21. Toulmin, S. Uses of Argument. Cambridge, England: Cambridge University Press, 1958, p. 99.
22. Toulmin, S., Rieke, R., & Janik, A. An Introduction to Reasoning (2nd ed.). New York: Macmillan, 1984, p. 86.
23. Ibid, p. 97.
24. Toulmin, S., et al. An Introduction to Reasoning, p. 97.
25. Toulmin, S. Uses of Argument, p. 103.
26. Govier, T. A Practical Study of Argument, Belmont, Calif.: Wadsworth, 1985, p. 13.
27. Copi, I. Introduction to Logic, pp. 482–483.
28. Ibid.
29. Ryle, G. If, So and Because, in Black M (Ed.), Philosophical Analysis. Ithaca, N.Y.: Cornell University Press, pp. 329–338.
30. Ryle, G. The Concept of Mind. London: Hutchinson's University Library, 1949, pp. 130–131.

Chapter 3

Fallacies

Study of this chapter enables the learner to:

1. Understand motives and reasons for committing fallacies.
2. Identify fallacies in nursing.
3. Avoid the use of fallacies in thinking critically.
4. Distinguish major types of fallacies.
5. Develop ways to prevent the use of fallacies.

INTRODUCTION

For one individual to say to another, especially in nursing and medicine, "You committed a fallacy" is generally regarded as a serious error in judgment. To say that one has committed a fallacy is to give a negative evaluation of an argument. *Fallacy* has a decidedly negative connotation. Reasons for identifying some forms of reasoning as fallacies extend beyond purely subjective considerations. Criteria show why one type of argument is fallacious and another is not. For example, Nursing Supervisor Brown says to Staff Nurse White, "We need you to work an extra shift. That's too bad about your college class. Patients come first. If you refuse, you won't be needed here anymore." In this statement, the supervisor is committing the fallacy of irrelevant appeal to force. Therefore, a reason to study fallacies is to expose and confront them.

Critical thinking spans various kinds of effective reasoning from everyday, informal logic to formal, deductive and inductive reasoning. In all of these types of reasoning, it is possible to commit fallacies.

THE MEANING OF A FALLACY

Fallacy has several meanings. It can mean a mistake, an error, an omission, a fault, a false belief, poor judgment, some form of wrong doing, or a conclusion that does not follow from its premises.

A fallacy is obviously not a good thing to commit. The fact that we can identify some form of reasoning as a fallacy shows that not everything is relative or subjective. Some arguments are valid, sound, or cogent, whereas others are fallacious. Terms of evaluation, positive and negative, such as calling an argument fallacious, show that critical thinking has an evaluative role in reasoning. Nursing is no exception. Some judgments are cogent, whereas others are fallacious. The term fallacy has a technical meaning as well, namely that a fallacy is an error in reasoning.[1] An important form of fallacy is a *non-sequitur,* which means that the conclusion of an argument does not follow from the premises. Strictly speaking, a logical fallacy occurs only when the premises do not imply the conclusion.[2] For example, a 64-year-old, 14-day postcoronary bypass graft surgical patient, expresses fear of going back to her trailer home. She also has a gastric ulcer. On these grounds alone, she is diagnosed as having "massive dependency needs."[3] Another example of a non sequitur is a nurse's statement that a patient, who lives in a mobile home, has a low income.[4]

WHY PEOPLE COMMIT FALLACIES

Some people commit fallacies because they are overcommitted to ideological, religious, political, and economic principles. As a consequence, they either refuse to listen to counter-arguments or they cannot understand alternative arguments for contradictory conclusions. Their minds are closed. The process of reasoning is unacceptable to them.

Some people regard any argument as warlike or quarrelsome behavior; and they identify the good life with peace, even peace at any price. So they accept the good or bad reasoning of others. Other people love to win a fight, physical or verbal. They will use, abuse, and twist words and concepts to make themselves and their cause seem good and their opponents and their arguments bad or stupid. Forever ridiculing their opponents, these fallacious reasoners prefer to win than to play by the rules of intellectual engagement. So they renounce or subvert critical thinking, logic, and rationality to meet their objectives. Some people who commit fallacies are intellectually untrained to identify fallacies or to know the difference between sound and fallacious reasoning. Other people know when they commit fallacies, and acknowledge that they made a mistake.

We can group fallacies in relation to motives or reasons for committing them: the drive for political or economic power or ideology, or being persuaded by the appeal of the powerful, cultural, or religious beliefs; ignorance or lack of education or training; or becoming lost in the beauty of the words of some passage that has no meaning. Plato (428–348 BC) in the *Phaedrus* distinguishes between rhetoric, sophistry, and philosophy. Rhetoric is the art of saying things beautifully, but not paying attention to the meaning of what is said. Sophistry consists in saying things to win people over, but without regard to truth or meaning. Philosophy aims to communicate what is meaningful and true.

To engage in rhetoric is to be unaware of the content of the message and to be prone to commit fallacies. The words of songs and poems, like sweet lullabies, amply illustrate the power to say and believe what may have no literal meaning or sense. In rhetoric, the poet or writer may produce artworks that communicate something beautifully, but these artworks may be empty of content. The audiences of art consumers are apt to believe literally what the artist expresses.

The sophist communicates something that is a fabrication, a deception, a lie. There is here the deliberate intent to deceive. There are also those to whom the deception is addressed, the unwary, the untrained, and the undereducated. Almost any type of cigarette or car advertisement illustrates sophistry. Some politician's messages are also sophistic. But everyone commits fallacies, even the educated and intelligent. We cannot always precisely identify motives, interests, or personal orientations that accompany or cause us to commit fallacies. That topic is closer to psychology than to critical thinking.

KINDS OF FALLACIES

A reason for studying fallacies is to detect, expose, and confront them. To study different kinds of fallacies is to be aware of them, and to be in a position to defend against them. Among the various ways of categorizing fallacies, six seem most useful to nursing.

• FALLACIES OF IRRELEVANT GROUNDS

Some arguments are fallacious on the grounds that their premises are irrelevant to their conclusions. For this reason, their conclusions do not follow. An example of irrelevant grounds is the slur against a minority nurse on the grounds that her people do not value life.

Appeal to Force

One irrelevant argument is the appeal to force to cause the acceptance of a conclusion. If Ruth's mother threatens to sue the hospital if Nurse A tells Ruth the truth about her condition, that threat is an appeal to force. If, however, Ruth's mother tells the nurse that Ruth's last days would be unhappy if she knew she were dying, such a reason may be inaccurate, but relevant to the issue of truth telling. If Dr. R orders a drug that is clearly wrong and Nurse A questions Dr. R, who says, "I'll see that you're fired if you question me," Dr. R is appealing to force to cause Nurse A to accept his or her decision. When a rational frame of reference is assumed, appeal to force is relevant only if it is shown to provide evidence for the conclusion. When a nurse says to a physically abusive psychiatric patient, "I have to give you this injection of tranquilizer," the appeal to force is relevant if there is evidence that the psychotropic medication is a necessary condition of the decision or conclusion to tranquilize the patient. When a mother yanks a child away from an oncoming car, the use of force is relevant to the decision, which is to save the child's life.

Abuse of the Person

Another pitfall of reasoning occurs if we substitute abuse of a person for relevant reasons of a decision. The abuse fallacy occurs in one of four forms. The first is personal abuse. Here the individual is criticized on grounds that have nothing to do with a conclusion or decision. If, for example, Nurse A wishes to resuscitate 5-year-old Sandy, who is dying of a brain tumor, Nurse B's argument, "You're just afraid of dying yourself" is no argument. Or if Dr. K tells a patient who refuses an x-ray, "You're just paranoid," the health professional is committing a personal abuse fallacy. There may be good reasons for not resuscitating Sandy or for not having x-rays taken, but they do not include irrelevant personal abuse.

A second form of abuse is *circumstantial abuse.* Here, in place of an argument, the person is chided into believing or doing X on the grounds of membership in a group that habitually does X. If, for example, Nurse A resuscitates Sandy and Nurse B says, "You're a Catholic," this may be true but irrelevant to the reasons Nurse A may have for resuscitating the child. Or if Nurse C says that what Dr. L did was magnificient, and Nurse D says, "Oh, you both work at Hospital H," Nurse D's statement is circumstantial abuse. It is not relevant to whether Dr. L. did or did not do a good job.

A third version of abuse is known as "You're another." If Nurse A finds Dr. S using drugs, and Dr. S retorts, "I've seen you use them," Dr. S's statement may be true, but irrelevant to the issue of Dr. S's drug use. A version of "you're another" (tu quoque) abuse fallacy is used in ethics in the principle that "two wrongs don't make a right."

A fourth and last version of the abuse fallacy is known as the genetic fallacy. Instead of accepting or refuting evidence on relevant grounds, the person is abused by casting doubt on his or her origins. A health professional, for example, tells a patient, "The reason that you're a drug addict is that you come out of the slums and nobody cared for you. Considering where you came from, no wonder you're an addict."

There is, however, a difference between the genetic fallacy and the genetic method. The latter is useful in medicine and the life sciences. A nurse's examination makes use of the medical history of a patient, and history is relevant and useful for diagnosis. The genetic fallacy occurs if someone's origins are used exclusively to draw a conclusion for abusive purposes. The origins are not necessarily relevant to the conclusion.

Appeal to Ignorance

Another form of fallacy appeals to ignorance as a form of evidence. For example, officials of cigarette companies stated publicly that there was no proof that smoking caused cancer. This created the impression and implied the conclusion that smoking does not cause cancer. The absence of complete proof for a conclusion, such as that smoking is a casual factor of cancer, does not mean that the evidence can be discounted. The fallacy of appeal to ignorance is committed by shifting the burden of proof for a conclusion to the other side and demanding complete proof for the opposite conclusion. Because complete proof is often impossible, the implication is that the opposite conclusion is true.

If a patient enters the hospital emergency room complaining of chest pain and, on the basis of an electrocardiogram and other tests, the health professionals find nothing wrong, the fallacy of the appeal to ignorance consists in saying, "We couldn't find anything wrong. Therefore, there is nothing wrong." In this situation, health professionals do not know the cause of the chest pain, possibly esophageal disease. The absence of evidence for a proposition does not establish the truth of the opposite conclusion.

Appeal to Populace

Appeal to the populace or appeal to a consensus is a further pitfall in making inferences. The fallacy consists in arguing that everyone else does something, therefore, it must be good. For example, an operating room supervisor says that all her colleagues are using antiseptic X for cold sterilization, therefore, it must be good. Popularity or consensus does not prove quality.

Appeal to Authority

A frequently used fallacy of irrelevant reasoning that occurs in health care is the appeal to authority. The appeal to irrelevant authority is that of a person with established authority in one field who tries to qualify as an expert in another field in which he or she is insufficiently prepared. For example, a psychiatric nurse of many years is generally not an expert in surgical nursing; therefore, that person's opinion on surgery is less than expert. Similarly, Nurse A commits the fallacy of appealing to authority if she recommends Dr. H, an eminent cardiologist, as an expert moral philosopher, economist, or political scientist.

Appeal to Pity

Another fallacy consists in the irrelevant appeal to pity to bring about the acceptance of a conclusion. For example, a drug addict on a detoxification unit appeals to Nurse A for morphine to relieve his or her distressing withdrawal symptoms, such as vomiting, convulsions, twitches, and severe abdominal pain, on the grounds that he or she is a drug addict. A particularly outrageous example of the fallacy of the appeal to pity is the trial of a youngster accused of murdering his parents with an axe. After being confronted with staggering evidence of his guilt, "he pleaded for mercy on the grounds that he was an orphan."[5]

• FALLACIES OF INADEQUATE OR MISSING GROUNDS

There are also fallacies that are made on insufficient ground for their conclusions. This type of fallacy also bears on statistical reasoning, as when figures and samples are misused to arrive at a conclusion that is not supported by the evidence.

Hasty Generalization

A fallacy, identified as an inductive fallacy, called hasty generalization, consists in making a universal statement on the basis of a limited sample. The example of one bad-smelling old patient cannot be generalized to the conclusion that all old patients smell badly. Sexist, racist, religious, or ethnic stereotyping also consists in generalizing about people of a particular sex, race, sect, or ethnic group on the basis of a small sample. If Nurse Jones treats Ms. Smith, a South American patient whom she sees smoking a cigar, and then infers that all South American women smoke cigars, she is committing the fallacy of hasty generalization.

There are two further versions of hasty generalization or induction. One is the slippery slope fallacy, which assumes that if one exception to a rule is allowed, the person granted the exception will ask for others in succession. This leads to an uncontrollable set of unwanted results. In courting behavior, some females in some cultures are cautioned by their parents not to let males "go too far." A kiss is said to lead to other sexual behavior, leading to an uncontrollable chain reaction with unwanted consequences, such as pregnancy, venereal disease or AIDS. Therefore, one is told not to allow the first kiss.

An antiabortion argument is that if abortion is morally and legally permissible, thus allowing the murder of a fetus, it will be followed by infanticide and then by the killing of children, the killing of the mentally ill and the nonproductive old. In time, killing of the unwanted will become morally permissible. Similarly, the slippery slope fallacy is committed in arguing that if euthanasia is allowed for one individual or group, there will be no way to stop the moral and legal permissibility of killing any unwanted person. Some hospital authorities who oppose collective bargaining for nurses similarly argue that if nurses are permitted to make salary demands, the hospital will go bankrupt.

The Heap Fallacy

A fallacy closely related to the slippery slope fallacy is known as the *heap fallacy,* which also presents a paradox of sorts. Imagine a beach of sand. Someone builds a little sand hill and then asks whether one more grain of sand will make a difference. The answer is No. What about adding two grains, or three or four, or even twenty five? Will they make a difference? No. At what point will they make a difference? The heap fallacy consists in inferring that little accretions do not or will not make a difference. Although those who commit this fallacy may recognize that 10 million grains of sand make a difference, their attention is on the little accretions of one grain of sand at a time that do not seem to matter. For example, a nurse may love to eat chocolates, ice cream, and steaks. As she puts herself on the scale and notices the weight gain, she tells herself, "I mustn't overdo it." As she gains more, she says, "What's another ice cream cone?" She's right. It's like adding a grain of sand to her collection. But the fallacy consists in thinking that by little accretions, there is never a point in the heap in which her added weight will show itself. Similarly, a cigarette smoker says, "What's just one more cigarette today?" Or a driver going a little beyond the speed limit who says, "What's a little extra speed?" There is a point where the heap shows, whether it is gaining weight by "just one more dessert," a drunken person having "having just one more drink," or a heavy cigarette smoker having "just a few more smokes."

Accident

The fallacy of accident, the converse of hasty generalization, consists in the indiscriminate application of a rule to every situation without regard to *accidental* variations or altered circumstances.[6] For example, a nurse believes in the Kantian imperative of always telling the truth. Her patient says, "If I have cancer of the breast with metastases, I will kill myself. I have no intention of dragging on for years in pain and in misery the way my mother did." This nurse then tells the patient that she has cancer of the breast with metastases, without counseling and preparing the patient for the bad news. If a physician orders an adult dose of Thorazine for all patients without questioning the variations of dosage in relation to the person's body weight, age, and degree of disturbance, the physician is committing the fallacy of accident.

Begging the Question

A serious fallacy of inadequate grounds is the fallacy of begging the question. To beg the question is to assume in the premises the very thing to be proved. To say, for example, that Beethoven is greater than Brubeck because persons of higher socioeconomic brackets prefer Beethoven begs the question at issue. To say a certain patient is incurable because experts agree that people with that disease are incurable begs the question of whether this particular patient is incurable. If Nurse Jones recommends Dr. Smith as a neurosurgeon and when asked "Why?" responds, "My friends in the operating room say he has the best sterile technique," this nurse is begging the question. The mortality rate of this surgeon's patients exceeds that of other neurosurgeons in similar circumstances. Or consider this further example: Nurse N. "Smith is telling the truth." Question: "Why do you say that?" Answer: "She wouldn't lie to me about this."[7]

The Is–Ought Fallacy

The *is–ought* fallacy consists in arguing that because X (some custom or practice, decision or policy) is in reality the case, therefore, it follows that X ought to be the case. For example, someone who says, "Nurses are physicians' handmaidens; so, nurses ought to be subordinate to physicians," commits the is–ought fallacy. Similarly, the statement, "Nurses give direct care to clients. So, nurses ought to stay at the bedside," also commits the is–ought fallacy. Another example of the is–ought fallacy is that "Nurses get low salaries, therefore, nurses ought to get low salaries." The desire of a physician, a patient, or a nursing supervisor to have her or his orders followed does not by itself imply that such orders ought to be followed. Just because some pre-Nuremberg medical experimenters conducted research without consent of subjects does not imply that doing so was or is morally permissible. The fact that nurses work overtime does not imply that they ought to do so or that it is a good thing that they do so.

A particularly subtle use of the is–ought fallacy arises when health care decisions are regarded as value-free. To regard choices among medical or nursing alternatives as value-free means that the values of patients and health professionals are denied. The implication is that health professionals decide exclusively what treatment to use without patient input. There are values in all sorts of health care decisions, such as the respect and worth accorded to the nursing role in a hospital or the way an injection is given. Values are embedded in decisions regarding the equipment a hospital purchases and maintains. Values are expressed or denied in the controls of health care, including educational standards of nurses and medical practitioners.

The relation of values to facts is, as the President's Commission reports, a dynamic interaction, not a static separation of facts and values. Smoking cigarettes, for example, is a cause of lung and heart disease. This is a fact, but it also has value implications of what a society and individuals in it ought to do. To avoid the is–ought fallacy, a further premise to the effect that lung disease and heart disease are undesirable is needed.

• FALLACIES OF DEFECTIVE OR FAULTY GROUNDS

Some fallacies are said not on inadequate or missing grounds, but on defective or faulty grounds. The premises of such arguments may not be irrelevant, but they go away from supporting their conclusions.

Forgetful Induction

Whereas the fallacy of hasty induction is a clear case of inadequate grounds, forgetful induction,[8] as its name points out, is a case of a lapse or omission. This type of fallacy occurs when a subgroup of a larger group is sampled, and on the grounds of the findings of the subgroup, the same relation is applied to the larger group. Other groups, therefore, are not studied. For example, an interviewer studies the tea drinking habits of English nurses and concludes that because they have a high rate of tea consumption, other European nurses have a similarly high rate of tea consumption. What the interviewer forgot or ignored is that French nurses, for example, may have a high rate of coffee consumption and a low rate of tea consumption.

Slothful Induction

The slothful induction fallacy consists in the refusal to allow any evidence to be considered that refutes one's conclusion. This fallacy is sometimes identified as holding a priori assumptions,[9] the method of tenacity,[10] or the use of self-sealers.[11] By whatever name, these expressions of slothful induction are ways of insulating against criticism. For example, the new staff nurse wants to discuss a forthcoming surgical case involving the amputation of the left leg of a frightened patient. The head nurse says, "Here at Hosptial R, only the surgeon talks directly to the patient about forthcoming surgery."

The dogmatic refusal to question the ways of a group is dramatically illustrated in efforts to burn people at the stake for believing that the earth was not flat or that the earth is not the center of the universe. Dogmatists and book burners have refused to allow others to believe that *Homo sapiens* could evolve from other animals, that sex could be a driving force in human nature, or that injecting a person with a disease could provide an immunity. Part of the education of the human race consists in exposing and confronting dogmas and the refusal to question wherever it occurs. An important freedom and an antidote to slothful induction is the right to inquire, no matter where the inquiry leads. A nurse or physician who refuses to question a particular treatment or diagnosis is committing the fallacy of slothful induction.

The Fallacy of Attribution

The fallacy of attribution is also known as the *fallacy of reading somebody's mind.* For example, if a nurse says to a patient, who has just been told she has cancer, "You must be feeling very angry," the nurse is attributing a state of mind to the patient that the patient may or may not have. Or if a nurse responds to a patient's complaint of pain shortly after giving the patient an analgesic, by telling the patient, "You're just imagining it," that nurse is committing the fallacy of attribution. Or if a nursing instructor says of a student who is frequently late or absent, "Mary is lazy," the nursing instructor is committing the fallacy of attribution. There may be other reasons for the student's lateness and absences.

The Pathetic Fallacy

The pathetic fallacy consists in attributing human qualities to non-human beings such as pets, structures, or machines. To say that a machine is purring, that the car is sick, or that "My car died on me," attributes human qualities to non-human beings.

The Apathetic Fallacy

The converse of the pathetic fallacy is the apathetic fallacy. This fallacy is committed if non-human qualities are attributed to humans. An example is a nurse's statement, "Patient X is like a rock, hard and immovable." It is said that Freud's id, superego, which supposedly orients the unconscious, resembles a hydraulic mechanism.

The Monte Carlo Fallacy

The Monte Carlo fallacy consists of supposing that because a certain event in a series has not occurred for a long time, the probability increases of its occurring the next time. For example, an obstetrical nurse who says, "We haven't had any deliveries all day. It's got to pick up tonight," is committing the Monte Carlo fallacy. The law of large numbers does not predict what will happen next; only that in the long run, the probability of any given event occurring is the same as it is for any other event in a series. Fallacies on defective grounds have premises that are off the point from the conclusion of the argument.

• FALLACIES OF INCONSISTENCY

There are several fallacies of inconsistency. A major violation in logic is called contradiction, as when someone says, "Your statement contradicted your earlier statement." In terms of formal logic, we may not have premises that assert a proposition P followed by a conclusion that asserts that P is not the case. P cannot be both asserted and denied. If a health professional says, "I was in Room 310 at 4 PM," and later denies it, the latter statement contradicts the first statement. To argue that abortion or euthanasia is wrong because these acts show disrespect for human life and to then argue for more nuclear weapons, a larger defense establishment, and more defensive military actions, shows disrespect for human life. To reduce welfare benefits to families with dependent children, the elderly, and other vulnerable groups, is inconsistent with respect for life. Also nurses who neglect or abuse patients are inconsistent with the core of nursing practice, which calls for giving care to people.

Category Mistakes

A category mistake consists in joining terms in a sentence that cannot fit into the same logical category or type. To say that "John sprained his ankle" is appropriate, but not "He sprained his brain."[12] This is not an ordinary mistake, but a logical mistake. Another example of a category mistake is to say that "Nurses engage in medical diagnosis." This is an inconsistent use of what nurses do, namely nursing diagnosis. The following examples are category mistakes. "Henry is an unborn child," "Albert, who just died, is resting in peace," "X, who died yesterday, took her last trip to the cemetery today." The reason these are category mistakes is that if taken literally, these expressions consist in the misallocation of terms that properly belong to one category and are treated as if they belong to another category. If a fetus is referred to as being unborn, he is not yet a child, nor does he have a name in normal locution. If Albert is dead, he is not resting in the way a person rests or sleeps. He is not at ease; nor is he restless. Categories that apply to Albert, while alive, do not apply to Albert when he is dead. To refer literally to a comatose patient as a vegetable commits a category mistake. Each of these sentences has fragments that do not logically fit with one another. These are, strictly speaking, self-contradictory sentences. Another illustration of a category mistake, according to G. Ryle, who developed this idea, is of a cricket team, with its batsmen, bowlers, wicket keepers. Someone then asks, "Who supplies the team spirit?"[13] It has to be pointed out that the team as a whole supplies the team spirit, not another specialized player. One could apply the same reasoning to any activity such as nursing. If a client is told that nurses care for the client at the bedside and give appropriate medications under physicians' prescriptions, and then asks, "Who provides for the patient's recovery, treatment, and cure?" the answer is that these are the activities that health professionals and patients do together.

An example of a category mistake, according to T. Szasz, is that there is no such disease as *mental illness,* which he calls a myth. The words *mental* and *illness* do not logically fit together.[14] Szasz says that illnesses are physical, and mental refers to cognitive and character functions. The two, he says, are not in the same category. On Szasz's account, it makes sense to say that there are physical illnesses and character disorders, but not mental illnesses.

• FALLACIES OF FAULTY AND UNJUSTIFIED ASSUMPTIONS

These fallacies occur if the assumptions on which arguments depend are faulty or unjustified. (e.g., A nurse assumes that a given patient is breathing without difficulty, that respirations are within normal limits, when in fact the patient's respirations are shallow and rapid.)

Complex Question

The complex question fallacy consists in asking a question whose answer depends on the affirmative answer to a prior question that, however, is not stated. The question, "When did you stop beating your wife?" presupposes the answer to two prior questions: "Do you have a wife?" and "Did you beat your wife?" If the person addressed was and is a bachelor, then the question does not arise. A health care example is the question to patients, "Do you want to have this surgery and live, or not have this surgery and die?" The unasked questions are "What other treatments are there?," "How long do I have to live?," "Will the surgery cure me?," and "How will I survive the surgery?"

Similarly, the question, "Are you part of the problem or part of the solution?" is a complex question, sometimes known as the fallacy of exclusive alternation or black or white thinking. If we are presented with two alternatives, it does not mean that they are mutually exclusive or that there are no other alternatives. If we suppose that there are only two alternatives, we commit the fallacy of black or white thinking. For example, a patient need not be a Christian or a Jew. The patient may be a Humanist, a Hindu, a Muslim, or a Buddhist. Similarly, if we say there are two alternative treatments for some cancers, chemotherapy and Laetrile, we commit the black or white fallacy. There may be other alternatives, or one of these may not be a real alternative.

A head nurse who asks Nurse A, "Why didn't you give Ms. R, the patient, digitalis yesterday at 8 PM?" commits the complex question fallacy if either Nurse A was not on duty at that time or Ms. R died before the time referred to in the question.

False Cause

The fallacy of false cause occurs when a speaker assumes that because two events have occurred in temporal sequence, the first is the cause of the second. Nurse A, for example, sees a patient, who had Laetrile after a cancer remission. Nurse A incorrectly concludes that Laetrile causes cancer remissions. Beating the drum and claiming that the rainfall is related to drum beating commits false cause. People who believe that walking under ladders causes bad luck also commit the fallacy of false cause.

The fallacy of false cause sometimes occurs if event A precedes event B. The fallacy is to conclude that A is the cause of B. The unwarranted assumption is that temporal precedence implies a causal sequence. If this version of false cause occurs, it is referred to as the *post hoc ergo propter hoc* fallacy. A health professional may infer that because an expert was at a sick patient's bedside, the patient will recover. The presence of the health professional does not assure the patient's recovery.[15,16]

• FALLACIES OF AMBIGUITY

Fallacies of ambiguity depend on a play on words. The same word is open to different interpretations.

Equivocation

Some fallacies depend on using the same term but with different meanings. In deductive, syllogistic logic, this is known as the four-term fallacy. A syllogistic rule is that the syllogism must have exactly three terms, a major, a minor, and a middle term. But in the *four-term* fallacy, one of the three terms is used in a second and different sense. Equivocation depends on two different uses of a word, where a shift in meaning has occurred. For example, a nurse says, "I'm a nurse. Therefore, I'll nurse this old car." A further example of ambiguity is:

> The end of a thing is perfection.
> Death is the end of life.
> ∴ Death is perfection.[17]

Equivocation is a frequent source of misunderstandings. For example, some people have wanted peace in their time, only to find that the conditions for peace, dictated by the powerful, often made lasting and worthwhile peace an elusive goal. Other terms that are often used equivocally include freedom, democracy, and happiness. These words may mean totally different things to the persons who use them. Minimizing the equivocation of terms, such as peace, fair wages, strike, health, nursing, and nursing process, depends on careful analysis of the conditions that make such terms clearly operative and functional.

Composition Fallacy

To argue that whatever applies to part of a thing applies to the whole is to commit the fallacy of composition. For example, Mr. Jones's leg ulcer is dirty; therefore, Mr. Jones is dirty. Or, to argue that "the cells of the body are microscopic, therefore, the entire body must be microscopic" commits the fallacy of composition.[18] Or "If all the parts of the machine are light in weight, therefore, the whole machine is light," again commits the composition fallacy.[19] If we argue that because each human being to date has lived less than 125 years, therefore, the whole human race lives less than 125 years, a composition fallacy is committed. We cannot automatically attribute the same attributes to its parts. Attributing life or death to whole civilizations also commits the composition fallacy.

Division Fallacy

The division fallacy is the converse of the composition fallacy, and occurs if the same property attributed to the whole is attributed to each of its parts. To say that nurses are well paid does not imply that each and every nurse is well paid. Just because hospitalization is very expensive does not mean that the patient's nursing care is also expensive. University Medical Center is a great institution. It cannot be implied, however, that each and every nursing and medical practitioner is also great. A particularly objectionable example of the division fallacy is committed by a hospital administrator who argues that nurses are the most costly item on the hospital budget. The implication is that each nurse costs and earns more than everyone else. The reason that nursing service costs more is that nurses are needed more than any other category of health professionals or hospital workers, and because nurses provide 24-hour care.

Fallacy of Accent

A further fallacy of ambiguity consists in shifting emphasis in written or oral presentations. For example, in the statement, "He should not have treated his wife that way in public,"[20] it is not clear whether he should not have treated his wife that way, or just that way in public; it is also ambiguous as to what "that way" refers to.

The fallacy of accent occurs frequently in advertisements, in newspaper headlines, and in magazine promotional schemes. A book cover that refers to Jacqueline Kennedy Onassis carried the headline "Jackie's true love revealed." One expects a shocking revelation. Instead we learn that her "true love is her children."[21] Another lure is to say "CANCER CURE." The article concludes with "the remote possibility of finding a cure for some types of cancer within our lifetimes."[22] Or "CANCER CURE" in big letters is followed by small print, "doubted by experts."

Amphiboly

Amphiboly is a fallacy of ambiguity that occurs as a result of grammatical construction. Amphibolous phrases depend on interpretation, some of which have "humorous aspects."[23] For example, one amphibolous bumper sticker reads, "Let's not meet by accident." Amphibolous statements also appear in literature. Shakespeare arranges for the witches in *Macbeth* to reassure Macbeth that no man of woman born will slay him. He feels reassured until Macduff, who was born through a cesarian birth, kills Macbeth. In health care practice, amphiboly can be committed by ambiguous orders, such as "Give two aspirins to four ward patients every day."

A humorous practice of experienced nurses was to dispatch naive students in nursing to "Fetch a fallopian tube."

EXERCISES

Cite the fallacy.

1. When will you stop cheating?
   Answer: Complex question. Presupposes that the person began cheating.
2. That nurse is a mindless evangelist. That doctor is a crazy scientist.
   Answer: Question-begging epithets.
3. If she doesn't believe in God, she won't go to Heaven, according to her priest.
   Answer: Appeal to force.
4. Touch therapy has never been disproved. Therefore it's apt to be true.
   Answer: Appeal to ignorance.
5. If I can't have a turn jump roping, I'll take my rope home.
   Answer: Appeal to force.
6. I went out last week with an intern from Jay Stewart hospital and he was dull. Yesterday, I dated another intern from Jay Stewart. He was even duller. So, don't bother with interns from Jay Stewart.
   Answer: Hasty generalization.
7. Your sandwich made me nauseous at 5 AM. Your sandwich was the last thing I ate before going to bed. So the last thing I ate was the cause of my nausea.[24]
   Answer: False cause.
8. The tomato is round. Therefore, its parts must be round.
   Answer: Division fallacy.
9. I can't find my medication. So, it's lost.
   Answer: Appeal to ignorance.
10. Columnist gets urologist in trouble with his peers.[25]
    Answer: Accent, with ambiguity about "his." Unclear whether "his" refers to columnist's or urologist's peers.
11. Ethiopians are becoming extinct. That man is an Ethiopian. So, that man is becoming extinct.
    Answer: Division fallacy. Moving from class to individual or part.
12. Because all humans are mortal, the human race will some day come to an end.
    Answer: Composition fallacy. Moving from individual humans to the class of humans.

13. All diploma schools are practically extinct. Mt. Care is a diploma school. So Mt. Care is becoming extinct.
Answer: Division fallacy. Going from the whole to the part.

14. Rev. Cook believes in God. You can't trust a clergyman to give you a rational argument about the existence of God.
Answer: Circumstantial *ad hominen* fallacy.

15. "Each person's happiness is good to that person, and the general happiness, therefore, is a good to the aggregate of all persons." J.S. Mill, *Utilitarianism.*
Answer: Composition fallacy. Going from individual to aggregate.

16. Mr. L is poor as a church mouse. Moreover, he loses whenever he plays cards. So, he is a poor loser.
Answer: Equivocation on the word *poor.*

17. Assumptions are basic principles often documented in the literature and assumed to be true.[26]
Answer: Begging the question fallacy. Using the same word to be defined in the definition.

18. A study of several thousand heroin users showed that 70 percent had used marijuana before they tried heroin. The investigator concludes that 70 percent of all marijuana users will go on to try heroin.[27]
Answer: Hasty generalization, insufficient sample.

19. Nurse Gree: "I couldn't find the antibiotics in the 'frigerator. So, they forgot to deliver them yesterday."
Answer: Fallacy of appeal to ignorance.

20. When did you stop smoking?
Answer: Complex question, presupposes that person had ever begun.

21. Dr. Little has a sharp mind. So, he cuts people up.
Answer: Equivocation on *sharp.* Being alert does not imply that Dr. Little does surgery.

22. If someone argues that 80 percent of nurses support a right to health care, therefore, 80 percent of the people support a right to health care, what fallacy is committed?
Answer: Forgetful induction: Forgot to notice percentage of physicians opposing a right to health care, and forgot to study other professional health groups.

23. School guidance counselor to Nora, 18, a high school senior, "To which schools of nursing will you be applying?"
Answer: Complex question. Nora may decide not to apply at any school of nursing.

24. If you don't like it in this hospital, go to another one and see how you like it.
Answer: Either–or fallacy. To reject one alternative does not imply acceptance of a second one as better.

25. Nurse Leslie: "A dozen newborns were normal. The next one is bound to be abnormal."
Answer: Monte Carlo fallacy.

26. Nurse Freeley: "I've always been lucky. I love Joe Smith, the new resident. He loves me. He looks so clean cut. I'm sure he hasn't had casual sex. Therefore, I think I'll have sex with him."
Answer: Fallacies of false cause and hasty generalization.

MINIMIZING AND AVOIDING FALLACIES

Fallacies are minimized and avoided by recognizing how they are detrimental to effective and clear thinking. We develop habitual training and skill in identifying them, and, in reconstructing arguments without fallacies, we learn to discriminate between cogent and fallaceous arguments. To develop these skills of intellectual criticism helps us to minimize and avoid being trapped by or using fallacious arguments.

Fallacies are pitfalls and booby traps in critical thinking. They are errors in reasoning to be avoided whenever possible. One way to do so is by identifying the fallacies, much as we recognize danger signals on the road.

Another way is to have a checklist,[28] such as a pilot uses before a take-off. Such a checklist will have questions of the following kind:

1. What are the grounds in the premises to support the conclusion?
2. Are these grounds relevant to the conclusion?
3. Are the grounds contained in the premises evidentially adequate to justify the conclusion?
4. Are the assumptions on which the argument depends themselves justifiable?
5. Are the premises and conclusion of the argument clear?

If, for example, one is asked "Are you a good hospital nurse or are you an academic nurse?" one needs to expose this question as an example of a complex question. One can then provide a rejoinder, such as "Yes, I'm a competent, intelligent, questioning, committed, practicing nurse with an academic degree." Or to the question, "Why did you fail to give the patient in Room 304 the needed medication (Digoxin 0.25 mg qd., HCTZ 250 mg bid, KCl 20 meg bid, Prednisone 40 mg),[29] which would have prevented his fatal cardiac arrest?" One may appropriately respond, "I didn't fail, since I was not on duty yesterday."

As with any other serious activity, practice with reasoning helps us to achieve intellectual guardedness, alertness, and mastery over the many fallacies we are apt to encounter on a daily basis. But as with other human activities, there is no panacea or definitive cookbook recipe, surefire immunization, or insurance policy on avoiding fallacies. One does not rest secure. To effectively minimize fallacies requires daily practice in distinguishing good from fallacious reasoning.

CONCLUSION

A central function of critical thinking in nursing is the identification, exposure, and attempted avoidance of fallacies. This chapter explains what fallacies are so as to be on intellectual guard against either committing fallacies or of being a victim of them. Although there are no "cures" against fallacies, being aware of fallacies, and being intellectually alert to them, may help to minimize their occurrence and help guard against the harm that can come from their indiscriminate use.

REFERENCES

1. Copi, I. Introduction to Logic (7th ed.). New York: Macmillan, 1986, p. 91.
2. Barker, S. Elements of Logic (4th ed.). New York: McGraw Hill, 1985, p. 197.
3. Tanner, C. Factors Influencing the Diagnostic Process, in Carnevali, D., et al (Eds.), Diagnostic Reasoning in Nursing. Philadelphia: J.B. Lippincott, 1984, pp. 64–65, 86–87.
4. Ibid, p. 65.
5. Copi, I. Introduction to Logic, p. 96.
6. Ibid, p. 99.
7. Toulmin, S., et al. An Introduction to Reasoning (2nd ed.). New York: Macmillan, 1984, p. 135.
8. Barker, S. Elements of Logic, p. 245.
9. Hospers, J. An Introduction to Philosophical Analysis (2nd ed.). Englewood-Cliffs, N.J.: Prentice-Hall, 1967, p. 186.
10. Peirce, C. The Fixation of Beliefs, in Klemke, E.D., Kline, A.D., Hollinger, R. (Eds.), Philosophy: The Basic Issues (2nd ed.). New York: St. Martin's Press, 1986, pp. 47–49.
11. Fogelin, R. J. Understanding Argument (2nd ed.). New York: Harcourt Brace, 1982, p. 186.
12. Hospers, J. An Introduction to Philosophical Analysis, p. 91.
13. Ryle, G. The Concept of Mind. London: Hutchinson's University Library 1949, pp. 11–23.
14. Szasz, T. The Myth of Mental Illness, in Edwards R. (Ed.), Psychiatry and Ethics. Buffalo: Prometheus, 1982, pp. 19–28.
15. Carnevali, D. The Diagnostic Reasoning Process, in Carnevali, D., et al, Diagnostic Reasoning in Nursing, pp. 48–49.
16. Tanner, C. Diagnostic Problem Solving Strategies, in Carnevali, D., et al (Eds.), Diagnostic Reasoning in Nursing, pp. 90–93, 95.
17. Copi, I. Introduction to Logic, p. 113.
18. Toulmin, S., et al. An Introduction to Reasoning, p. 172.

19. Copi, I. Introduction to Logic, p. 117.
20. Toulmin, S., et al. An Introduction to Reasoning, p. 170.
21. Ibid.
22. Toulmin, S., et al. An Introduction to Reasoning, p. 171.
23. Copi, I. Introduction to Logic, p. 115.
24. Toulmin, S., et al. An Introduction to Reasoning, p. 159.
25. Ibid, p. 197.
26. Seaman, C.H., & Verhonick, P.J. Research Methods (2nd ed.). East Norwalk, Conn.: Appleton-Century-Crofts, 1982, p. 33.
27. Salmon, M.H. Logic and Critical Thinking. San Diego: Harcourt Brace, Jovanovich, 1984, p. 62.
28. Tanner, C. Factors Influencing the Diagnostic Process, in Carnevali, D., et al (Eds.), Diagnostic Reasoning in Nursing, p. 96.
29. Toulmin, S., et al. An Introduction to Reasoning, p. 179.

Part II
DYNAMICS OF PRACTICAL ARGUMENTS IN NURSING

Chapter 4

Use of Critical Thinking in Scientific Reasoning

Study of this chapter enables the learner to:

1. Understand the significance of scientific reasoning in the development of knowledge.
2. Distinguish between the senses of knowledge, including belief, intuition, revelation, and authority.
3. Identify the conditions of knowledge, including the meaning of truth and evidence.
4. Evaluate the arguments for one, none, or many methods of scientific reasoning.
5. Use the essential features of the process of scientific reasoning in analyzing and evaluating arguments.

INTRODUCTION

Nurses benefit by learning scientific reasoning. Nursing is increasingly involved in scientific practice, methods, technology, research, and achievements. Modern hospital nursing occurs primarily in university affiliated teaching hospitals. These institutions, in turn, draw their resources, power, and direction from research in the sciences.

Similarly, community nurses are caring for patients in their homes. These patients are in need of scientific teaching, monitoring, and highly technological care, such as peritoneal dialysis. Dialysis patients must be observed and monitored for fluid and electrolyte imbalance, signs and symptoms of fluid deficit or overload, renal insufficiency, side effects of powerful drugs, exercise and activity, and nutritional intake. Scientific reasoning is essential in this practice area as well.

A second term closely associated with scientific reasoning is empirical knowledge. In a strict sense, science means knowledge. An important aim of this chapter is for the nurse to learn to apply critical thinking to claims of knowledge. In this way, the nurse can distinguish bona fide from bogus knowledge. A further objective of this chapter is to distinguish truth from belief, and either of these from the sources of knowledge. The goal is to help nurses achieve justifiable judgments with which to guide nursing actions and decisions.

Why do we value knowledge? To know is among the highest marks of intellectual achievement in most cultures. So highly celebrated is knowledge that it is the basis for individuals achieving advanced degrees. Academic diplomas attest that the degree recipients have the required knowledge to practice their professions effectively. For a nurse to be identified as one who knows, distinguishes her or him from others who may know less or not at all what is required to help a patient. So exhalted and useful is knowledge as a goal of learning and of social activity that we occasionally claim to know more than we actually know. At times, nurses and physicians claim to know more than they can demonstrate. Nurses may claim to know on the basis of various sources of knowledge, which are sometimes confused with knowledge itself. These sources of knowledge include experiences, reason, faith, intuition, revelation, sense impressions, and authority. Even though nurses can trace their knowledge to these sources, they still may not know.

SCIENTIFIC REASONING IN NURSING

Science is all about us. Science and scientific reasoning influence our health practices, occupation, life-style, and even recreation. The practice and theory of nursing is heavily influenced by science. Nursing theory, research, and practice is based on scientific reasoning as is medicine and allied health professions.

Scientific reasoning exerts powerful influences on everyday nursing decisions. A decision is operationally defined as choosing to do something, a choice of action selected from among competing actions. Few decisions are as simple as "Stop smoking or risk lung cancer." These decisions depend on empirical knowledge based on investigation and inductive forms of argument that can never yield certainty. Empirical knowledge, as the outcome of research, is accumulated data that is probable but not certain. Critical thinking is an indispensable tool in evaluating such decisions.

In this work, scientific reasoning is a broadly defined approach covering what is commonly called problem-solving and scientific method. The nursing process itself can be viewed as one variation of the scientific method. The nursing process is regarded as appropriate for clinical judgments and decisions related to particular clients. In contrast, the problem-solving approach is regarded as the systematic attempt to define a problem, to search for explanations and solutions, to redefine the problem when indicated, and lastly, to eliminate the problem. In comparison, the nursing process begins with the assessment of the patient, identifies problems, formulates nursing diagnoses, sets goals, puts these into motion, and evaluates outcomes in relation to specific nursing interventions. Use of the nursing process tends to be restricted to patient care, whereas the problem-solving approach is, in general, used for patient, staff, management, and administrative problems. Both schema can be viewed as possibly simplified variations on the more rigorous, more generalizable method of scientific reasoning.

VALUE OF METHOD

Modern science and technology, now at the core of health care delivery, depend on methods of proceeding from the initiation of a process to its conclusion. In nursing there are methods for achieving desirable results for patient care. The nursing process and its documented applications attest to the value and importance of method.

We value method because it shows us a reliable way to achieve predictable, desirable results. Avoid decubitus by turning the patient in specified ways and frequencies. Following a method usually achieves the desired results. We can use critical thinking where it is needed and leave to methods much of the task that is required of anyone doing something for the first time. Using method means we do not have to "re-invent the wheel." The use of method(s) shows us what others have learned. The use of methods, therefore, saves energy for learning new things and from which further methods will be developed.

IS ONE METHOD SUFFICIENT?

John Dewey is the modern advocate of the so-called scientific method. His view was that scientific reasoning can be reduced to six steps including identifying the problem, looking for hypotheses, and trying them out. Dewey's confidence in method was not his alone. Philosophers, such as R. Descartes (1596–1650), Spinoza (1632–1677), and Leibniz (1646–1716), held a similar view of method. Essentially, Descartes's method consists of four rules: (1) doubt everything, including one's own customs, country, teachers, and parents; (2) start with the simplest ideas, those that are clear and distinct and that cannot be doubted upon reflection. Here Descartes comes to the famous "cognito ergo sum," "I think, therefore, I am."[1] (3) Move in an orderly progression from the simplest to the most complex ideas; and (4) make reviews so general as to omit nothing.

Descartes's method, as Dewey's scientific method later on, appealed to professional decision makers such as physicians, nurses, biologists, chemists, teachers, lawyers, pilots, and bankers. The use of a method, however, cannot substitute for years of accumulated knowledge gained through work in a discipline stressing cognitive processes.

There are, however, other views of the idea of method. One view is that there is no method of success in science or in any other field. The question persists: What do we expect from a method or process? One answer is that use of a method or process may provide specific steps leading to a particular outcome as in a cookbook recipe. Follow the steps as given and bake a pie, assemble furniture, operate a computer, or calculate a drug dosage. In these examples, learning the method goes hand-in-hand with doing the specific activity; never in isolation from the materials within a field or specific domain.

Another response to the question of one, several, or no methods, is that of William James and the American physicist, Percy Bridgman. A method, they said, is "doing your best to succeed, with no holds barred."[2] Another view is that of Paul Feyerabend, who holds that there is no method, "Anything goes."[3] To Feyerabend, the only thing that counts, and that distinguishes science from voodoo, is results. According to Feyerabend, slavish addiction to a method, process, or a set of steps does not give people in a field sufficient freedom to gain the knowledge and effective decision making they seek.

A further distinction regarding method made by Ernest Nagel, an American philosopher, is the difference between the methods of discovery and the methods of corroboration. Learning the standards of inquiry is helpful. There are, however, no shortcut methods toward discovery of new knowledge. Insights, inferences, or hunches are not self-guaranteeing, self-certifying, or self-evident. Standards of inquiry, such as those used in the nursing process, data collection, inferences, hypotheses, diagnoses, and intervention, are in need of testing and corroboration. Caution regarding a problem-solving method is expressed by Ernest Nagel's concern to look to "habits of scientific workmanship" in place of a hardened, codified, mechanized routine. According to Nagel,

> What is loosely called scientific method, is generally a habit of workmanship that skilled investigators possess, and not a codified set of principles which they explicitly acknowledge.[4]

Appeal to the scientific method may nevertheless have value as a rallying symbol and protocol representing the commitments of nursing to the generalized aims, methods, attitudes, and procedures of science. Critical thinking offers guidelines for distinguishing several senses of scientific reasoning and showing how these apply. To emphasize the form and content distinction, the scientific reasoning process helps to organize the content in logical, sequential, analytic forms that can be corrobated. But there is no substitute for knowledge of the content of nursing as the basis of discovery.

The use of only one method of reasoning in nursing, such as the nursing process or a problem-solving approach, may be an instance of premature closure and ultimately damaging to the continuing development of the theoretical base of nursing. The ability to think critically about other methods and approaches to problems is more helpful to individual and collective development than the gain in security from relying primarily on one method of reasoning. A second justification for thinking critically is its usefulness to personal spheres of life and living. The student or nurse practitioner who recognizes the value of critical thinking to all of human activities is more likely to achieve mastery of multiple modes of reasoning.

SOURCES OF KNOWLEDGE

All methods of arriving at knowledge invariably depend on sources in human nature. These include sensory impressions, such as looking, hearing, touching, and feeling. These sources of knowledge also include appeal to intuition, reason, authority, faith, and revelation. These sources of knowledge are important and helpful in arriving at knowledge. But they are sometimes confused with knowledge itself.

To be a living, thinking human being is to be bombarded by sensations, perceptions, feelings, experiences, opinions, beliefs, intuitions, faith, mysticism, revelation, and authority. A function of critical thinking is to discriminate among these sources of data by seeking to separate knowledge from impressions and opinions.

"How do you know the patient is coughing?" one nurse asks another. "Because I hear him and see his facial contortions, his chest heaving," says another nurse. "How do you know Mrs. S is in pain?" Look at her clutching her abdomen and yelling." These are audible, visible signs of pain and of coughing. We claim to know on the basis of sense impressions. Sense impressions are sources of knowledge and are frequently reliable clues. But if someone can say, "I feel the patient's pulse, but I could be mistaken in my counting," then that person can no longer correctly say, "I know the rate and quality of the patient's pulse." If we cannot be sure that what we claim is true or if we cannot produce sufficient evidence, then we lack two conditions for saying correctly "I know."

How do we know that what we believe is true? How does a nurse know that what she or he asserts is in fact true? How do nurses know the conditions of their patients? How does a nurse know what interventions to use with a particular patient? And, sometimes equally or more importantly, how does a nurse know what not to do or to avoid? Sense experience, the use of reason, resort to authority, intuition, revelation, and faith are commonly used paths to knowledge, but often without sufficiently critical thought to their strengths and limits.

The road of sense impression as a way to knowledge is well-traveled as it is used in nursing, in medicine, in science, and in daily living. We depend on our senses to see, hear, touch, taste, and smell for our very survival. Our senses collect experiences that we then classify and judge. Perceptual errors, such as failing to recognize cyanosis, jaundice, or pallor, reflect faulty judgments rather than defects in the senses. The correction of faulty judgment based on sense–experience is to collect further sense–experience and to test it before making a judgment. The nurse who is not sure that the patient's sclera are jaundiced can unobtrusively hold up a white wash cloth or paper handkerchief next to the patient's eyes. The adequate collection of sense—experience is significant in the assessment phase as the basis for nursing diagnosis.

No matter how meticulous and comprehensive the assessment phase is conducted, ultimately, the nurse must judge whether the patient's breathing pattern is dyspnea, orthopnea, Cheyne-Stokes respiration, or normal. To spend hours carefully observing a patient is not enough. Sense experience requires judgment, reason, and correct inferences. In nursing, judgment can be a nursing diagnosis related to the goals and interventions of the nursing care plan, a judgment related to the medical diagnosis and treatment, or to the health mission of the institution. To make that judgment, the nurse needs knowledge: concepts of normal breathing patterns, normal skin tones and deviations, and nursing frameworks that connect sense experience to nursing knowledge. Sense experiences without rational judgments are not very meaningful, because they are merely subjective sensations and perceptions. Moreover, sense impressions are not infallible.

In contrast, internal states of feeling, moods, attitudes, pleasure, and pain are based on experiences. We can make assertions about our internal states of mind and emotions and know them to be true. For example, a nurse may say, "Joan Smith is exactly the kind of nurse I'd like if I got seriously ill and hospitalized." Or Mary Green may assert "I have painful menstrual cramps." If the question "How do you know this?" was asked, the answer might be simply "I feel it." If, however, the nurse says, "I feel that John Black is going to be transferred to the surgical services," the nurse is talking about a state of affairs in the world. These two statements and what they assert are distinguishable. The nurse who asserts that she feels painful menstrual cramps is talking about her internal feelings. The truth of the proposition, "John Black will be transferred" is not related to feelings expressed in the first person, but to actual state of affairs of the world that are open to testing and verification. Moreover, the word *feeling* is ambiguous because it can be confused with opinion, touch, belief, hope, or thought. In the first person declarations of feeling, as in "I have menstrual cramps" or "I am happy," the person speaking is the final authority. But in second and third person statements, independent verification is required as a condition of knowledge.

A second distinction in sense experience is what J. Hospers calls the difference between an occurrent state and a dispositional state.[5] Nurse Green, who runs to a patient's room in response to a cry of help from a colleague is in an occurrent state. Her concern and running activity occurs at a given time. This same nurse, however, has an attitude, a commitment, and an internal state that disposes her toward helping and caring for people in every way possible. Hospers calls this a dispositional state. Given the circumstances of someone else's pain, discomfort, or need, Nurse Green is disposed to help, given the appropriate circumstances. We make this distinction when we say "He is not in love with her since he is not disposed to treat her with consideration, tenderness, generosity, empathy and so on." The person may say, "I'm madly in love," but if he is not inclined to show it, we tend to doubt such words. To show care on a rare occasion is an occurrent rather than a dispositional state. "An impartial examination of . . . behavior over an interval of time" reveals the difference between an occurrent and a dispositional state.[6]

To make claims on the basis of feelings of inner experiences is to go beyond that experience. Evidence is required to support the truth in this assertion. To say that "I have menstrual cramps" is a statement about a person's feelings, which are self-authenticating; and is different from saying "I have a lump in my breast." The latter is empirically verifiable.

Reason

There are two kinds of reasoning—deductive and inductive (or scientific). Deductive reasoning is a source of knowledge that does not depend on sense experience. The nurse who calculates the proper dose of a drug, such as aspirin (Acetylsalisylic Acid) or chlorpromazine, for a 10-year-old child is reasoning. Reasoning is also used when one statement implies or is the basis for making other statements. In deductive reasoning that is valid, the conclusion logically follows from the premises. For example:

If it is raining, the streets will be wet.
It is raining.
∴ The streets will be wet.[7]

This argument is valid because the conclusion follows logically from the premises. The premises need not be true to have a valid argument, as this example illustrates:

All nurses are gifted persons.
I am a nurse.
∴ I am a gifted person.

This, too, is a valid argument, because the conclusion follows logically by virtue of the form rather than the content of the argument. In contrast to valid or invalid arguments, propositions or statements are true or false. First, we must know if the argument is valid. Second, we inquire about the soundness of the argument or the truth or falsity of the premises and conclusion. The first feature concerns the form of the argument, the second concerns the content. For a conclusion to be true means the premises must be true. If these conditions are fulfilled, we have a valid and a sound argument. An example of a valid argument is:

> If a nurse is practicing as a licensed professional nurse, she will have passed state board examinations.
> Mary Ann is practicing as a licensed professional nurse.
> ∴ She passed the state board examinations.

The point is that deductive reasoning may give us valid arguments, but they may be empty of content. Thus, deductive reasoning as a source of knowledge cannot by itself yield scientific truths.

Inductive Reasoning

In inductive reasoning, we may know the truth of the premises, but we still do not know that the conclusion is true—"the premises provide evidence for the conclusion, but not complete evidence."[8] The conclusion is not certain but probable. For example, the most common chracteristics of diabetes mellitus are "increased appetite . . . increased thirst, and increased urine volume . . ."[9] This does not mean that each individual with diabetes mellitus has this cluster of symptoms. It does mean that if 10,000 diabetes cases were screened and each showed these symptoms, it does not follow that the next diabetic will have these symptoms. The probability is high that these symptoms indicate diabetes and that diabetics have these symptoms, but it is not certain. As with other sources of knowledge, inductive reasoning is not by itself a complete method of arriving at knowledge.

Intuition

Whereas intuition is also a source of knowledge, it, too, does not guarantee knowledge. According to R. F. McCain,

> Nursing . . . is primarily intuitive. Unlike the professions of law, engineering and medicine, nursing has not developed a precise method of determining when nursing intervention is needed.[10]

Some nurses believe that the practice of nursing is largely intuitive, an art rather than a science. These nurses, when faced with the question "How do you know Mrs. Y is anxious?" will answer in terms of their intuitions.

"He makes me anxious." Intuition is said to be like the turning on of a flashlight; something is made clear that was not apparent before. The issue becomes "the acceptability of intuition when it is made to underwrite a claim to knowledge."[11] The claim that "human beings are more than and different from the sum of their parts"[12] is made by M. Rogers. Rogers' work is rich with intuitions regarding the relations of wholeness, openness, four dimensions of space and time, principles of reciprocity, synchrony, helicy, resonancy, and homeodynamics of humans in a simultaneous interaction with the environment.[13] This nursing model is filled with propositions in need of support from scientific reasoning, empirical studies, and critical reasoning. Although Rogers' intuition that the wholeness of humans is the proper study of nursing, it disregards the individual's susceptibility to hereditary deficits and to the disease process. Her theory may be viewed as intuitive; and as with other intuitions, there is a need for independent evidence to sustain their credibility.

Whatever problems there may be with the nursing process, such as expecting it to be a panacea for health care problems, it does show that an intuition or feeling—an immediate apprehension about a process—cannot be self-certifying or self-evident. Rather, every hunch, intuition, feeling, is subject to further, independent reflection, appropriate corroboration, and validation. The nurse who uses self-sealing arguments or closed-minded assumptions does not show that his or her intuitions are sound. Intuitions may be correct. But intuitions can also be a substitute for lack of knowledge. Nurse A, for example, has an intuition that Mr. Baxby, 77 years old, down the hall with gastric tubes and intestinal cancer, will die within the next day or two. Nurse B intuits that Mr. Baxby is having a remission and will live six months. If, in actuality, Mr. Baxby does not die in the next few days, or go home and live six months, what can we say about either Nurse A's or Nurse B's intuitions? They both could not be right. In fact, they both were wrong. Or if Nurse A intuits that Mr. Baxby wants to die and Nurse D intuits that Mr. Baxby is clinging to life, how do we decide who is right? Even if one nurse's intuition is right, there is the equal possibility that it could have been mistaken. That no intuition is self-authenticating is sufficient to show that a nurse's intuition is not knowledge.

Faith

A similar claim to knowledge is through the path of faith. The disagreements among world religions about the identity or existence of a supreme being, as either Jesus, Jehovah, the Messiah yet to come, Allah, Buddha, or some humanistic or atheist view, illustrates the difficulties of validating such claims. When in daily living we say, "I have faith in that nurse," we mean to say that she or he deserves our confidence. The grounds we give are that the nurse is competent, trustworthy, and caring. This confidence comes about by observation, experience, and evaluation of that nurse's performance through sense–experience. Hospers defines faith "as a firm belief in something for which there is no evidence . . . We only speak of faith when we wish to substitute emotion for evidence . . . But if faith is an attitude . . . then faith cannot be a source of knowledge."[14]

People have been known to appeal to faith to save them. But faith, if unaccompanied by wisdom, can also lead to disaster, as shown by the followers of Reverend Jones in Guyana in the 1970s. His followers believed his propositions of alien invaders to be true. The faith of "true believers," of any fanatic grouping, cannot be trusted as a faith that can justify claims to knowledge.

Some nurses have faith primarily in the spiritual healing power of a religion; other nurses place their faith in the recovery power of the patient along with the curative power of modern medicine. Nurse A could say, "I have faith in Allah." Nurse B could say, "I have faith in Christ." Nurse C could say, "I have faith in Buddhism." Nurse D could say, "I have faith in Taoism." And Nurse E could say, "I have faith in modern medicine and the patient's will to live." The point is that these different faiths cannot all be true.[15] Faith is not cognitively strong enough to warrant or justify saying that faith is knowledge.

Authority

A further source of knowledge is an appeal to authority. We all depend on authority for giving powerful medications and complex, technological care to patients. We trust authorities, perhaps far more than we should. Some people trust the authority of Dr. Linus Pauling's claim that vitamin C has vast curative powers. Since the Roe versus Wade Supreme Court decision (1973) entitling a woman to decide on an abortion in the first trimester, that decision is regarded as the authoritative law of the land, along with other Supreme Court decisions. But as everyone may know who appeals to the authority of Supreme Court decisions, a different group of justices may well come to a different ruling in a future decision. And Dr. Pauling's claim needs independent verification to establish its credibility.

The nurse also appeals to authority who says, "I know it's true because I read it in a medical journal" or "I know it's true because Dr. Z said so." In realistic terms, an ordinary life span is not enough time to check out the truth of each assertion that comes our way, even those that are important to our survival. As an expedient, we accept as true articles that appear in *Nursing Research, the New England Journal of Medicine,* or the *Journal of the American Medical Association,* or the word of someone who has supposedly read it with understanding.

Hospers suggests several precautions regarding the use of authority. (1) Only experts speaking strictly to their field of expertise are authorities. Persons with reputations of authority in one field are not authorities in a different field.[16] In cases of disagreement among authorities, judgment is suspended until agreement is reached.[17] (3) Statements of authority are public in the sense that the person's statements can be checked as true or false. A nursing diagnosis can be checked by colleagues; likewise so can a medical diagnosis or a scientific proposition. A statement that claims that Jehovah is the only true God cannot be checked, even if it comes from a world authority on religion, because it cannot be known by any means other than authority. For that reason, "authority cannot be a primary source of knowledge."[18]

Revelation

The use of revelation as a path to knowledge rests on the claim of divine intervention. The statement about an unfortunate event, "Oh, but it was God's will" substitutes the authority of the speaker for the authority of an expert. But even here, there are no experts who can judge whether a given revelation is true or false. Although each person may declare the other's claim to be false, the criteria for distinguishing true from false revelations are absent.[19] The basic question "How do you know what you claim to know?" remains unanswered.

The point in reviewing these sources of knowledge is that appeal to each of these, reason, intuition, faith, authority, and revelation, is not self-certifying. None of these sources assures that our knowledge claim is secure. To secure knowledge claims, we look instead to conditions and criteria of knowledge.

CONDITIONS OF KNOWLEDGE

We find secure foundations for knowledge by examining three conditions of knowledge: truth, belief, and sufficient relevant evidence.

Conditions and Senses of Truth

The first characteristic of any proposition considered to be knowledge is for it to be true. If a nurse says "I know that Mr. X is experiencing shortness of breath," the nurse is really saying "Mr. X's experiencing shortness of breath" is true. A simple check of Mr. X's breathing, position, bodily movements, and demeanor will suffice to assert that this is a true proposition. Or if someone says, "There is a nursing shortage in this hospital," this statement is either true, false, or meaningless. Because this statement asserts a state of affairs that is verifiable, it has meaning. The statement is true or false. The truth or falsity of this statement can be established by calculating the ratio of patients to nurses on each shift and comparing these numbers to accepted standards. The assertion of a nursing shortage in this hospital is either true or false on these grounds. The individual stating the proposition may not, however, find this process satisfying. That person may really mean, "There is a nursing shortage in this hospital since the number of professional nurses with academic degrees on each shift and service is inadequate to insure high quality patient care, patient teaching, and discharge planning." A nurse who interprets "nursing shortage" in this way appeals to a different criterion, one with different outcomes to measure the adequacy of the ratio of nurses to patients.

Correspondence Theory of Truth

A major concept of truth is for any statement, such as "Ms. Golden has hypertension," to be judged as true, means that there is a one-to-one correspondence between the statement and the state of affairs referred to. The blood pressure can be measured by a sphygomonometer and compared with the norms for Ms. Golden's age, sex, present condition, and past history. If a nurse says "Laetrile cures cancer," she can only be said to know this statement if the statement is true. The statement is true only if there is a one-to-one correspondence between the nurse's statement and the state of affairs to which the statement refers.

Beliefs About Truth

A nurse may believe that a proposition, such as "Laetrile cures cancer," is true even if it is false, which is documented by the research literature. The assertion that "The earth is flat" was once believed to be true,[20] until Columbus refuted that assertion by sailing around part of the earth. The strong beliefs of a few, even the majority of people, in the cancer curing properties of Laetrile does not determine the truth or falsity of its effectiveness. If, in fact, Laetrile did cure cancer, then we could correctly say that the proposition was true. Because the facts are based on great quantities of published research evidence that Laetrile does not cure cancer, we cannot correctly believe that the proposition "Laetrile cures cancer" is true. The facts are the critical factor, not our beliefs.

It is equally fallacious to say "I believe in touch therapy as a cure for disease until it is proved false" or "I believe touch therapy as a cure for disease to be false until it is proved true." Instead, a rational belief is one that is in proportion to the amount and quality of evidence that favors it.

Subjective Uses of Truth

One response to the question "What is the truth?" is to say, "Well, at least as far as I'm concerned, it's true."[21] We cannot maintain that a proposition is true and, if it is shown to be false, claim that somehow we only believed it to be true. Therefore, we are excused from responsibility for the truth of our beliefs.[22] An example is one nurse saying of another, "One narcotic is missing and as far as I'm concerned, Jane took it for her own use." If the speaker is shown to be wrong, she answers, "Well, I only thought that."

We may vary this response by saying "To me it's true, to you it may not be."[23] This answer begs the question "Is it true or isn't it? . . . The same proposition cannot be both true and not true."[24] Truth cannot be the possession of a single individual in contradiction to the facts. Nurses who assert that to them Laetrile and touch therapy are both cures for cancer, but that others may not share this version of the truth, are flying in the face of the facts; and they are also going against the process of critical thinking. They are begging the question "Is Laetrile effective or not for curing cancer?" and "Is touch therapy effective for curing cancer?" This is different from Nurse A saying, "I have a backache from turning Mr. Smith," which is an expression of personal truth. When Mr. Smith says "I have a backache from lying in this position for so long," this is a different proposition of personal truth. It does not mean that Nurse B has a backache from moving Mr. Smith. "The word *I* refers to a different person every time it is used by a different speaker . . ."[25]

Statements of belief differ from statements of truth. If Nurse A says, "I believe that Mr. Z is abnormally suspicious" and Nurse B says, "I believe that Mr. Z is just a very sharp, critical thinker," their statements do not contradict each other for both are disagreeing in attitude. Whether Mr. Z is paranoid, however, is a true or false assertion, and different from statements of belief or attitude about whether Mr. Z is or is not abnormally suspicious.

Phrases, such as "to me" or "as far as I'm concerned," add nothing to the content of the claims or propositions to which these phrases are attached. The addition of these phrases may be intended to protect the speaker's statements from critical examination; but examining such phrases shows that this move does not succeed. If we make statements that are intended to be true, such statements are not *personal truths* or *subjective truths,* but real truths.

A variaton on the phrase "true to me" is that some statements are true for a certain time, but not forever. This view that truth varies with time also needs analysis. If "Florence Nightingale's research demonstrated that sanitation, hygiene, and nutrition lowered mortality rates during the Crimean War of 1854" was true at that time, then that statement is true at any other time. Truth and falsity do not vary with time. The earth was not flat at one time and round from the time of Columbus on. If an event occurred at time t_1, such as "The Declaration of Independence was signed in 1776," then that statement is true for all time. The truth value of this statement does not change with the passage of time, or because historical circumstances change. The only basis for changing the truth value of a statement is if the objective evidence points to a different direction.

Coherence Theory of Truth

A second major concept of truth is coherence. According to the coherence view, every statement in a system of statements must fit together to form a unified whole. An example of coherence is the statement that the nurse treats the whole patient. The coherence view of truth implies a field theory or a systems approach to knowledge, a grand scheme, "the big picture." The correspondence theory implies a one-to-one relation between statements and states of affairs. To use the correspondence theory is slower, less elegant, and less poetic than the more dashing coherence theory. But the correspondence theory is also more precise and thorough. The use of the correspondence theory of truth points to the strengths of careful analysis of wholes into their parts. The use of the coherence theory points to synthesis, speculation, theory, conjecture, guess, and the bold inference.

Both theories fit together as follows: The coherence view points to the ideal with no way to locate huge missing fragments. The correspondence view offers practical day-to-day guidance in finding how the small parts fit, but with little inspiration or vision as to the relatedness of all things to one another. No grand scheme is there in turning to correspondence between statements and the data of the world presented by our senses.

The Truth Is What Works

Hospers points to still another definition of truth as "truth is what works, and a true proposition is one that works."[26] To engage in critical thinking is to look at counter-examples of this generalization. If, for example, a nurse's car fails to start on an extremely cold morning, we can say that the failure of the car is due to the cold, to a weak or dead battery, or to a defective ignition. If electrical energy is transmitted to the battery from another car and the motor starts, we still do not know if the cold or a weak battery was at fault. We can only be sure that the battery was not totally dead or the ignition defective. Similarly, a depressed, debilitated, elderly man, a recently widowed client, is admitted to the psychiatric unit of a hospital. This patient receives excellent psychiatric nursing care in a therapeutic milieu, a high vitamin, high protein, high caloric diet, appropriate rest and activity, and antidepressant medication. After four weeks of treatment, the patient shows remarkable improvement. Was it the nursing that "worked," was it the drugs, the client, the therapeutic milieu of the psychiatric ward, or simply the passage of time and the lessening of loss and depression after his wife's death? As this example illustrates, it is best to confine the use of the concept "truth is what works" to things that are working.[27]

The formula "what works" is apt to reduce to the correspondence theory. One of the features of correspondence is that "it works." If the correspondence between statement and data does not work, as when a nurse says, "Mr. Jones is having Cheyne-Stokes respirations" when he is not, then a person using the correspondence view says, "That's not true, he's breathing normally."

A feature of the correspondence view of truth is that we can use true or false about our statements. We cannot attribute true or false in the coherence theory. Coherence means that the parts all fit together to make up the whole. The parts, however, have on this account no truth value.

Only the whole does. And the whole story is still quite incomplete as is the use of some leading nursing theories that espouse coherence. The coherence view, therefore, makes true or false statements unusable in daily nursing judgments. The correspondence view of truth also makes a direct link to the basis for asserting that one statement is true and another false, namely the evidence that makes it so.

The Belief Condition

A second condition of knowledge is belief. One who knows also believes. To know is to have good reasons to justify a belief. Knowledge is justified, true belief. A major difference between knowledge and belief is justification. Only those scientific beliefs that are supported by good scientific reasoning are justified.[28]

A second difference between belief and knowledge is that a statement must be true to be known.[29] A belief may be true or false. No matter how strongly a belief or conviction is held or how good the reasons for holding the belief are, if the statement is false, then the claim to know is wrong.[30] As for the truth, according to R. Giere, a philosopher of science,

> There is nothing one can do to ensure that any particular scientific hypothesis is true. The best one can do is to make sure that those hypotheses one believes to be true are justified in a way that provides some reliable connection between hypotheses that are so justified and those that are in fact true.[31]

According to Giere, the grounds for claiming to know a statement are:

1. The person believes the statement to be true.
2. The person is justified in that belief.
3. The statement is true in fact.[32]

Justification, supported by scientific reasoning, is critical to claims to knowledge in all fields, including nursing.

The Evidence Condition

The most difficult requirement to fulfill for justifying claims to knowledge is to provide sufficient relevant evidence for the conclusions. The evidence condition is not satisfied by appealing to the testimony of our friends or with those who agree with the conclusion we hold. Evidence refers to rigorous objective standards of independent testing and corroboration. A person strengthens a claim to knowledge by having or being in a position to refer to relevant evidence. Such strength gives a person justifiable grounds for claiming to know. Knowledge generated from experiments in the laboratory, that can be replicated and evaluated, is one example of claims based on justifiable grounds.

To Know That, To Know How, and To Know Why

There are various ways of interpreting knowledge of different kinds. We adopt a distinction made by G. Ryle between *know-that* and *know-how.*[33] Know-that refers to propositional knowledge, such as "I know that a sign of increased intracranial pressure is bradycardia and a rising blood pressure."[34] Other examples include: "I know that George Washington was the first U.S. President," "I know that the earth is an oblate spheroid," "I know that drinking unclean water spreads infection," "I know that Mt. Everest is the tallest mountain on earth," and "I know that rusty sputum, temperature 38.8C (102F), respiratory rate 45, and lethargy confirms a diagnosis of bronchial pneumonia."[35] Know-that statements are verifiable.

Differentiated from know-that propositional knowledge statements are know-how procedural knowledge statements. They are characterized by skills, abilities, propensities, capacities, dispositions, knacks, flairs, and aptitudes. Here are some examples: "I know how to position a patient," "I know how to provide range of motion exercises," "I know how to insert a needle into a patient's vein," "I know how to calculate dosages of drugs," "I know how to change intravenous solutions," "I know how to change sterile dressings," "I know how to suction a patient," "I know how to read electrocardiograms," "I know how to read vital signs on the monitor," "I know how to teach a postoperative cardiac patient the most effective coughing technique," "I know how to teach a patient crutch-walking," and "I know how to apply renal dialysis to patients."

Know-how statements are also verifiable, but they refer to a different kind of knowledge from propositional knowledge. Both are important grounds for effective nursing judgments.

Some critical thinking scholars also refer to a third kind of knowledge, *know-why.* This refers to knowing about or having insight into explanations and justifications. But some critical thinking writers prefer to identify know-why as a subtype of know-how. Arguments can be mounted on both sides of this issue. On balance, we prefer to distinguish the three kinds here. But this is a debatable issue. Verification of adequate relevant evidence is a condition for establishing all three types of knowledge claims. For example, Nurse Adler knows why Mr. Roberts, a patient with a carcinoma of the esophagus who has an esophagoscopy, will experience hoarseness and a sore throat.[36]

Exercises

For each of the examples, state whether the statement is known or how it can be known.

1. How well do you know your anatomy?
   Answer: Correspondence view.
2. Keeping the blood glucose at more normal levels may improve sexual functioning of diabetics.[37]
   Answer: Correspondence view.

3. If a patient is immobile, if the patient is elderly, and if the patient's nutritional status is poor, then the probability of decubitus is 95 percent.[38]
   Answer: Correspondence view.
4. Analyze the following meanings of *true* or of *truth.*
   a. The truth is I got a high grade in mathematics.
      Answer: Correspondence.
   b. Is it true that Dr. H is a gifted surgeon?
      Answer: Correspondence theory.
   c. Ms. A, the head nurse, is a true professional.
      Answer: Value endorsement.
   d. She is a true friend.
      Answer: Value endorsement.
   e. Ms. Golden has hypertension.
      Answer: Correspondence view.
5. In which of the following statements do feelings imply knowledge?
   a. I feel a toothache coming on.
      Answer: One knows oneself. First-person statement.
   b. I feel you have a toothache coming.
      Answer: No knowledge.
   c. Mrs. L. has diabetes.
      Answer: Correspondence view.
   d. I have a heart.
      Answer: Correspondence view.
   e. I know that my son is in pain 12,000 miles away.
      Answer: Feeling statement: Intuition, with no basis in knowledge.
6. Which kind of *know* is the following?
   a. Do you know how to give morphine to the patient?
      Answer: Know-how.
   b. You don't know what death is like until you die.
      Answer: Know-that, no evidence.
   c. The symptoms of hypoglycemia include clammy skin.[39]
      Answer: Correspondence view.
   d. I know that if myasthenia patients don't get their prostigmin right on time, they begin to develop muscle weakness.[40]
7. How is the term *know* used here?
   a. How well do you know your patient?
   b. How well does your patient know you?
   c. How well do you know your medications?
      Answer: Know-that.
8. In the following, do you know or believe?
   a. Patients with advanced myasthena gravis require tube feeding and frequent nasopharyngeal suctioning.[41]
      Answer: Believe.

b. Patient X has 100 percent probability of experiencing preoperative anxiety. With teaching, Patient X has 50 percent chance of having his anxiety reduced.[42]
Answer: Belief.

c. It is important for the nurse to observe what the patient and family know about the disease and its implications.
Answer: Know-that.

d. Does the patient know the names of the medications she or he is taking?
Answer: Know-that, correspondence theory.

FORMAL AND EMPIRICAL STATEMENTS AS BUILDING BLOCKS OF SCIENTIFIC REASONING

Satisfying the conditions of knowledge enables us to construct statements that satisfy truth conditions. These statements include definitions and empirical statements. The appropriate uses of definitions and empirical statements are crucial to effective scientific reasoning.

Although different scientific disciplines emphasize distinct aspects, scientific reasoning falls into a general pattern of arguments as justifications for conclusions.[43] Statements are the basic units of reasoned arguments.

Statements: Truth and Falsity

A statement is a sentence that makes an assertion, unlike a question, command, or request. Statements of assertion are either true or false. The truth or falsity of a statement is objective in its freedom from individual or group desires.

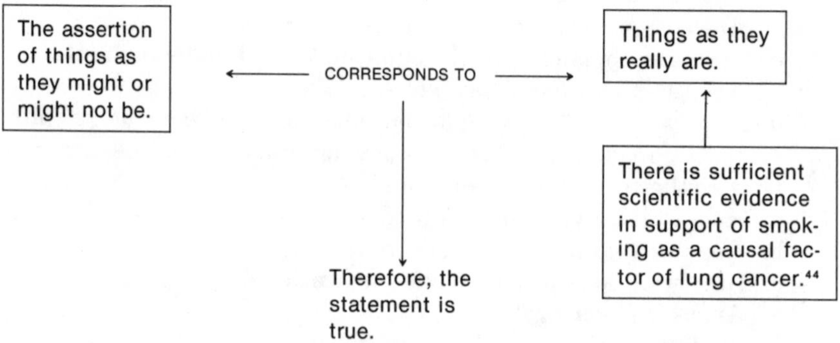

Figure 4-1. An example of the correspondence theory of truth. Statement: Smoking is a causal factor of lung cancer.

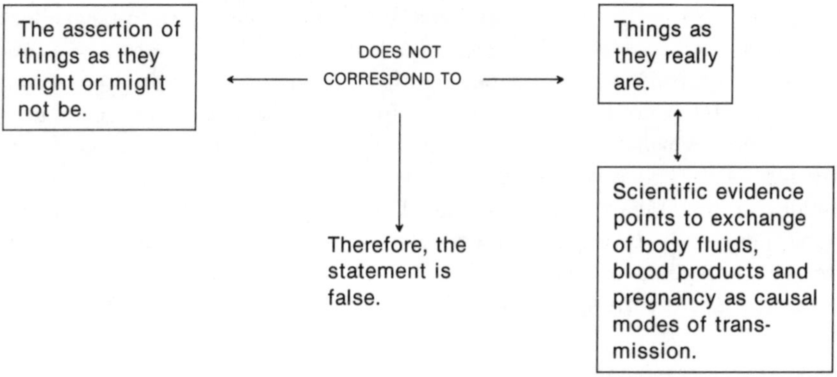

Figure 4–2. A second example of the correspondence theory of truth. Statement: Acquired immune deficiency syndrome (AIDS) is transmitted by airborne virus.

The correspondence theory of truth (see Figs. 4–1 and 4–2) is used by most practicing scientists.[45] This theory holds that the statement is true that corresponds with the way things really are. . . . "Smoking causes lung cancer" is true if smoking does cause lung cancer, and false if it does not.[46]

Key Concepts
A statement asserts the way things might or might not be.
A True statement asserts the way things are.
A False statement is a statement that is not true.[47]

Definitions

Definitions in science are different from the descriptive or prescriptive definitions in a dictionary. Definitions arise from new knowledge and become the use of new words or the use of old words in new ways.[48] The American Nurses' Association (ANA) defines nursing as "the diagnosis and treatment of human responses to actual or potential health problems."[49] This is an example of a stipulative, persuasive, and also theoretical definition.

Critical thinking requires that stipulative, persuasive, and theoretical definitions to be distinguished from reportive definitions. The ANA definition of nursing, therefore, cannot be considered a scientific statement or a true or false statement, as it was stipulated by the Association without correspondence with an actual state of affairs in the world. Nevertheless, this definition of nursing plays an important role in the profession's development of its theory and practice. This definition of nursing cannot yet be found in general dictionaries, because it is stipulative. Organized attempts to make the definition both descriptive and prescriptive are made by educators and practitioners who seek to distinguish nursing as a science based on nursing theory and research. Nursing theorists and researchers use the stipulative definition to create new concepts as the basis of scientific investigation. New concepts require "creating new words or giving new meanings to old words."[50] As a stipulative definition, one that uses old and new words in new ways, this definition is neither true nor false, but serves as the basis for further statements about nursing and for legislating new meanings in nursing. The nurse engaged in critical thinking will carefully distinguish between empirical, scientific statements that are verifiably true or false, and definitions that are stipulative or persuasive and without correspondence with the states of affairs as they really are.

COMPOUND STATEMENTS

Compound statements are two statements put together to form a more complex statement. One form is a conjunction of two statements connected by the word *and*. For example, "Nurses and physicians administer antibiotic drugs to control specific infections." Clearly this statement is the conjunction of two statements. "Nurses administer anitbiotic drugs to control specific infections" and "Physicians administer antibiotic drugs to control specific infections." If both parts of the statement are true, then the whole conjunction is true. If either or both parts are false, then the whole conjunction is false. For example, the conjunction "Nurses and physicians are licensed to practice nursing" is false, as a physician is not licensed to practice nursing, but licensed to practice medicine. Similarly, the conjunction "Nurses and physicians are licensed to practice medicine" is false, because a nurse is not licensed to practice medicine, but to practice nursing. A nurse engaged in critical thinking is aware of such false conjunctions as "Licensed practical nurses and licensed associate degree registered nurses practice at the technical level and should be titled 'Associate nurses.'"

Disjunctions are complex statements connected by the word *or*. The word *or* can be used in the inclusive sense meaning that either or both disjuncts are true.[51] For example, "Either the nurse or the physician can give antibiotic drugs by injection." This is a true disjunction in the inclusive sense.

The second use of the word *or* is the exclusive sense meaning that EITHER BUT NOT BOTH of the disjuncts are true. For example, "Either the nurse or the physician is qualified to determine the nursing needs of patients," is a true disjunction (in the exclusive sense) because one component "The nurse is qualified to determine the nursing needs of patients" is true. Because the other disjunct, "The physician is qualified to determine the nursing needs of patients" is false, the disjunction can be interpreted in either sense, the inclusive or exclusive, as both parts are not true.

Generally false disjunctions are "regarded as false only when BOTH components are FALSE."[52] Nurses, therefore, need to think critically about the following disjunction, because, although one of its parts is false, it will generally pass as a true disjunction, as one of its parts is true. "Psychiatric nurse clinical specialists *or* psychiatric social workers are qualified to manage a client's psychotropic drug regimen" This statement falsely contends that a social worker is as qualified as a nurse to manage psychotropic drugs. Statements made questioning the value of academic preparation for nurses suggest that nursing functions can be performed by a nurse *or* anyone else who is a compassionate, dedicated individual, willing to give physical care and carry out physician's orders.

A NEGATION is a sign or statement that denies an initial assertion. As a sign it means NOT. As a statement, it denies what a statement asserts. The statement that "Nursing did not evolve from medicine" is the negation of the initial assertion "Nursing evolved from medicine." The statement that "Medicine did not evolve from nursing" is the negation of the statement "Medicine evolved from nursing." The relations between a statement and its negation are direct. "If the ORIGINAL statement is TRUE, its NEGATION is FALSE. If the ORIGINAL statement is FALSE, the negation is TRUE."[53] A double NEGATION, the negation of the negation of a statement, is simply a return to the original statement. For example, P. Watzlawick, a psychiatric theorist, postulates that "You CANNOT NOT communicate."[54] Watzlawick simply restates for emphasis the original statement "You are continuously communicating."

CONTINGENT STATEMENTS

Most scientific claims are couched in the form of contingent statements. A contingent statement is one that "both might be true and also might be false."[55] Its truth or falsity does not depend on its logical structure or the meaning of its words, but is dependent on empirical data; therefore, it is contingent on evidence. A nursing example of a contingent statement is, "Nurse midwives practicing in poor rural areas can significantly lower the maternal and neonatal mortality and morbidity rate." Only carefully compiled evidence can determine the truth or falsity of this contingent statement.

COGNITIVE STATES

Cognitive states may be defined as the relationship between statements and the individual, somewhat like "a state of consciousness," a "state of mind," or an "emotional state."[56] Cognitive states, however, are especially important because they involve knowing or believing. In thinking critically, it is important to distinguish between belief and knowledge.

The following nursing example rests on the author's strong belief in the truth of what she writes. Carolyn Clark advocates "creative visualization" as a self-care practice to increase one's own healing potentials. Clark writes that the nurse's values and beliefs listed below must be concordant with practice for creative visualization to be effective.

> I can see how creative visualization could be used as a self-care practice.
> I can picture myself teaching a client how to use creative visualization.
> I believe creative visualization should be part of my nursing skills.
> I believe creative visualization can help to shrink tumor cells.
> I believe creative visualization can be used to lower blood pressure.
> I believe creative visualization can be used to decrease pain and increase healing.
> I believe creative visualization can be used to decrease glaucoma.
> I believe I could use creative visualization myself to promote my own healing.[57]

Clark cites the work of the Simontons

> . . . that shows people (medically incurable and terminal) can influence the course of their cancer through visualizing their cancer cells as weak, mushy hamburger and visualizing their white blood cells as strong, flexible and adaptable . . . (that) demonstrated that their patients lived an average of 2 years longer than patients receiving traditional treatment alone (that) more than 51% of their patients maintained a high quality of life, as measured by level of activity, prior to and after diagnosis.[58]

Clark's strong belief in the power of creative visualization to help shrink tumor cells, lower blood pressure, decrease pain, decrease glaucoma, and increase healing, and the truth of these claims is more a reflection of her state of mind, her cognitive state, than conditions as they really are. There is research evidence linking mental states of stress, such as fear and anger, with physiological states affecting vital signs, blood counts, blood chemistry, brain waves, and the like. These and smaller empirical findings are far from the evidence needed to support Clark's concluding statement that "This (reported findings) provides evidence that we are what we think and feel."[59] There is in Clark's article a significant and critical distance between her beliefs and the knowledge needed to support those beliefs.

One characterization of scientific reasoning is as a means to reach true or rationally justified beliefs.[60] The term *belief* is used in different ways to mean different things. The word belief may be used to characterize an individual's attitude in regard to the truth of a specific statement, as Clark's belief in the truth of the work of the Simontons in the previous example.

A second use of the term belief refers to the extent of confidence in the truth of a particular statement. In this view, one believes by degrees, more or less.[61] To think critically is to recognize that belief and truth are not directly connected. We may or may not share Clark's strong belief that creative visualization shrinks tumor cells, lowers blood pressure, decreases glaucoma, decreases pain, and increases healing independently of its truth or falsity.

Someone cannot be said to know what Clark claims is true. An obvious example of the difference between belief and knowledge is the once strongly held belief that the earth was flat. We now know that the belief was always false. Likewise these may be true statements as yet unknown or currently disbelieved.

The uniquely personal approach of the statement, "that's true for me but maybe not for you" is not rationally acceptable, because a particular statement cannot be both true and false, true for one person, but false for others.[62] A statement must be either true or false for everyone.

UNCERTAINTY

The concept of certainty and the acceptance of uncertainty is expressed in everyday language in very imprecise ways. For example, one nurse may say "I am certain that therapeutic touch is healing." That nurse may hold the strongest possible belief that her statement is true. A second nurse may say, "I know for certain that antibiotics cure most bacterial infections." The second example differs from the first in that the second belief regarding antibiotics is justified by strong evidence showing that the statement is true. To claim to know is to provide a guarantee that the statement is true without a chance of its being false.[63]

Clearly, this is not possible. Antibiotics do not cure all bacterial infections. Scientific claims are stated in contingent terms, as previously discussed. No method or investigator can guarantee the absolute truth or freedom from error of any statement, no matter how strong current evidence is in support of a conclusion. Later evidence may negate it. Science cannot provide absolute truth; nor are there any absolute justifications. To engage in critical thinking is to distinguish carefully between justifying reasons that are better and those that are worse.[64]

JUSTIFICATION OF HYPOTHESES

The goal of inquiry and research is to provide *justification* for believing that a scientific statement, a hypothesis, or the conclusion of an argument is either true or false.[65] To determine whether or not an hypothesis is justified, knowing the relationship between statements that justify the hypothesis and the hypothesis itself is useful. In some contexts the hypothesis is the conclusion of the argument; the other statements are the premises of the argument. In other contexts, the hypothesis may function as a leading premise.

- *Example 1* (Hypothesis I). Perceived susceptibility to breast cancer is positively and significantly associated with frequency of breast self-examination practices.[66]

- *Example 2* (Hypothesis II). Perceived benefits of breast self-examination are positively and significantly associated with frequency of breast self-examination.[67]

- *Example 3* (Hypothesis III). Perceived barriers to breast self-examination are negatively and significantly associated with frequency of breast self-examination.[68]

- *Example 4* (Hypothesis IV). Age is negatively and significantly associated with breast self-examination.[69]

- *Example 5* (Hypothesis V). Self-concept is positively and significantly associated with frequency of breast self-examination.[70]

These examples illustrate the relationship of the argument to the hypothesis. In example 1, the hypothesis functions as a premise of the argument. In example 2, the hypothesis may function as the conclusion of the argument. In example 3, the hypothesis may function either as a premise or the conclusion of the argument. In example 4, the hypothesis appears to be a premise of the argument. In example 5, the hypothesis is most probably a premise of the argument.

The argument can be reconstructed as in the following example; however, the argument can be reconstructed in still different ways related to how the premises themselves are justified.

- *Premise 1.* Perceived susceptibility to breast cancer is positively and significantly associated with frequency of breast self-examination practice.[71]
- *Premise 2.* Age is negatively and significantly associated with breast self-examination.[72]
- *Premise 3.* Self-concept is positively and significantly associated with frequency of breast self-examination.[73]
- *Premise 4.* Perceived barriers to breast self-examination are negatively and significantly associated with frequency of breast self-examination.[74]
- *Conclusion.* Perceived benefits of breast self-examination are positively and significantly associated with frequency of breast self-examination.[75]

The preceding argument was complex. The form of a simple argument is generally that of two premises followed by a conclusion that may be used as an hypothesis to be tested.

First premise
Second premise
———————
Conclusion

Analysis of this simple form suggests that one justification for believing in the conclusion of an argument is that the premises of the argument themselves are justified.[76]

First premise: Infections caused by pneumococcus bacteria respond to penicillin.
Second premise: Mr. X has an infection caused by pneumococcus bacteria.
———————
Conclusion: Therefore, Mr. X's infection caused by pneumococcus bacteria responds to penicillin.

Because the premises of an argument provide grounds for believing the conclusion, the premises themselves must be justified. Unjustified premises do not justify a conclusion.

Example:
AIDS is cured by penicillin.
Baby Doe has AIDS.
∴ Baby Doe will be cured by penicillin.

Another failure in providing justification for the conclusion of an argument is from an insufficient connection between its premises and its conclusions.[77]

Example:
Intelligent people prize good health.
I prize good health.
∴ I am intelligent.

Although these premises may seem acceptable, there is insufficient connection between the premises and the conclusion. In this case, the middle term *good health* is undistributed; therefore, the argument is invalid. The premises do not justify the conclusion, as they lack an appropriate connection.

Example:
AIDS is a lethal disease.
Persons with AIDS are alive.
∴ AIDS is not lethal.

The use of logic reveals whether or not a particular "argument has the right sort of connection to provide a justified conclusion from justified premises."[78] This argument also is invalid, even though each of the premises is true. One reason this argument is invalid is that affirmative premises cannot imply a negative conclusion. Another reason this argument is fallacious is that *lethal*, the predicate of the conclusion, is not distributed in the major premise. (For further analysis, consult Chapter 9.)

If, however, the issue becomes justification of the premises, for example, in research, it becomes a matter of scientific knowledge. To settle the issue of the justification of a particular hypothesis, both the argument and the plausibility of its premises must be considered.[79]

SCIENTIFIC METHOD APPLIED TO NURSING

The view taken here is that *scientific method* is one approach to problem-solving activity. Scientific reasoning occurs within the nursing process and problem solving. There is a strong likelihood that all forms of scientific reasoning lead to decision making; and all such activity needs to be subjected to critical scrutiny.

An example of the general pattern of scientific method is Copi's seven-step model (Table 4.1). Copi's version is selected because of its operational quality and emphasis on the processes and habits of workmanship.

The Problem

Before an investigator can begin working, there must be a perceived problem. A problem may be facts, events, or situations that lack explanation or that are incongruent with accepted beliefs, expectations, or precon-

TABLE 4-1. COPI'S SEVEN-STEP MODEL OF THE SCIENTIFIC METHOD

1. The problem
2. Preliminary hypotheses
3. Collecting additional facts
4. Formulating hypotheses
5. Deducing further consequences
6. Testing the consequences
7. Application[80]

ceptions. Without expectations and beliefs, life holds no surprises and no problems.[81] Problems often come ready made.

A nurse investigator saw that the administration of intramuscular medications was followed by adverse effects of pain and cutaneous, subcutaneous, and intramuscular lesions from frequent injections, as a ready-made problem for nurses.[82] The intramuscular injection of medications is a therapeutic measure universally performed by nurses. Despite the frequency of reports of adverse effects of injections in specific patients reported in the literature, M. Keen found insufficient documentation of systematic studies of the actual occurrence of adverse effects or of ways to prevent such events.

Preliminary Hypotheses

The preliminary hypothesis step is especially important because in nursing there may be too many facts, too much data, and too many distractors for the reasoner to use effectively. Charles Darwin, the author of the theory of evolution, made this statement about data collection ". . . All observation must be for or against some view, if it is to be of any service."[83] This means simply that the investigator must have a strong hunch, a preliminary hypothesis, a working hypothesis, against which to collect and to reject data. As the investigation by Elstein and co-workers on the diagnostic reasoning of experienced physicians revealed, physicians generate specific diagnostic hypotheses long before the bulk of the data is even available in most cases.[84]

A preliminary hypothesis is simply tentative, incomplete, possibly insufficient, but based on previous knowledge, belief, and expectations. Preliminary hypotheses may be rejected as the data collection process advances. They may differ greatly from the solution to the problem; nevertheless, preliminary hypotheses are essential for inquiry to proceed.[85] Keen's study provides nursing examples of preliminary hypotheses. From the review of the literature and her experience, Keen hypothesized that the actual frequency of adverse effects secondary to injection therapy is probably higher than documented. A further preliminary hypothesis was that the population at highest risk consists of patients repeatedly injected over days or weeks. A further preliminary hypothesis was that needles used are too short with deposit of the injected solution into the subcutaneous tissue rather than in the muscle. A further preliminary hypothesis was that the injected solution leaked into the subcataneous tissue after the withdrawal of the needle because of the use of a straight injection pathway.[86]

Collecting Additional Facts

Every serious inquiry begins with a fact or set of facts considered to be problematic that suggest preliminary hypotheses to the investigator.[87]

These initiate the search for additional facts that will provide clues to the solution of the problem.[88] A search that is careful, systematic, and complete facilitates the accomplishment of the goal.

In Keen's nursing investigation, a complete review of the literature provided additional facts that helped formulate her testable hypotheses. For example, one researcher demonstrated, by the use of x-rays, that standard intramuscular injections of heavy metals, such as bismuth, enabled the injected solution to flow back along the injection path. This researcher also demonstrated by x-ray that the Z track method, a broken injection pathway, would prevent the injected solution from flowing back.[89] Additional facts came from Robert's (1975) unpublished study of the frequency of skin reactions and discomfort of hospitalized patients receiving prescribed injections. Roberts reported prolonged discomfort noted in one-third (20 of the 60 subjects), and 88 percent (53) subjects with a defined injection site lesion. Patients at highest risk for unacceptable reactions were those who received repeated injections for days or weeks.[90] These additional facts were helpful toward moving from preliminary hypothesis to the formulation of a testable hypothesis.

Formulating Hypotheses

At this stage, working hypotheses account for all the data, retained or rejected. Working hypotheses account for the original set of facts that made up the problem and the additional facts needed to consider preliminary hypotheses.[91] Criteria for evaluating an explanatory hypothesis are its relevance to the problem, its testability, its compatibility with other well documented positions, and most important of all, its predictive power. Keen's explanatory hypotheses were that the incidence and degree of severity of patient discomfort will be less after administration of the drugs using the Z track intramuscular injection technique than by administration by standard intramuscular injection technique. Keen's second working hypothesis was that the incidence and degree of severity of injection site lesions would be less using the Z track intramuscular injection method than the use of the standard technique.[92]

Deducing Further Consequences

A really good hypothesis is one that accounts for the facts contained in the original problem, explains others in addition, and then points in the direction of new and unsuspected facts.[93] The verification of those further consequences will add further confirmation to the hypothesis upon which they are based.[94] Because the importance of an hypothesis is in its explanatory or predictive power, an hypothesis is adequate only if additional facts can be deduced from it. Once a prediction is deduced from the hypothesis, it must then be tested to be confirmed.[95]

In Keen's nursing study, hypotheses predicted that the incidence and degree of severity of both patient discomfort and injection site lesions will be less using a Z track technique of intramuscular injection instead of a standard technique. This prediction was then tested.

Testing the Consequences

The consequences of a hypothesis, the predictions based on it, can be tested in various ways ranging from observation to the most intrusive and radical of experiments. In Keen's nursing investigation, the utmost care was taken to select patients free of interfering illnesses or tissue abnormalities, but with the same prescribed medications to be given by intramuscular injections. Painstaking measurement scales for postinjection severity of discomfort and the character and size of lesions were used. A pilot study on eight patients tested the interrater reliability. The procedure for injection control was fastidious. The results of the investigation of 240 injections to 50 subjects were found to be statistically significant in support of the explanatory, predictive hypothesis.

Application

Because the ultimate function of the scientific method is to solve problems, the practical application of testing and either confirming or disconfirming hypotheses is important. In Keen's nursing study, the clinical applications are that by using the Z track intramuscular injection method, nurses can decrease the severity and incidence of lesions and discomfort at the injection site for all solutions. Keen's study points to the particular helpfulness of the Z track injection method to those patients receiving frequent injections for extended periods.[96]

This particular nursing investigation fulfilled all of Copi's steps in his suggested model of scientific reasoning, and illustrates the application of critical thinking to its formulation.

Another example of nursing research, less rigorous, in which the investigator used both deductive and inductive kinds of arguments, for both qualitative and quantitative methods of research, is M. Fenton's report of her attempts to measure humanistic nursing behavior.[97] The stated purpose of the study was the development of a reliable, theoretically based scale for measuring the extent of humanistic health care in hospitals as perceived by nurses. The scale was to be used as a diagnostic aid and an instructional tool. Some of the inductive and deductive arguments used to support the research are:

- *Premise 1.* The nature of the interaction between patient and health care, the environment in which it occurs, influences physical and psychological outcomes of illness.
- *Premise 2.* Nursing provides humanistic care in an environment that is concerned and supportive of physical and psychological outcomes of illness.
- *Conclusion.* The unstated conclusion of the argument may be that nurses are qualified judges of humanistic care.

These statements are believed to be true by the researcher based on experience, general opinion, and some evidence. These statements are presuppositions or preliminary hypotheses given the problem of the need for improvement of the quality of patient care.

An example of an if–then conditional statement from the same investigation is "If a concerned, supportive, humanistic approach to providing care improves patient health outcomes, (then) it is important to develop methods to identify the level of humanistic care in nursing care settings."[98] This statement could be the problem or, because it presumes many presuppositions or assumptions, it could be the working hypothesis.

A further deductive argument was the definition of humanistic care itself.

- *Premise 1.* "Humanistic care enhances the dignity and autonomy of patients and health profession alike . . . ."[99]
- *Premise 2.* The dignity and autonomy of patients and health professionals are reflected in the amount of individual freedom of choice.
- *Conclusion.* Therefore, individual freedom of choice is enhanced by humanistic care.

The actual scale surveyed responses that were self-reports reflecting the presence or absence of J. Howard's eight theoretical components of humanistic health care delivery: irreplaceability, holistic selves, freedom of action, status equality, shared decision making and responsibility, empathy, positive effect, and inherent worth.[100] A tremendous amount of work went into compilation of 192 statements describing patient and nursing staff behavior, testing, revision, retesting, establishing reliability and validity, selecting study populations and sites, data collection from 316 respondents, and data analysis. In the concluding discussion, the investigator reports the probabilistic nature of her findings and the importance of an unsettled issue: "whether the main effect of personalized humanistic care may depend more on the characteristics of individuals who staff a unit than on the overall type of hospital and its administrative policies."[101] Thus, the investigator ends her report on an appropriate note of probability and uncertainty. These are examples of critical thinking and scientific reasoning.

CONCLUSION

Scientific reasoning is a key to effective critical thinking. To understand what scientific reasoning involves calls for a distinction between the sources and conditions of scientific knowledge. Health professionals make use of sources of knowledge in patient treatment, but to check on their ideas, hypotheses, judgments, and hunches requires that these judgments be submitted to appropriate testing and corroboration.

To achieve the goals of making scientific reasoning an essential part of nursing education means nurses are trained to distinguish between certainty and uncertainty; and to use deductive reasoning and scientific reasoning, both aspects of critical thinking, to enhance nursing theory and practice.

REFERENCES

1. Descartes, R. Meditations, 1641, Lafleur, L. (Trans.). New York: Liberal Arts Press, 1951, p. 22.
2. James, W. The Will to Believe. Boston: Dover, 1957.
3. Feyerabend, P. Against Method. Atlantic Highlands, N.J.: Humanities Press, 1975, p. 23.
4. Nagel, E. Sovereign Reason. Glencoe, Ill.: Free Press, 1954, p. 300.
5. Hospers, J. An Introduction to Philosophical Analysis (2nd ed.). Englewood Cliffs, N.J.: Prentice-Hall, 1967, pp. 125–127.
6. Hospers, J. An Introduction to Philosophical Analysis, p. 127.
7. Ibid, p. 128.
8. Ibid, p. 131.
9. Thomas, C.L. (Ed.). Taber's Cyclopedic Medical Dictionary (14th ed.). Philadelphia: F.A. Davis, 1981, p. 396.
10. McCain, R.F. Nursing by Assessment—Not Intuition, in La Monica, E.L. (Ed.), The Humanistic Nursing Process. Belmont, Calif.: Wadsworth, 1985, p. 103.
11. Hospers, J. An Introduction to Philosophical Analysis, p. 136.
12. Rogers, M.E. An Introduction to the Theoretical Basis of Nursing. Philadelphia: F.A. Davis, 1970, p. 46.
13. Ibid.
14. Hospers, J. An Introduction to Philosophical Analysis, p. 141.
15. Ibid.
16. Ibid, p. 135.
17. Ibid.
18. Ibid, p. 130.
19. Ibid, p. 139.
20. Ibid, p. 118.
21. Ibid, p. 119.
22. Ibid, p. 119.
23. Ibid.
24. Ibid.
25. Ibid, pp. 115–120.
26. Ibid, p. 117.
27. Ibid, p. 118.
28. Giere, R.N. Understanding Scientific Reasoning (2nd ed.). New York: Holt, Rinehart and Winston, 1984, p. 27.
29. Ibid, p. 26.
30. Ibid, p. 26.
31. Ibid, p. 27.
32. Ibid, p. 26.

33. Ryle, G. The Concept of Mind. London: Hutchinson's University Library, 1949, pp. 28–29.
34. Desharnais, A., et al. Appleton's Review of Nursing For the New State Board Examination (2nd ed.). E. Norwalk, Conn.: Fleshner Publishing, 1986, p. 127.
35. Ibid, p. 129.
36. Ibid, pp. 153, 171.
37. Tanner, C. Factors Influencing the Diagnostic Process, in Carnevali, D., et al (Eds.), Diagnostic Reasoning in Nursing. Philadelphia: J.B. Lippincott, 1984, p. 63.
38. Blainey, C.G. Care of Persons with Diabetes Mellitus, in Carnevali, D. (Ed.), Diagnostic Reasoning in Nursing, p. 153.
39. Tanner, C. Factors Influencing The Diagnostic Process, in Carnevali, D. (Ed.), Diagnostic Reasoning in Nursing, p. 63.
40. Ibid, p. 61.
41. Ibid.
42. Ibid, p. 63.
43. Giere, R.N. Understanding Scientific Reasoning, p. 11.
44. Ibid, p. 18.
45. Ibid.
46. Ibid.
47. Ibid.
48. Ibid, p. 19.
49. ANA Nursing: A Social Policy Statement. Kansas City, Mo.: The Association, 1980, p. 9.
50. Giere, R. Understanding Scientific Reasoning, p. 19.
51. Ibid, p. 21.
52. Ibid.
53. Ibid.
54. Watzlawick, P., Beavin, J.H., & Jackson, D.D. Pragmatics of Human Communication. New York: W.W. Norton, 1967, p. 49.
55. Giere, R. Understanding Scientific Reasoning, p. 23.
56. Ibid, p. 24.
57. Clark, C.C. Creative Visualization as a Self-Care Practice, in New Directions for Nursing in the 80s. Kansas City, Mo.: American Nurses Association, 1980, p. 69.
58. Ibid, p. 70.
59. Ibid.
60. Giere, R. Understanding Scientific Reasoning, p. 24.
61. Ibid, p. 24.
62. Ibid.
63. Ibid., p. 28.
64. Ibid.
65. Ibid, p. 32.
66. Rutledge, D.N. Factors Related to Women's Practice of Breast Self-Examination. *Nursing Research* 1987; 36(2):117–121, March/April.
67. Ibid.
68. Ibid.
69. Ibid.

70. Ibid.
71. Ibid.
72. Ibid.
73. Ibid.
74. Ibid.
75. Ibid.
76. Giere, R. Understanding Scientific Reasoning, p. 34.
77. Ibid, p. 35.
78. Ibid, p. 36.
79. Ibid, p. 36.
80. Copi, I. Introduction to Logic (7th). New York: Macmillan, 1986, pp. 492–501.
81. Ibid, p. 493.
82. Keen, M.F. Comparison of Intramuscular Injection Technique to Reduce Site Discomfort and Lesions. *Nursing Research* 1986; 35(4):207–210, July/August.
83. Cohen, M.R., & Nagel, E. An Introduction to Logic and Scientific Method. New York: Harcourt Brace, 1934, p. 197.
84. Elstein, A. Shulman, L.S., & Sprafka, S.A. Medical Problem Solving. Cambridge, Mass.: Harvard University Press, 1978, p. 64.
85. Copi, I. Introduction to Logic, p. 496.
86. Keen, M.F. Comparison of Intramuscular Injection Techniques to Reduce Site Discomfort and Lesions. *Nursing Research* 1986; 35(4):207–210, July/Aug.
87. Copi, I. Introduction to Logic, p. 496.
88. Ibid.
89. Keen, M.F. Comparison of Intramuscular Injection Techniques to Reduce Site Discomfort and Lesions, p. 207.
90. Ibid.
91. Copi, I. Introduction to Logic, p. 498.
92. Keen. M.F. Comparison of Intramuscular Injection Techniques to Reduce Site Discomfort and Lesions, pp. 207–210.
93. Copi, I. Introduction to Logic, p. 498.
94. Ibid.
95. Ibid.
96. Keen. M.F. Comparison of Intramuscular Injection Techniques to Reduce Site Discomfort and Lesions, pp. 207–210.
97. Fenton, M.V. Development of the Scale of Humanistic Nursing Behaviors. *Nursing Research* 1987; 36(2):82–87, March/April.
98. Ibid.
99. Howard, J., et al. Humanizing Health Care: The Implications of Technology, Centralization and Self-care. Medical Care 5 Supplement, 15:11–26, 1977.
100. Ibid.
101. Fenton, M.V. Development of the Scale of Humanistic Nursing Behaviors. *Nursing Research* 1987; 36(2):87, March/April.

Chapter 5

The Role of Critical Thinking in the Nursing Process

Study of this chapter enables the learner to:

1. Use the nursing process as a variation of scientific reasoning and justify nursing judgments and interventions.
2. Employ critical thinking to make relevant, valid, and sound uses of the nursing process.
3. Apply critical thinking to an analysis of nursing concepts such as those involved in the nursing process.
4. Use critical thinking to make valid, sound, and relevant uses of the nursing process.

INTRODUCTION

The aim of this chapter is to apply critical thinking to the nursing process, both in its entirety as an integral part of professional nursing, and to the inferences made in the phases of the nursing process.

The nursing process is defined as a variation of scientific reasoning and is used by nurses "to diagnose and to treat human responses to potential and actual health problems." Making of inferences is like leaping from what is known, the data, into what is unknown, a hunch, a preliminary hypothesis, or an inference. Making inferences includes the aspect of using the data to guess or to speculate about a patient's dysfunctional patterns or to make a generalization about the patient's functional state of health and to corroborate or verify that inference. Thus, an inference can be viewed as a preliminary or working hypothesis that is either confirmed or disconfirmed by further data until a nursing diagnosis is reached. Nursing diagnosis includes both the classification of a dysfunctional pattern and its etiology as the basis for nursing intervention and evaluation of the outcomes.

The whole of the nursing process can be viewed as a series of means–ends relationships. The means are the nurse's accurate assessment, diagnosis, and treatment of the patient and the ends are the patient's increased level of function and well-being.

CRITICAL ANALYSIS OF THE NURSING PROCESS

Critical thinking about the use of the nursing process raises issues that are the source of continuing controversy. One issue is that the nursing process is but one variation of scientific reasoning used by nurses to organize, systematize, and conceptualize nursing practice. A second issue is that through the use of the nursing process, nurses seek to differentiate spheres of nursing practice from those that are medical practice. In turn, the use of the nursing process may facilitate identification of spheres of health care delivery that require collaborative nursing and medical activity. Stevens regards the nursing process as incomplete nursing theory. A complete nursing theory has the further requirement of context and form. Stevens views nursing diagnoses as attempts to provide form to the nursing process. Without nursing diagnosis, the process is the same as processes used by physicians, social workers, and teachers.[1] Stevens outlines the parallel between the use of process in medicine and nursing as follows:

Medical Term	**Nursing Term**
Patient examination	Patient assessment
Diagnosis	Nursing diagnosis
Prognosis	Goal setting
Prescription	Nursing Care Plan
Therapy	Nursing intervention
Evaluation	Evaluation

(Source: Ref. 2.)

Despite the clear similarity between the nursing and medical processes, their application presents different challenges. There are nursing theorists and practitioners who struggle to differentiate between a medical diagnosis and a meaningful nursing diagnosis, a patient/client goal that is a mutually agreed upon outcome of a nursing care plan and nursing intervention, and evaluation that is able to separate nursing from medical outcomes.

On this view, the nursing process is a general approach to client systems of individuals, families, groups, or communities. Because of its generality, the nursing process can be used to extract, deduce, or infer from data analysis exclusively to those spheres of practice that apply to nursing. Also correlated to its generality, the nursing process can be used in the context of various nursing standards and concepts that are competitive and contradictory at points. Because the intention of nurses is to identify and treat "human responses to actual or potential problems of health," the nursing process can be used to diagnose, treat, and evaluate client systems comprehensively and in considerable depth.

The American Nurses' Association (ANA) *Social Policy Statement* explains the broad mandate of nursing as "diagnosing and treating human responses to actual or potential health problems . . ."[3] but not the health problems themselves. The *Statement* notes that although human responses to health problems are less discrete or circumscribed than medical diagnostic categories tend to be,[4] there is "an intermeshing and complementarity of the distinct foci of the practices of nursing and medicine . . ."[5] Admittedly, nursing intersects with other health care professions and at "these interprofessional interfacings, nursing extends its practice into the domains of other professions."[6] The critical inference made here is that the *Statement's* proclaimed adherence to nursing as *diagnosis and treatment of human responses to health problems* but not the health problems themselves, contradicts the *Social Policy Statement's* assertion that "Nursing's boundaries and intersections with other professions should not be limited or fixed but should allow for expansion and flexibility."[7] Medicine is the profession most problematic and challenging to nursing expansion. On this view, these statements reflect a dilemma of nursing regarding its relation to the domain of other professions, especially medicine. Critical reasoning is in conflict with the claim that nursing is unique.

DEFINING CHARACTERISTICS OF NURSING

The ANA *Social Policy Statement* identifies the four characteristics of nursing as "phenomena, theory application, nursing action, and evaluation of effects of action in relation to phenomena."[8] The phenomena of concern to nurses are the human responses of individuals and groups to actual health problems, to related self-care needs, and to potential health problems.[9] Diagnosis is the effort to "objectify a perceived difficulty or need by naming it, as a basis for understanding and taking action to resolve that concern."[10]

Theory used in nursing is acknowledged to be partly self-generated and partly taken from other fields.[11] Because nursing is primarily an applied field, the selection of theory consists of nursing research that tends to be specific to the discipline and nonnursing theories useful to the explanation of phenomena of concern to nursing.[12] Consequently, the range of theories used in nursing is as broad as needs to be to explain all the possible interpretations of the phenomena of concern to nurses, "the diagnosis and treatment of human responses to actual or potential health problems."[13]

The following recommendations by J. Griffith and P. Christensen are adapted from Hardy. These are useful when selecting a specific theoretical framework or model to apply to the nursing process.

1. Which theoretical framework is most useful in dealing with the variables of concern to the health professional in the client situation? Griffith and Christensen suggest the use of Aguilera's crisis intervention theory for a victim of rape and a theoretical framework of family development for expectant parents.[14]

2. Which theoretical framework has variables or concepts that focus on improving clients' health status and situations? The examples given by Griffith and Christensen suggest the use of Satir's family model, which focuses on dysfunctional communication, and E. Erickson's developmental model, which addresses children's psychosocial behavioral problems.[15]

3. Which theoretical framework supports the primary focus of change and provides direction for nursing strategies? Griffith and Christensen suggest Roy's adaptation model as the basis for strategies helpful to clients with physiological alterations, and systems theory for change at the community level.[16]

Using this concept, because each client, whether a single person, family, group, or community, presents a unique situation of health, the practitioner needs familiarity with the spectrum of theoretical approaches as the basis for selection. The collection of basic information about the client is the recommended basis for the selection process. The selected theoretical approach is then used to guide additional data collection and analysis of data. Using this concept, therefore, the theoretical model is selected on the basis of the nurse's knowledge of the client's situation and judgment of the most effective model for change through nursing interventions. Theories, theoretical frameworks, conceptual models, and guiding principles identify and classify phenomena and guide the assessment, analysis, and implementation phases of the nursing process. Theoretical approaches are seen in this view as the means for justifying each phase of the nursing process and the nurse's accountability to clients.[17]

By the terms of this definition of nursing, nurses are to restore and promote health and prevent illness.[18] The choice of actions and their implementation need to be theoretically justified. Evaluation of the effects of these actions is intended to benefit the recepient of nursing and to provide evidence of the effectiveness of particular nursing actions in relation to specific phenomena.[19]

The ANA *Social Policy Statement* holds that these concepts are contained in the nursing process when used as the framework for organizing nursing practice.[20] The nursing process is regarded as a systematic approach to assessment, planning, implementation, and evaluation that includes patient, family, and nurse participation. These steps may be taken all at once and reconsidered as necessary. The ANA's *Standards of Nursing Practice,* developed by psychiatric, maternal–child, medical and surgical, and community health nurses, reflect the use of the nursing process and the ANA's defined characteristics of nursing as basic to practice. Thus, the nursing process has achieved wide acceptance in nursing circles despite its generality and incompleteness of context and form. Moreover, the debate in nursing circles surrounding the relative merits of particular conceptual frameworks and nursing process schema continues at an intense level. Nursing practitioners, educators, researchers, and administrators, therefore, are free to choose among competing and sometimes conflicting models of nursing.

SUPPORT FOR THE USE OF THE NURSING PROCESS

For the practitioner to succeed in using the nursing process, the user must operate within a set of interrelated assumptions or concepts as a frame of reference. Otherwise, the practitioner is like the captain of a ship trying to navigate unknown waters without a map or chart. To be useful, data collection must be made in reference to the intended purpose of nursing and in relation to the client's health problems. These interrelated concepts are the presuppositions upon which data are gathered, analyzed, and synthesized. These concepts are the basis for nursing judgments in the form of diagnosis, nursing plans, implementation, and evaluation. To use the nursing process model without a framework of nursing purpose, goals, expectations, knowledge, beliefs, and values is similar to driving a car without purpose or destination.

The difference, however, among nursing theorists regarding goals and the use of nursing process schema results in a variety of steps and phases. In the 1983 edition of Yura and Walsh's book, *The Nursing Process,* the authors still recommend a four-step nursing process of assessment, evaluation, planning, and evaluation along with an elaborate human needs theory as the basis of assessment.[21] Carnevali and co-workers, in contrast, use a diagnostic reasoning process that they describe as generic. These steps are: the search for data and diagnostic possibilities; hypothesis activation; hypothesis evaluation; prognosis and treatment; and evaluation and revision.[22]

Reasons for Supporting the Use of the Nursing Process

Currently only four components of the nursing process, assessment, including diagnosis, planning, intervention, and evaluation, have met with universal acceptance and incorporation into the ANA *Standards of Nurs-*

ing Practice, 1973, and the ANA *Social Policy Statement*, 1980. The nursing process, however, is couched in sufficiently abstract terms to be usable for nursing and even nonnursing conceptual frameworks. Within the broad steps of the nursing process, assessment tools related to the concepts of client, health, nurse, and environment are specified or suggested by each conceptual framework. The assessment, diagnosis, planning, intervention, and evaluation of data become quite different, however, when viewed from different conceptual frameworks, even though the broad steps of the nursing process remain constant. It is the conceptual framework, or the theoretical model that gives "purpose and direction to nursing process and particularly, to diagnosis."[23]

Some practitioners prefer to use a social work or medical model.[24] Other nurses use a problem-solving, decision-making model, or some variation thereof as a basis for practice. A few nurses simply use their own variation of the scientific method. Whatever the conceptual model used, every nurse, physician, social worker, or scientist must collect, analyze, and synthesize data on the basis of preconceived notions, however inexplicit of purpose, method, function, and goals. "Even implicit, unrecognized models influence perception and judgment."[25] This use of unrecognized conceptual models may lead to unsystematic, and faulty reasoning processes resulting in false and erroneous conclusions. Errors in reasoning can lead to professional ineptness and frustration as well.

The assessment phase of the nursing process includes two steps. The first step is the collection of data from primary and secondary sources. The second step is the analysis of the data as the basis for nursing diagnoses.

The critical issue for the data collector becomes that of asking fundamental questions, purpose, goals, and intent underlying the use of the data. Even if the purpose of data collection is to use the nursing process to arrive at a nursing diagnosis and treatment plan that can then be implemented and evaluated, the data still need to relate to the client's perceived needs and health problems, goals, values, and life-style. A common practice of nurses is to collect voluminous data, especially psychosocial data that are interesting but remotely relevant to the health problem at hand. For example, sexual patterns, marital relationship, and financial status of a client with an acute abdomen, facing surgery, are of little or no immediate consequence. These issues may never be relevant to nursing diagnoses and treatment in this person, as the hospitalization and nurse–patient interaction period are brief. Similarly, the patient's weight, height, and nutritional status, if not grossly deviant, may be of little or no immediate concern when the presenting problem is one of thought disorders, such as delusions of impending destruction or command hallucinations to kill a family member.

To be useful, data collection, as Charles Darwin observed, must be for or against a particular hypothesis. Hypotheticodeductive reasoning has been demonstrated by Elstein and co-workers as the most productive method of arriving at a medical diagnosis.[26] The outcomes of research with expert physician diagnosticians, conducted by Elstein and associates, revealed medical diagnosis to be a problem-solving process that begins with the patient's chief complaint, a known starting point, and moves toward an unknown diagnosis and treatment decision. In their example, physicians generated early hypotheses, long before most of the data were available in a specific case. More hypotheses were generated as the physician's medical knowledge linked the problem to long-term memory.[27] These operations can only be done with patient-related content from the data collection and stored prior knowledge as the basis of hypothesis generation. Elstein and co-workers claim that "the generation of hypotheses and utilization of a hypotheticodeductive method seems to be a nearly universal characteristic of human thinking in complex (poorly) defined environment . . . the problem must be represented cognitively in the mind of the problem solver."[28]

From their research experience with expert physician diagnosticians, Elstein and colleagues recommend the technique of changing the open system of inquiry into a series of hypothetically closed systems that are systematically explored. This can be managed by creating a few end points and then testing the appropriateness of different ways of reaching these hypothesized end points. These physicians collect data, as do nurses, through patient interviews and histories, physical examinations, and laboratory findings. This information is the basis for generating hypotheses used in interpreting data as the diagnostic process continues. These hypotheses define the boundaries of the problem and the possible solutions. As the data increase, however, it is used to evaluate these hypotheses. Some are discarded. New ones are generated. Because each hypothesis implies a limited number of probable features, data can be evaluated by their correspondence with or the lack of it, to the features of each hypothesis.[29] Hypotheses are considered on the basis of their "probability, seriousness, treatability, and novelty."[30] Elstein's model of diagnostic inquiry is shown in Table 5–1. Elstein and co-workers give this example of the solution of a problem using the hypotheticodeductive process.[31]

- *Case:* A single, sexually active, 21-year-old woman suddenly became paralyzed
- *Cue acquisition:* Overdue menstrual period. Sexually active, upset, demanding, and uncooperative, suddenly paralyzed
- *Hypothesis generation:* Conversion hysteria, 20 out of 23 physicians; neurological condition
- *Cue interpretation:* Multiple sensory losses, transient blindness in one eye, critical cue. Conversion hysteria ruled out
- *Hypothesis evaluation:* Multiple sclerosis or brain tumor to be confirmed

TABLE 5-1. ADAPTATION OF ELSTEIN'S HYPOTHETICODEDUCTIVE MODEL FOR DIAGNOSTIC INQUIRY

Cue acquisition	Includes both normal and abnormal findings
Hypothesis generation	A continuous process of testing in which some hypotheses are discarded and new ones evolve. Early hypotheses are usually general, whereas later hypotheses are more specific
Cue interpretation	Cues weighted as positive, negative, or noncontributory for each hypothesis. Sufficient and relevant data needed to confirm or rule out each hypothesis. Data can be evaluated by their correspondence with the features of each hypothesis
Hypothesis evaluation	Hypothesis is ranked in relation to probability, seriousness, and treatability. Hypothesis is evaluated in relation to a verifiable explanation that can lead to action and solution

Source: Ref. 32.

MAKING INFERENCES

All data collection and diagnostic reasoning processes make use of inferences. Inferences are defined as the movement of thought that proceeds from something given, a cue or data, to a conclusion as to what that data means or signifies. For example, a common nursing occurrence is the care of a 25-year-old male homosexual patient in the intensive care unit apparently dying of AIDS. The patient is now semicomatose and abandoned by friends and family. The patient arrests. Nurse A infers that as the patient cannot recover, resuscitation is futile. Therefore, she does not call a Code. Nurse B is committed to the position that human life is so precious as to warrant all efforts to save it. She infers that the young patient's life can be saved by resuscitation. Therefore, Nurse B calls for cardiopulmonary resuscitation. Some inferences, such as the ones that deal with handicapped or repulsive clients, can be stereotypes of individuals as no more than a disability.

Writers on the nursing process emphasize the point that the phases of the nursing process call on the nurse to make inferences.

> The level of inferences is dependent on the experiences, perceptivity, and theoretical knowledge of the nurse. Initial references, which are based on incomplete data about a patient, may be of low level. As the nurse continues to collect data and verify meaning with the patient, her inferences become more accurate.[33]

U. K. Carrieri and J. Sitzman continue with the role of inference as follows:

> The nurse infers, usually without sufficient data, that a certain type of problem exists for the patient. An awareness on the nurse's part that

> she is using the inference process, with its reliance on intuition as well as theoretical knowledge, in making decisions about the nature of her patient's problems should be a caution to her that she may . . . be functioning without sufficient data, and thus lead her to seek additional information before acting on the problem as she perceives it.[34]

If we seek a strong knowledge base to support nursing diagnoses, we may find that knowledge of medicine, physiology, biochemistry, and physics is helpful to expand nursing practice.

According to M. Gordon, the diagnostic process comprises four activities: collecting information, interpreting information, clustering information, and naming the cluster.[35] "Underlying these activities," according to Gordon, "are decision making, inference, conceptualization and judgment."[36] Gordon identifies the logical–formal model for all inferences, "in which the inferential process is explicit." The formal model clarifies the rules, whereby conclusions follow validly from premises. Here, the truth is inconsequential. Reasoning is examined only for structure or form . . . and is expressed in a syllogism. A common example is: All men are mortal (premise). Socrates is a man (observation). Therefore, Socrates is mortal (conclusion).[37] According to Gordon, formal logic tests "the validity of a conclusion."[38]

Gordon next defines "statistical inference" in which "the truth value of premises influences the accuracy of the inference drawn." For example, 93 percent of a large random sample of American newborns weigh more than 5.5 pounds; therefore, there is a high probability (93%) that American newborns weigh more than 5.5 pounds.[39] According to Gordon, the statistical conclusions from large scale research, if available, "can be applied in clinical inference."[40] Clinical inference applies both to the formal model of inference along with the statistical mode of inference, using probabilities.[41]

In addition to the use of inferential processes, there is no substitute for both scientific and nursing knowledge as the basis for all assessment. All nursing frameworks must function on a solid foundation of knowledge. The differences between nursing paradigms, such as the ones of Johnson, King, Orem, Rogers, Roy, are not yet sufficiently developed as to preclude the use of a common assessment approach. Assessment tools abound. The essential issue becomes the use, the interpretations, the inferences, and the hypotheses generated from the data. Each nursing framework proposes a somewhat different perspective for analyzing and using data. There is a general need to incorporate medical data in the assessment approach to clients in nursing conceptual frameworks. The struggle to maintain a clear and absolute separation between nursing diagnosis and medical diagnostic reasoning and treatment can be an unnecessary expenditure of energy as it cannot usually be done. Orem is an exception. She identifies categories of health deviation self-care requisites as "genetic constitutional defects, human structural and functional deviations and their effects, and medical diagnosis and treatment."[42] From assessment of these areas, the therapeutic self-care needs and self-care actions can be determined.

Gordon argues strongly for agreement at the concrete level regarding the common areas of information needed in nursing assessment.[43] She regards the assessment of nutritional metabolic patterns to be vital to the conceptual frameworks of Rogers, Roy, or Orem. She argues that standardization of assessment structure does not imply a standardization of the interpersonal approach, analysis, and synthesis of data, or of the goal of nursing and client relationships. Instead, standardization provides a minimal accountability of the profession to the public it presumably serves.[44]

THE USE OF CRITICAL THINKING IN THE NURSING DIAGNOSIS

After assessment comes analysis, which is the ordering, sorting, and organization of data into various groupings and patterns. According to C. Shannon and colleagues,[45] analysis leads to or implies nursing diagnosis. Shannon and co-workers cite the case of Mrs. A, a 32-year-old woman, 5 feet 8 inches, 145 pounds, who was admitted

> into the acute care psychiatric unit of a general hospital. She complained of inability to concentrate, fatigue, nervous and shaky feelings, mild inability to get her work done, increased use of alcohol. . . .[46] Mrs. A. quarrels frequently with her husband whom she married three months ago. She has two stepsons, Tom, 18, and Bob, 16, with whom she also quarrels. Mrs. A is a secretary and hopes to quit in six months. She feels that when she can stay home everything will be fine.[47]

On this basis, she is given a nursing diagnosis of 'depressive illness,' 'depressed mood,' 'anxiety,' 'diminished attention span related to depression,' 'increased use of cognitive defense mechanisms related to anxiety,' and 'alteration in gastrointestinal function as a result of emotional distress.'[48] The problems in the diagnosis of Mrs. A are: How do we know the cause or etiology of Mrs. A's increased anxiety, depressed mood, altered gastrointestinal functioning? Can we rule out alcoholism, diabetes, hypoglycemia, or anemia or some other physical cause to account for her problems? How different is this nursing diagnosis from the medical diagnosis except that it is made by a nurse?

According to Webster's dictionary, diagnosis is "the art or act of identifying a disease from its signs and symptoms."[49] The term *diagnosis* is derived from two Greek words *dia* and *gnosis,* meaning two way, as in a two-way conversation or dialogue. This presumably means either between patient and health professional or between signs and symptoms and inferential judgment. Dia also means to distinguish or discriminate and gnosis means to know. In connection with both aspects of diagnosis, the philosopher L. Wittgenstein remarked that "an 'inner process' stands in need of 'outward criteria.' "[50] Mrs. A's diagnosis is in need of outer criteria, as the inner process can be related to several other criteria, such as "disturbance in role performance" or work-related problems. But how can we tell which it is?

We see a patient coughing blood, a sign of an inner process. The unseen inner process or cause of this sign needs an outer criterion, a sound, verifiable inference in the form of knowledge as to what accounts for that internal process. The same is true of a submarine commander. He wants to know what is going on above his submarine. He observes to some extent; but he also infers the rest; and the lives of his companions may rest upon the acuity of his inference. Science, medicine, nursing, and daily life follow a similar course. In making inferences, one searches for something missing that links the data to a diagnosis.

Nursing diagnosis is not only classification, but inference to an unknown, unseen process, one that has outward verifiable criteria, thus making the inner process known. Identifying a flower as a rose or a car as a Ford is not a diagnosis. Diagnostic inference is more than naming or classifying. Diagnosis is a search for and the verifiable discovery of the missing aspect of the cause or etiology of an inner, sometimes unseen, disorder. More knowledge, experience, and insight is called for in diagnosis than in classification into existing groupings. The meaning of the *inner process* may be outside of the existing groupings, or the inner process, sometimes the inner part of a patient's body, is sometimes not easily accessible and may be more complex than the classification provides.

The important point of contact and overlap between the nursing process and diagnosis is that both involve an if–then inference from the problem and data of signs and symptoms presented to a well-informed guess as to what the cause of the trouble is, whether illness or disease. To lay people, sniffles, running nose, and frequent coughing indicate a cold. Presumably, a nursing diagnosis is somewhere between a lay person's guess and a medical diagnosis.

Some nurses say physicians deal with disease whereas nurses deal with "levels of wellness" or with health and well-being of the whole patient. In practice, however, there are overlaps between medical and nursing diagnoses, and between disease and "levels of wellness."

B. Stevens writes that "nursing diagnosis is still problematic. There is still no agreement on just what a nursing diagnosis is."[51] Stevens cites five different sorts of entities we could refer to in discussing nursing diagnoses.

> (1) States of being experienced by the patient and possibly inferred by the nurse (e.g. pain, anxiety, confusion). (2) Physiologic deviations from

> the norm (e.g. irregular bowel functions, impaired mobility). (3) Patient behaviors perceived as problematic by the nurse (e.g. noncompliance, manipulation). (4) Altered relationships by the patient on which value judgments have been placed by the nurse (e.g. alteration in faith in God, altered relation with self and others). (5) Reactions of another party (e.g., significant others' adjustment to patient's illness).[52]

Although the notion of nursing diagnosis may convey the idea that the field of nursing has a unique domain, any analytic view of concepts, such as "fracture of femur," would seem to imply "limitation of mobility," with the former being structural and the latter functional. Limitation of mobility may be a necessary but insufficient diagnosis because it fails to explain the etiology or imply the treatment or nursing intervention. But, if we successfully make the case that nursing diagnosis is autonomous, we would have to show that the nursing diagnosis is not dependent on the medical diagnosis, but completely independent. The nursing diagnosis of "limitation of mobility" is incomplete without an explanation of the reason for the loss of function to plan nursing interventions. If we make the case that nursing diagnosis is autonomous, we would have to show why only a nurse, trained in nursing, could show that if there is a fracture of the femur, then there is limitation of mobility. Moreover, physicians are not precluded from inferring that if a femur is fractured, there is limitation of mobility.

The effort to apply a scientific method to the nursing process and to the nursing diagnosis, in particular, calls for appropriate indications of what the nursing process can and cannot achieve. The steps of the nursing process, when formulated, provide a set of directions for nurses to follow, somewhat like an airplane pilot is taught to follow a checklist of buttons and switches before take-off. According to Anderson and Yoder, the nursing process provides "organization and direction to various elements of nursing practice. . . .Nursing process is a way of thinking about nursing care. It provides a more rational basis for nursing practice than intuition."[53]

But Anderson and Yoder go on to assert that the "nursing process is a rational, scientifically based framework for nursing,"[54] that the nursing process provides "an accurate means of predicting outcomes."[55] Furthermore, the "nursing process provides a method for establishing standards of nursing care. These standards constitute a means for judging the quality of nursing services. Thus, the quality of nursing care is monitored on the basis of objective data and scientific criteria."[56]

These and other writers on the nursing process may be holding out more of a hope and promise than a reality. Although we may assert that the nursing process provides a general direction for nursing actions, there is no evidence of the nursing process providing "an accurate means of predicting outcomes." Nor is the nursing process by itself an adequate basis for "establishing standards of nursing care."

Critical thinking is concerned with the correctness of the completed process rather than with the psychology or the formulated stages of the nursing process. Criteria of critical thinking, such as the rules of validity, soundness, and rigor, apply to the four phases of the nursing process. For a patient to be teary eyed, downcast head, curled up in bed, may imply that a patient is depressed, frightened, or in pain; but more evidence would seem to be indicated before inferring that these signs and symptoms imply either of these conclusions. A basic principle of critical thinking is that we may not conclude with more than there is in the premises. Claims for what the nursing process can predictably achieve seem to go beyond the evidence as to what such a process has achieved to date. A promising programmatic feature is not a substitute for evidence. This includes claims made on behalf of the nursing diagnosis.

J. Kaufman distinguishes medical from nursing diagnoses, and commends Gordon's definition of nursing diagnoses as "made by professional nurses, which describe actual or potential health problems, (and) which nurses, by virtue of their education and experience are capable and licensed to treat."[57] But Kaufman concedes that "in acute settings, both diagnoses, medical and nursing, may be the same . . . For example, respiratory distress (or the nursing diagnosis 'Breathing pattern ineffective'), may be indicative of the medical diagnosis of status asthmaticus."[58] The treatment will be different. But according to Kaufman, a nurse may clearly identify pulmonary edema or ventricular fibrillation as the patient's problem.[59] But according to Gordon these are not nursing diagnoses as the nurse is "not licensed to treat them."[60] However, Kaufman contends, "the nurse may implement therapy, and collaborate with the physician . . . In this situation, it is difficult to draw a clear-cut line between what a physician and nurse should do. Collaboration is mandatory."[61]

Several questions arise about nursing assessment. Stevens' notion that a nursing diagnosis is a "mimicry" of medical diagnosis seems borne out by Kaufman's examples. Indeed the two types of diagnoses seem to provide grounds for three sets of circles as shown in Figure 5–1.

If a logical argument can be sustained that a fracture of the femur implies impaired physical mobility, then the inclusive model of diagnosis seems to win the day. The rebuttal might be that the nursing diagnosis "Mobility, Impaired Physical" might have etiologies other than medical, such as lack of transportation. Such examples, however, lead to the charge that this nursing diagnosis is trivial and begs the question of a professional need for intervention. Kaufman's examples of ventricular fibrillation and pulmonary edema also favor the inclusive model, one that houses nursing diagnosis within medical diagnosis. The claim for nursing diagnosis, however, is that it is autonomous and different from medical diagnosis in accordance with the exclusive model. Although both medical and nursing diagnoses are involved with the maintenance, promotion, and restoration of health, and few nursing examples support the exclusive model, there

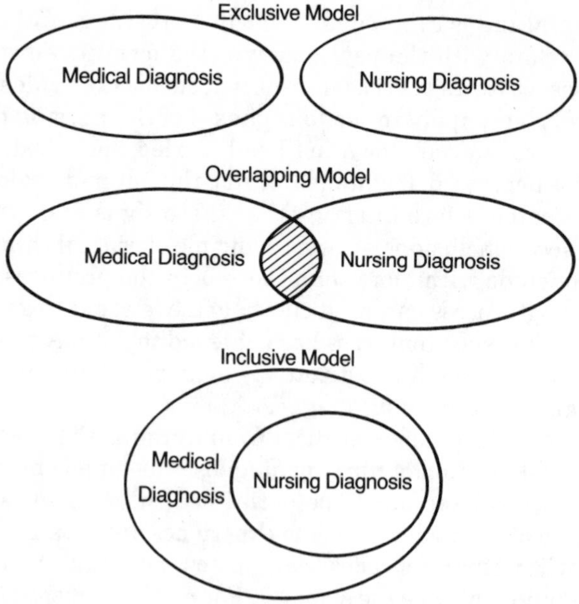

Figure 5-1. Relationship of nursing and medical diagnosis models.

does not seem to be much ground for the exclusive model at this time.

If nursing care is successfully differentiated from medical cure, there may be a case for the overlapping model. But even here, the medical diagnosis does not entail cure, but rather treatment, and treatment entails care. The way to cure, which is a health care objective, is through treatment and care. A case can be made, however, for nursing care as the primary objective of clients with incurable chronic ailments for whom medical care is largely minimal, routinized, and palliative. Nursing care makes the positive difference in the functional level and well-being of these individuals.

Again, invoking the task–achievement distinction previously mentioned, cure is an achievement and a success, whereas treatment and care are tasks and processes. Health care providers, whether nurses or physicians, are not miracle workers, but practical scientists, artists, and humanists. Nurses and physicians are concerned with such concepts as *recovery, restoration, healing,* and *convalescence,* which are implied by care and treatment. On these grounds, the inclusive model of medical and nursing diagnosis, along with the overlapping model, has more of a rational basis than the exclusive model.

M. Thomas and R. Coombs support the overlapping model of the nursing process. They ask the question of how nursing diagnosis is "similar to and different from the diagnosis made by other professions."[62] They give this answer:

> There are similarities. Every diagnosis begins with the gathering of facts. The facts may be a hemotocrit of 30%, the location of a stray bullet, the

> inability to add a column of figures, or the report that the father of a large family has lost his job.[63]

After fact gathering, "the practitioner in a given field recognizes a pattern"[64] that he or she states in the form of premises and conclusion of an argument. People vary in their ability to see a *pattern,* because diagnosing is a task and not an automatic achievement. Some diagnoses are clearly superior to others. For some human conditions and diseases, the entire human race has not come to a diagnosis that is the right or true answer.

The possibility of a diagnosis being faulty shows that in venturing to diagnose, whether in medicine, nursing, or some other profession, diagnosing is a process that is error prone, about which "trial and error" are appropriate. So, too, is the nursing process. Yet we find, sometimes more in tone than in outright assertion, that the faith placed in the nursing process or its next of kin, the problem-solving method, or more recently "decision making" have all the apparent brandishes or earmarks of success.

The implied message in the nursing process is that if we will only travel through the tunnel or method, the end of it results in solutions, successes, and achievements. But to think of the nursing process as necessarily implying success is to misconstrue what it can do in and for nursing. To place undue faith in method is to regard it as deductive. Rather, diagnosis is prone to trial and error; and being a process rather than an instantaneous success, diagnosis is largely inductive and uncertain. If the slogan "Nursing diagnosis is essential to nursing" is to be useful, its distinctiveness from medical diagnosis needs to be established. The tentative character of any diagnosis and process also needs to be carefully noted in place of the magic sometimes associated with the nursing process.

Thomas and Coombs endorse L. Hall's conception of nursing with its three overlapping aspects:

> 1. The nurturing aspect—a close interpersonal relationship concerned with the intimate bodily care of patients;
>
> 2. The medical aspect shared with the medical professional and concerned with assisting the patient through his medical, surgical and rehabilitative care;
>
> 3. The helping aspect, shared with all professional persons involving therapeutic interpersonal skills to assist the patient in self-actualization.[65]

Thomas and Coombs define a nursing diagnosis as the "recognition of a pattern."[66] Yet they too cite example after example of nursing diagnoses that fit into the inclusive model. For example,

> Mr. T mentions that his barium enema showed a "mass" in his abdomen. On his history it is noted that he had a cancerous lesion removed from his lip four years previously. . . . The diagnosis may become '*Fear and*

> *anxiety concerning the possibility of cancer.'* Could he be concerned about a recurrence of cancer?[67]

Another example is that

> A nurse observes that Ms. E's newly applied cast is saturated with a blood stain measuring one inch in diameter. Fifteen minutes later we find the blood stain is two inches in diameter. Information concerning the possibility of hemorrhage may be sought by measurement of the blood pressure . . . by inspection of skin color, and by consultation with the physician about his expectations regarding bleeding . . . Gradually or suddenly our thought process draws the facts into a pattern, culminating in 'the recognition of a pattern.'[68]

The thought process by which these facts are related to the possibility of hemorrhage is influenced by knowledge of and past experience in nursing, a foundation of scientific knowledge, and of acquaintance with medical practice. The nursing diagnosis may be the same as a medical diagnosis: hemorrhage and cardiac arrest. More often, a nursing diagnosis attempts to focus on an individual patient's response to illness or to reflect the progress of an individual in coping with physical and psychobiological trauma. The task is to establish a scientific basis for nursing practice.

In the philosophy of mind, one account of the mind–body relation is provided by what is termed *epiphenomenalism,* meaning that an object leaves a trail or impression on a person's mind. The relation between medical and nursing diagnosis may be similar to epiphenomenalism. The medical diagnosis exhibits the structural features of a disorder and the nursing diagnosis presents a follow-up trail or impression. If this analogy has weight, it supports the inclusive model of medical and nursing diagnoses.

Thomas and Coombs conceded that the nursing diagnosis may be the same as the medical diagnosis. We may note the epiphenomena in the two kinds of diagnoses cited by Thomas and Coombs.

> The medical diagnosis may become 'ventricular fibrillation' or 'myocardial infarction' and the nursing diagnosis may become 'ineffective cardiac output' or 'fear of pain.'[69]

The first of these terms, the medical diagnosis, implies the second, the nursing diagnosis, as a trail or epiphenomena. If the epiphenomenal view of the relation of medical and nursing diagnosis is correct, this gives a further argument on behalf of the inclusive or overlapping model of medical–nursing diagnosis.

An important difference between the nursing process and the medical diagnosis may depend on the primary method of logic used by each. Experienced practitioners and diagnosticians in either profession are likely

TABLE 5-2 GORDON'S TYPOLOGY OF ELEVEN FUNCTIONAL HEALTH PATTERNS

Health perception–health management pattern
Nutritional-metabolic pattern
Elimination pattern
Activity–exercise pattern
Cognitive–perceptual pattern
Sleep–rest pattern
Self-perception, self-concept pattern
Role–relationship pattern
Sexuality–reproductivity pattern
Coping–stress–tolerance pattern
Value–belief pattern

Source: Ref. 70.

to use both inductive and deductive logic in arriving at a diagnosis. The nursing assessment and diagnosis phase, however, are often approached inductively, that is, by the sheer compilation of data until a pattern or problem emerges, without reference to particular norms, concepts, or schema. Gordon has attempted to remedy this deficiency by proposing concrete guidelines for assessment usable as approaches to abstract nursing conceptual frameworks (Table 5–2). Gordon's identification of patterns "as a sequence of behavior across time . . . rather than isolated events," (or normal and abnormal signs and symptoms) are the data used in clinical inference and judgment.[71]

In seeking to explain the etiology of a dysfunctional pattern, scrutiny of one or more of the patterns is essential. Understanding of, and correct application of, logical notions of cause and effect, and necessary and sufficient conditions and probability, previously discussed in this text, are essential in justifying the etiological factor as the cause of a dysfunctional pattern. That procedure is, in turn, the basis for the prediction of nursing outcomes and the choice of nursing interventions.

The use of Gordon's typology of functional health patterns is largely done inductively by the accumulation of specific information relevant to each pattern. Data may soon suggest what Gordon calls "diagnostic hypotheses."[72] The logical method then becomes "hypotheticodeductive,"[73] meaning that the search is then focused on those "defining signs and symptoms . . . the relevant cues that support or negate a hypothesis."[74] Here, Gordon switches to a diagnostic model, hypotheticodeductive, and to terminology, signs, and symptoms, similar to that used by physician diagnosticians as demonstrated in Elstein's work.

Elstein and associates investigated the diagnostic reasoning process of medical problems by two groups of experienced physicians, one group recommended by peers and the other not. The data indicated that diagnostic problems were solved by a hypotheticodeductive method.[75] This means that diagnostic problems were solved by generating hypotheses, followed by verification. Hypotheses were consistently generated early in the work-up even on the basis of very limited data.[76] These early formulations were subject to revision or to rejection if further data collection failed to confirm them. Some initial hypotheses were correct.

These hypotheses functioned as forms or methods for organizing long-term memory. They helped long-term memory by narrowing the

> size of the problem space that must be searched for solution . . . Hypotheses serve to transform an open medical problem (What is the patient's illness?) into a set of closed problems that are much easier to solve (Is the illness X? or Y? or Z?). Means–ends (previously discussed in this work) is used to reduce the difference between end points and the state of affairs existing at any time.[77]

A nursing example of the hypotheticodeductive method is that of a nurse who observes a newly admitted patient on a medical ward moaning, crying, and pacing. The nurse can transform a global problem regarding the cause of the patient's behavior into a set of hypotheses that reduce the size of the problem space. The nurse hypothesizes that:

1. The patient is in physical pain and in need of relief, or that
2. The patient has been given bad news concerning diagnosis and is expressing psychological distress, or that
3. The patient is fearful and anxious concerning this first hospitalization and impending surgery and is expressing emotional distress, or that
4. The patient has a serious social or family problem aggravated by the illness condition, or that
5. The patient is experiencing an emotional crisis related to her illness.

Nurses would proceed in the assessment process of this problem. According to Elstein's investigation, physicians collected data through patient interviews and histories, physical examinations, and laboratory procedures. This information provided the basis for generating hypotheses and interpreting the data in relation to these hypotheses as the assessment process continued. The problem space is defined by these hypotheses, usually three to five at a time. Some hypotheses were rejected, others kept, and some revised as the accumulating data either corresponded to or departed from the specifications of the diagnostic hypothesis. A completely inductive method until a solution appears was never used since the problem space would be too big and unyielding. Diagnostic problems were solved by a hypotheticodeductive method.[78]

This model of diagnostic inquiry centered on the cognitive activities of "cue acquisition, hypothesis generation, cue interpretation, and hypothesis evaluation."[79] The cues presented from the patient are both normal and abnormal. Each abnormal finding must be explained. The task of the diagnostician is to work out a verifiable explanation that can lead to action and solution.

This study showed that diagnostic problems in medicine are solved through the generation and verification of hypotheses. Hypotheses were ruled out by lack of supporting data and by growing support for other hypotheses. The same data made it possible to test several hypotheses at once, thereby narrowing the problem space. The ultimate diagnostic decision was made on the basis of physical findings and the results of tests. The accuracy of the solution depended on generating sufficient hypotheses, using knowledge to recognize the kind and amount of data needed to confirm or rule out each hypothesis, securing the required data, and making accurate interpretations and decisions based on the evidence. Multiple solution problems were more difficult to solve than single solution problems. Statistical models of diagnosis inadequately handle patients with more than one disease. Disorders, such as anemia, caused by a variety of connected and unconnected sources, are also difficult problems for clinical logic. The challenge becomes knowing when to cluster probabilistic cues and when to treat them as separate causal implications (Table 5–3).[80] Anticipations direct problem-solving behavior. Thus the work-up is in part a guided search for the findings that each hypothesis implies.

A further example of a hypotheticodeductive method for diagnosis is the use of artificial intelligence. The enormous capacity of computers for storing data and for rapid mathematical computation underlie the growing use of artificial intelligence for diagnosis. As Buchanan and others have maintained

> Discovery in science and medicine can be profitably viewed as systematic exclusion of hypotheses. . . . Two necessary conditions are that the space of relevant hypotheses is definable and that there exist criteria of rejection and acceptability. Because the space of hypotheses is immense for most interesting problems, it is also desirable that there exist criteria for guiding a systematic search.[81]

The diagnostic reasoning process using a hypotheticodeductive model is in the phase of further development in nursing. The work of the North American Nursing Diagnosis Association is toward classifying and identifying the defining characteristics of a nursing diagnosis.

TABLE 5–3 ELSTEIN'S MODEL OF PHYSICIAN DIAGNOSTIC REASONING (ADAPTED)

Cue acquisition	Collect data
Hypothesis generation	Generate preliminary and probable general hypotheses
Cue interpretation	Discard, reformulate, or generate new hypotheses on the basis of data, cues, and findings
Hypothesis evaluation	Observe certain findings if hypothesis is true

Atkinson and Murray recommend that the nursing diagnosis begins to follow the identification of a problem focus area from the patient's data base. They have identified a framework of 13 basic needs that represent problem focus areas. These are oxygen needs, nutritional needs, needs for temperature maintenance, fluid needs, elimination needs, rest and sleep needs, needs for pain avoidance, sexual needs, safety and security needs, love and belonging needs, spiritual needs, self-esteem needs, and self-actualization needs.[82] After data collection, the problem area is located and the nursing diagnosis is made on the basis of the closest correspondence between the set of defining characteristics and the patient's data base.[83] The etiology is related to the individual patient. An interesting example of their adaptation of the North American Nursing Diagnosis Association classification of spiritual distress includes a definition, etiology, and 13 defining characteristics. The definition is presented as a disruption in the life principle that pervades a person's entire being and that integrates and transcends his or her biological and psychosocial nature.[84] The etiology presented is that of "separation from religious and cultural ties and challenged belief and value system."[85] The 13 defining characteristics range from expressed concern and conflicts regarding the meaning of life, existence and death or belief system (starred as a critical defining characteristic), anger toward God and religious representatives to alteration in behavior or mood with crying, withdrawal, hostility, apathy, and so forth.[86] Such a classification lends itself to the use of a hypotheticodeductive model. Based on this needs classification of diagnosis, the nurse collects data and hypothesizes or infers the diagnosis from the data base. After data collection, the nurse can discard, reformulate, or generate new hypotheses as the data are interpreted. Thus, the moaning, crying, pacing patient can be diagnosed as having spiritual distress. Hypothesis evaluation occurs in the process of accounting for all the data, either accepted or rejected.

CRITICAL THINKING IN THE PLANNING, IMPLEMENTATION, AND EVALUATION PROCESS

Once nurses establish the diagnosis and the etiology, they set out to correct the malady by intervention. They usually plan for a patient's recovery, although planning for a good death is a worthy goal for a terminal patient. In doing so, nurses set out with a health goal that is either the restoration, maintenance, or promotion of health. The nursing goal orients the plan; and the plan is set in motion by the nursing analysis or diagnosis. The planning phase involves strategies and means–ends thinking. Once the ends of a patient's diagnosis, situation, and recovery program are set, the means, such as the required nursing interventions, patient self-care, or nurse–patient transactions, are put into motion.

Nursing implementation or intervention normally follows the planning phase, and consists in a methodical, systematic, scientifically based patient care plan. For example, Ms. A, being seen and helped by a psychiatric nurse clinical specialist and a psychiatrist several times a week may comprise part of a nursing implementation.

The last phase, evaluation, is concerned with how effective the initial assessment, the diagnosis, the planning, and the implementation were. In this evaluative process, standards and procedures of critical thinking play an important role. This phase reminds us of the need for objectivity as implied by the appeal to scientific reasoning. One of the hard earned lessons of human inquiry is the role of self-corrective feedback, implied by appeal to objective standards of inquiry, and these include appropriate methods of verification.

CONCLUSION

The components of the nursing process are presented in a variety of steps. In 1973, the ANA included the steps of the nursing process in the *Standards of Nursing Practice* as follows:

1. Nursing assessment
   a. Data collection
2. Analysis/Synthesis of data
   a. Nursing diagnosis
3. Nursing plans
   a. Goals and objectives
   b. Plans for implementation
   c. Scientific rationale
4. Nursing implementation
5. Evaluation.[87]

The nursing process provides scope for the independent, interdependent, and dependent roles of the nurse and as a means to demonstrate nursing accountability. Griffith and Christensen view the nursing process as an adaptation of the "scientific method" to nursing.[88] As in other disciplines, the scientific process is used by nursing along with theoretical frameworks to collect data, seek knowledge that is relevant, and that guides practice effectively. This theory-based, scientific approach provides a "method and focus for data collecting; analysis of client health patterns, and diagnosis of client concerns or problems (and) . . . selection of nursing implementation strategies."[89] In this conception, each step of the nursing process lends itself to the systematic application of scientific theories, theoretical frameworks, and conceptual models.

This work takes the position that nursing is a dynamic, evolving field moving in many directions. Until nurses formulate a theoretical basis for practice that is distinctly nursing, however, disagreement among leading theorists about basic frameworks will continue.

Technology will profoundly influence the theory base and practice of nursing. Aspects of nursing will become increasingly technical, and drawn into the orbit of medicine. Other aspects of nursing may fulfill the hopes of independent practice focused on client's self-care and optimum levels of "wellness" and function.

At this time, there does not seem to be sufficient agreement on professional goals, purposes, and methods for one theory to be used as a basis for practice, research, and education. Many methods, therefore, as with many flowers, must be allowed to bloom. The use of critical thinking, however, with whatever theory or process selected, will enhance the validity, reliability, and worth of nursing outcomes to clients, patients, and practitioners.

REFERENCES

1. Stevens, B.J. Nursing Thecry: Analysis, Application, Evaluation (2nd ed.). Boston: Little, Brown, 1984, p. 76.
2. Ibid, p. 107.
3. American Nurses' Association. Nursing: A Social Policy Statement. Kansas City, Mo.: The American Nurses' Association, 1980, p. 10.
4. Ibid.
5. Ibid.
6. Ibid, p. 16.
7. Ibid.
8. Ibid, p. 9.
9. Ibid, pp. 9–10.
10. Ibid, p. 11.
11. Ibid.
12. Ibid.
13. Ibid, p. 9.
14. Griffith, J.W., & Christensen, P.J. Nursing Process. St. Louis: C.V. Mosby, 1982, p. 8.
15. Ibid.
16. Ibid.
17. Ibid, p. 9.
18. American Nurses' Association. A Social Policy Statement, p. 12.
19. Ibid.
20. Ibid.
21. Yura, H., & Walsh, M.B. The Nursing Process (4th ed.). Norwalk, Conn.: Appleton-Century Crofts, 1983, pp. 156–164.
22. Carnevali, D.L., et al (Eds.). Diagnostic Reasoning in Nursing. Philadelphia: J.B. Lippincott, 1984, pp. 36–52.
23. Gordon, M. Nursing Diagnosis: Process and Application. New York: McGraw Hill, 1982, p. 77.

24. Ibid.
25. Ibid.
26. Elstein, A., et al. Medical Problem Solving. Cambridge, Mass.: Harvard University Press, 1978, p. 299.
27. Ibid, p. 64.
28. Ibid, p. 65.
29. Ibid, p. 66.
30. Ibid, p. 66.
31. Ibid, pp. 75–77.
32. Ibid, pp. 278–281.
33. Marriner, A. (Ed.). The Nursing Process (3rd ed.). St. Louis: C.V. Mosby, 1983, p. 2.
34. Carrieri, U.K., & Sitzman, J. Components of the Nursing Process, in Marriner, A. (Ed.), The Nursing process, p. 9.
35. Gordon, M. Nursing Diagnosis: Process and Application, p. 13.
36. Ibid, p. 14.
37. Ibid.
38. Ibid.
39. Ibid, pp. 14–15.
40. Ibid, p. 15.
41. Ibid.
42. Orem, D. Nursing Concepts of Practice. New York: McGraw Hill, 1980, p. 41.
43. Gordon, M. Nursing Diagnosis: Process and Application, p. 80.
44. Ibid.
45. Shannon, C., et al. The Nursing Process, in Beck, C.M., et al (Eds.), Mental Health Psychiatric Nursing. St. Louis: C.V. Mosby, 1984, pp. 216–217.
46. Ibid, p. 230.
47. Ibid.
48. Ibid, pp. 232–233.
49. Webster's New Collegiate Dictionary. Springfield, Mass.: G. and C. Merriam, 1974, p. 313.
50. Wittgenstein, L. Philosophical Investigations. Oxford: Blackwell's 1953, p. 153.
51. Stevens, B.J. Nursing Theory, p. 108.
52. Ibid.
53. Anderson, J., & Yoder, K. Nursing Process, in Phipps, W.J., et al (Eds.), Medical–Surgical Nursing. St. Louis: C.V. Mosby, 1979, p. 87.
54. Ibid.
55. Ibid.
56. Ibid.
57. Gordon, M. Nursing Diagnosis and the Diagnosis and the Diagnostic Process. *American Journal of Nursing* 1976; 76(8):1298, August.
58. Kaufman, J. Assessment Process: Data Collection and Analysis, in Phipps, W., et al. (Eds.), Medical–Surgical Nursing, p. 112.
59. Ibid.
60. Ibid.
61. Ibid.
62. Thomas, M.D., & Coombs, R.P. Nursing Diagnosis: Process and Decision, in Marriner, A. (Ed.), The Nursing Process, p. 99.
63. Ibid.

64. Ibid.
65. Ibid, p. 99.
66. Ibid.
67. Ibid, p. 100.
68. Ibid, p. 101.
69. Ibid.
70. Gordon, M. Nursing Diagnosis: Process and Application (2nd ed.). New York: McGraw-Hill, 1978, p. 93.
71. Ibid, p. 92.
72. Ibid, p. 190.
73. Elstein, A., et al. Medical Problem Solving, p. 64.
74. Gordon, M. Nursing Diagnosis: Process and Application, p. 214.
75. Elstein, A., et al. Medical Problem Solving, p. 113.
76. Ibid.
77. Ibid, p. 114–115.
78. Ibid, p. 115.
79. Ibid, p. 66.
80. Ibid, p. 71.
81. Buchanan, B.G. Steps Toward Mechanizing Discovery, in Scheffner, K. (Ed.) Berkeley: University of California Press, 1985, p. 94.
82. Atkinson, L.D., & Murray, M.E. Understanding the Nursing Process (3rd ed.). New York: Macmillan, 1986, Appendix B, iii–iv.
83. Ibid.
84. Ibid, Appendix B, pp. 61–62.
85. Ibid, pp. 61–62.
86. Ibid, pp. 61–62.
87. American Nurses' Association. Standards of Nursing Practice. Kansas City, Mo.: The American Nurses' Association, 1973.
88. Griffith, J.A., & Christensen, P.J. Nursing Process, p. 4.
89. Ibid.

Chapter 6

Critical Thinking in Decision Making

Study of this chapter enables the student to:

1. Apply skills of critical thinking in reaching decisions.
2. Select a decision procedure suitable to a particular problem, personal style, goals, and context.
3. Use a problem-solving method of decision making appropriately.

INTRODUCTION

Making a decision is the end point of using critical thinking and scientific reasoning in problem resolution. All thoughts and actions culminate in some kind of a decision. Even "no decision" is a decision, because, in effect, it supports the existing state of affairs.

One practical method is a six-phase cycle. This method begins with problem identification and moves through steps of gathering information, generating, testing, and evaluating conclusions, and reaching decisions. Thinking critically throughout each phase is essential since the conclusion may open up possibilities for several different decisions. For example, Ms. Jablowski may conclude that nursing employment in Hospital X is highly desirable for obvious important reasons such as the working conditions, the learning opportunities, and other benefits. Yet Ms. Jablowski decides to remain at Hospital Y because she is at an administrative level or has only five more years before qualifying for a retirement plan. Or, on the basis of the same conclusion, Ms. Jablowski may decide to resign from Hospital Y, despite loss of salary and status, so that her last years in nursing may be satisfying and pleasurable. Or Ms. Jablowski may decide to actively participate in improving the conditions of nursing employment at Hospital Y through her administrative position and influence as the culmination of her long nursing career.

Each step in the decision process needs critical appraisal with respect to the soundness, accuracy, and adequacy of the unstated premises or presuppositions of the problem statement. Information gathered must be relevant, accurate, and adequate. Possible conclusions need to be tested as arguments by logical cannons of validity, soundness, and importance. If–then conditional statements need critical appraisal so that the conclusion is a valid and sound argument. Few decisions have only two options; "black and white" and "either–or" thinking often denies the options.

Decisions are also value laden, as the example of Ms. Jablowski's future employment illustrates. Giere's value matrix is based on "a set of possible actions, a set of possible states of the world, and a corresponding set of outcomes . . ."[1] Each possible outcome is either assigned an arbitrary number in a value ranking scale or the value is measured on an actual scale, such as dollars and cents.

Giere also identifies categories of decision strategies related to the availability of information. Definite knowledge of the state of the world, as Ms. Jablowski knows Hospital Y after 25 years of employment there, is called "decision making with certainty."[2] When nothing is known about the state of the world, Giere calls that "decision making with uncertainty."[3] The middle case is based on knowledge of the probabilities or statistics of each state's occurrence. This category Giere calls "decision making with risk."[4]

Clearly, nurses ought to participate in decision making on the basis of critical thinking, cannons of logic, value choices, and degrees of certainty and risk. Nurses have countless opportunities to make important decisions significant to the lives of patients, families, groups, organizations, communities, and themselves in the course of their personal and professional lives. The use of critical thinking in this process offers nurses the opportunity to decide wisely and in behalf of the well-being of others as well as their own benefit and happiness.

A PRACTICAL METHOD OF DECISION MAKING

A useful procedure in making practical decisions is to apply a six-phase cycle of critical scrutiny to the problem (Table 6–1). Phases of the cycle may proceed concurrently, and be repeated. Thinking critically throughout the process of completing all the steps, however, is the best assurance of a sound solution.

TABLE 6-1. PHASES IN DECISION MAKING

Phase 1.	Recognizing and defining a problem
Phase 2.	Gathering relevant information
Phase 3.	Generating possible conclusions
Phase 4.	Testing possible conclusions
Phase 5.	Evaluating conclusions
Phase 6.	Reaching decisions

Source: Ref. 5.

Phase 1. Recognizing and Defining a Problem

Some problems are self-proclaimed. A problem of understaffing, for example, announces itself because it is so irritating, painful, or frustrating to everyone concerned. Nurses, patients, and families are made uncomfortable by the conditions of scarcity. Because the problem seems obvious, the solution appears to be equally simple—securing more staff and more money to pay more staff. Therefore, the problem disappears from everyone's thinking.

As in most human enterprises, problems are not always what they appear to be. To engage in the process of critical thinking is to search for what is behind or what comes before what appears to be the real problem. Unstated, hidden, or suppressed premises, propositions, or assertions of fact or belief may be the real problem underlying the obvious symptomatic manifestations that cry for attention. To state the problem of understaffing on the medical unit to be a nursing shortage in Hospital X, for example, without critically examining the unstated, hidden, or suppressed premises regarding nurse autonomy, staffing pattern, patient characteristics, salary scales, housing, and transportation affecting nurses, may misidentify the problem. Problem misidentification leads to wrong decisions and no solutions.

How can thinking critically help to define the problem more accurately? One suggestion is that a problem definition should not be too general.[6] To define a problem in terms of a nursing shortage is to define the problem in global terms beyond solution and beyond investigation. Another suggestion is to avoid a problem definition too specific as it effectively restricts alternative solutions.[7] To define the problem as a nursing shortage on the medical unit due to the resignation of four staff nurses is to ignore the unstated, missing, suppressed premises that staff nurses resigned because of intolerable working conditions.

A third suggestion is that the definition itself is identified as a *solution* to the problem.[8] Typically, the problem of nursing shortages is used as the solution to understaffing. This is a circular definition, a tautology, that fails to inform or to move the problem forward toward a solution.

A fourth suggestion is to identify missing, unstated, or suppressed premises that are better candidates for the problem statement than the actual problem definition. For example, to state the understaffing on the medical unit in Hospital X as the "nursing shortage" is to deny the unstated, missing, suppressed premises of intolerable working conditions, substandard salaries, unavailability of affordable housing, and poor public transportation, any or all of which could be the problem definition of understaffing. Instead, an uncritical acceptance of the problem of understaffing is *solved* by reference to a nationwide nursing shortage as the cause.

This is an example of the fallacy of slothful induction; also called the fallacy of an a priori assumption, the method of tenacity, or the use of self-sealers.[9] The user of this fallacy refuses to allow evidence to be considered that contradicts a previous conclusion. These are defenses against possible criticism.

Assumptions are statements that are taken for granted without question. Assumptions can be hidden, implied, or ignored, but operate in a powerful manner. In the above example, some hidden assumptions are:

- Nurses' salaries are lower in Hospital X than in comparable facilities.
- Nurses' salaries support a low standard of living.
- Nurses' salaries do not reward experience.
- Affordable, decent housing is unavailable or scarce.
- Working conditions in Hospital X include serving a poor population with multiple problems and inadequate human and material resources.
- Hospital X is in an obsolete plant with outdated equipment in poor repair.
- Public transportation is inconvenient and expensive.
- The neighborhood is unsafe, especially for nurses on evening and night shifts.

By engaging in the process of critical thinking, hidden assumptions are converted into explicit assumptions that must be taken into account in reaching a decision. Suppressed or unstated assumptions are highly influential in leading the uncritical thinker to the wrong conclusion as the basis of a faulty decision.

Phase 2. Gathering Relevant Information

In principle, the more information gathered about a situation, the better the quality of the decision. In reality, the amount of data available regarding most subjects is often overwhelming. The challenge becomes one of sorting out and selecting data that are relevant to the investigation leading to a decision. A clear definition of the problem is useful to delineate its boundaries and categorize it as primarily a management, nursing, medical, social, or fiscal problem. Once the primary focus of the problem is defined, information can be gathered that bears directly on its core and disposition. For example, the primary focus of the nursing shortage in Hospital X is the interrelationship of all the factors—salary, policies, staffing, housing, transportation, plant conditions, and patient population—that make employment there undesirable.

Phase 3. Generating Possible Conclusions

A common problem that follows the gathering of information is that of deciding what to do with the data and how to use it most effectively. Several tests may be useful. The test of adequacy asks if there is sufficient data upon which to make inferences as the basis for generating possible conclusions. In the understaffing example, is sufficient data available regarding staffing patterns to allow for inferences to be made? Is reliable information regarding each of the identified variables gathered through surveys and exit interviews available? An inference may be characterized as a bridge or railroad track that permits movement from one place to another place; that is, to move from a statement, proposition, or judgment considered true to another statement, proposition, or judgment considered true that follows from the former.[10]

What criteria are useful in appraising sufficiency, accuracy, and relevance of information? One test of sufficiency of information about understaffing is to ask every departing nurse questions regarding the sufficiency of staffing and other variables of employment.

The data base might look like this:

- Nurses are paid lower salaries for comparable work than in other nearby hospitals.
- Fringe benefits, such as tuition reimbursement and sick days, are less liberal in Hospital X than in comparable hospitals.
- Flexible work hours to suit individual preferences are unavailable in Hospital X.
- Subsidized housing for nursing staff is unavailable in Hospital X.
- Public transportation to Hospital X requires transfers and double fares for most employees.
- Employee parking is insufficient in Hospital X.
- Hospital X is physician and research centered.
- Nurses are without voice in policy formulation.
- Staffing patterns are insufficient to provide effective care to acutely ill patients with multiple, complex problems.
- Nursing care is provided in an obsolete plant with outdated equipment in poor repair.

Possible inferences regarding employment in Hospital X that follow from this data are:

- Nurses are better paid in other hospitals.
- Fringe benefits are better in other hospitals.

- Work hours are more flexible to suit individual preferences in other hospitals.
- Subsidized housing is available in other hospitals.
- Public transportation is better in other hospitals.
- Employee parking is available in other hospitals.
- Nurses participate in policy formulation in other hospitals.
- Nurses exercise more autonomy in other hospitals.
- Staffing pattterns are better in other hospitals.
- Patient populations are more varied in other hospitals.
- Plant and equipment are more modern and plentiful in other hospitals.

A second test of information is that of accuracy. Information that is inaccurate, vague, or ambiguous is worse than useless as it can lead to an inaccurate conclusion and to a wrongful decision.

A third test of the worth of information is its relevance. Even though information is accurate, it may simply be irrelevant to the problem at hand. It may even obscure the directness and the clarity of decision making. For example, to survey the reasons for termination of employment in the past 10 years for every nurse once affiliated with Hospital B is irrelevant. Current conditions in nursing are now so different as to raise doubt regarding the relevance of findings more than a few years old.

Inferences based on data generate tentative conclusions. On the basis of information that is adequate, accurate, and relevant, inferences can be made regarding the salaries, housing, transportation, fringe benefits, and working hours of nurses at Hospital B in comparison to the same conditions at similar facilities.

These inferences are the basis of possible conclusions. Using the argument form modus ponens explained in Chapter 10 on the use of arguments, "If P then Q, P so Q," we can draw these conclusions:

If P (large salary increase, then Q (staffing increase),
P (large salary increase),
So, Q (staffing increase).

We can use the same argument forms for each of the variables as follows:

If P (preferred flex time), then Q (increased nursing staff),
P (preferred flex time),
So, Q (improved staffing).

If P (nurses' subsidized housing), then Q (increased nursing staff)
P (nurses' subsidized housing),
So, Q (increased staff).

If P (safe, accessible, convenient transportation), then Q (increased nursing staff),
P (safe, accessible, convenient transportation),
So, Q (increased nursing staff).

Logically, each of the above arguments is valid, because the premises imply the conclusion. Moreover, each conclusion could serve as the basis for a positive decision regarding increased salaries, subsidized housing, transportation, and flex time. We are only committed "to the claim that the conclusion follows from the premises. False claims have consequences, just as well as true claims."[11]

Phase 4. Testing Possible Conclusions

The objective of phase 4 is to critically assess the reliability of all possible conclusions. Because conclusions are reached by the process of reasoning, the validity, soundness, and usefulness of arguments used need critical scrutiny as the basis for reliable decisions.

The test for the validity of an argument is based on premises that imply the conclusion. A valid argument can have true premises and true conclusions, or false premises and false conclusions (but not true premises and a false conclusion). Therefore, the validity of an argument does not guarantee the truth of its conclusion. Because decisions in everyday life are expected to be reliable, that is, based on the truth of premises and of conclusions, an argument needs to be sound. The test for an argument that is sound is that it is both valid and based on true premises and true conclusions to be reliable as the basis for decisions.

A third test of possible conclusions is the criteria of usefulness. To test conclusions regarding understaffing of nurses 10 years ago at Hospital X is useless as it begs the question of possible conclusions related to present understaffing conditions at Hospital X. The conclusion that the problem of understaffing at Hospital X is caused by a national nursing shortage also begs the question and is, therefore, useless.

A further principle of critical thinking is that all conclusions are tested for reliability. To exclude some conclusions from testing is to protect beliefs and values from critical appraisal.[12] Such exclusions also serve to deny and conceal biased thinking. Testing all conclusions is an effective way to reduce mistaken decisions.

Phase 5. Evaluating Conclusions

The aim of phase 5 of the cycle is to determine what solutions among those tested are workable. The reliability of conclusions tested calls for critical appraisal. The evidence upon which the premises are based and the conclusion is inferred is subjected to intense scrutiny. We must consider whether the evidence for the conclusion is true beyond any reasonable doubt. Even if the evidence is highly probable in contrast with evidence with a low probability, we also consider whether the conclusion is sufficiently reliable to justify a decision. If the evidence in the premises is insufficient and the conclusion thus unsound and unreliable, clearly the cycle is repeated.

A further consideration in evaluating conclusions is to consider underlying value assumptions. For example, there is substantial evidence that increased salaries, benefits, and improved working conditions attract and retain nursing staff. The value placed on other workers in Hospital X, however, prohibits a disproportionate use of resources for nurses at the expense of all others. Moreover, if carried to its furthest point, nursing care could become prohibitively expensive. Similarly, the spread of acquired immune deficiency syndrome (AIDS) could be largely contained by testing and isolating carriers and victims of this dreaded disease. Such a conclusion, however, denies basic human rights of choice, privacy, and confidentiality. It would subject identified victims to stigma, rejection, isolation, and possibly cruel and unusual punishment. Society could become dichotomous, irreparably split into the haves and the have-nots of AIDS and its related conditions.

Phase 6. Reaching Decisions

After critical appraisal of each of these phases of the cycle, the decision is seemingly an obvious inevitable sequela of the process. Such a view of decision making omits consideration of those human characteristics that comprise our individuality. Each person's frame of reference includes an organized body of knowledge, experience, and beliefs useful to understand and interpret new experiences.[13] Each frame of reference contains what is known or believed to be true of the world—its contents and its dynamics, past and future. Each individual's frame of reference functions to gain new information and to decide what to do with what it knows.

No one's frame of reference is either totally accurate or complete.[14] Everyone has vast gaps in knowledge and understanding, and is, therefore, susceptible to many errors in decision. Our frame of reference also limits our perception. Like the visitor to a foreign land, we fail to *see* and to *hear* that which is obvious—simply because it is not within our frame of reference.[15] Or, we see people, things, and events and interpret them wrongly, as does a wealthy patient who fails to grasp the concept of self-care and who perceives her private nurse to be a personal maid to bathe and dress her and manage the environment.

A more serious limitation of our frame of reference is in the inability to recognize problems.[16] These limitations may occur because of lack of knowledge, as in the case of a newly graduated nurse in the intensive care unit for the first day. Because of lack of knowledge, that nurse is limited in the ability to acquire new knowledge. For example, the nurse without knowledge of the significance of blood gases and other blood chemistry values would be severely handicapped in learning to care for patients in cardiac intensive care units as signs and symptoms would be meaningless. "Knowledge is necessary to acquire knowledge."[17]

Inadequate frames of reference are a distinct handicap in reaching sound decisions. False information, such as belief systems that deny the power of science and medicine to cure an otherwise fatal disease, is a serious or even a fatal flaw in our ability to think critically and make appropriate decisions. A sound education is necessary for a healthy, well-developed frame of reference. Nevertheless, even a well-developed frame of reference is immeasurably enriched by the addition of critical thinking skills. The addition of objectivity, that is, the ability to think clearly and critically without distortion about self and the world, increases the effectiveness of thinking and decision making. Objectivity is necessarily incomplete and uneven because it springs from a less than perfect frame of reference. Sexist personal values and inadequate self-concepts may distort a nurse's perception of the significance of the professional role. Threats to an individual's established self-concept can seriously distort objective perception of reality and lead to defensive behavior and poor decisions. We may resort to deception as a defense of our perception of self-reality, however distorted that defense may be. Because frames of reference are value laden, values are intertwined with frames of reference.

The subjective and the objective also intersect. Threats to an idea or to a value become a threat to our frame of reference and ultimately to our sense of personal worth. New ideas that threaten the status quo tend to be resisted as current controversies regarding "entry into practice" issues demonstrate. Another threat to the status quo is the concept of nursing diagnosis, the expanded role of the nurse, and the independent nursing practice with third party payment as encroachments on the practice of medicine.

Values are sometimes expressed as statements containing *ought* or *should.* Values are distinctly different from frames of reference concerned with the way things are or are seen to be. Value judgments are implicit, if not explicit, in all thinking, critical and uncritical, behavior and actions. Decisions are always value laden even though nurses may believe that their actions are solely determined by scientific considerations. The nurse who calls for cardiopulmonary resuscitation on every patient is expressing the concept of life under any and all conditions as a primary value. The nurse who seeks to identify the patient's real wishes concerning cardiopulmonary resuscitation and to carry them out is supporting the concept of rights to one's own body as the primary value. Such decisions can be and often are in conflict.

Disputes surrounding values cannot be avoided. In practice, decisions are sometimes made without sufficient consideration for the underlying value premises. Implementation of such decisions may be stormy and cause considerable turmoil among those charged with carrying out such decisions.

An example in nursing may be the closing of units and the reassignment of staff. The explicit values expressed may be the good of the institution as a whole and the conservation of jobs. Unexpressed but implicit values are the considerable savings achieved from reducing the number of supervisory and managerial positions in nursing and the expected resignations of nurses with seniority who are dissatisfied with new and different assignments. Explicit but unacknowledged institutional values may be that nursing experience and nursing degrees are worth less on the salary scale than is working an evening or night shift. The downgrading of academic qualifications in nursing undermines the efforts of nurses to give quality care to patients. The identification of nursing as subordinate to or dependent on medical care is a further example of a value judgment that is pervasive in society and harmful to the development of nursing as an independent profession based on nursing theory and research.

The concept of self-worth is a basis for making judgments and an integral part of our frame of reference. To view nursing as an indispensable and universal human activity focused on care of the sick and promoting, maintaining, and restoring health to be based on scientific and humanistic knowledge is to grant the profession of nursing an importance appropriate to its contribution. This applies to any person's frame of reference. Such a definition grants high positive values to the practice of nursing. Nurses who regard themselves as competent, committed, and caring practitioners, who make a significant difference to the well-being of human beings, have a positive sense of self-worth that influences decisions. Such individuals have a clear sense of their competencies, talents, roles, and of the respect, dignity, and rewards due them.

USE OF CRITICAL THINKING IN EVERYDAY NURSING PRACTICE

Thinking critically is relevant to every decision made throughout every day of our lives. To choose a course of action is to make a decision. To choose one course of action means to eliminate others. Making distinctions between the structure of the decisions and of the process will be useful.

Few decisions have only two options; therefore, a preliminary step is to determine all the possibilities. Freedom from an attitude of "all or nothing at all" or "black and white" thinking is useful to approaching decisions with an open, flexible attitude.

The second step is to organize options so that the choices are mutually exclusive (free from repetition) and exhaustive (containing all possibilities).[18] For example, Nurse Jones either chooses to teach Mr. and Mrs. Green about colostomy care on Tuesday or not teach because she has the next day off. Nurse Jones may choose to demonstrate colostomy care by doing it herself or she may instruct Mr. Green as he irrigates himself in the presence of Mrs. Green. Or Mr. and Mrs. Green may view an instructional videotape made by nurses for patients with a colostomy as often as they choose. Or Nurse Jones may call on the services of an ostomy nurse clinical specialist to do all of the instruction. Or Nurse Jones may suggest to the patient and his wife that they contact the cancer society for help or the local visiting nurse association.

Nurse Jones' choices whether to teach or not teach colostomy care to Mr. Green are mutually exclusive. The choice of method is not mutually exclusive since more than one method may be used on the assumption that one method reinforces another. Realistically, the options presented are exhaustive of those courses of action available to Nurse Jones. To refrain from teaching Mr. Green because of insufficient time, staff, or resources is also a decision and a course of action. The choices may be plotted as shown in Table 6–2.

The outcome of Nurse Jones' decision is significant to the patient and his spouse in terms of his goals for self-care. This outcome is of great value to them.

The increasing number of infected persons and deaths from acquired immune deficiency syndrome (AIDS) and AIDS-related diseases, has forced sexually active individuals to reconsider their sexual practices and sexual partners. A recent article highlights the dilemma of a 38-year-old divorced woman seeking safer sex. She was torn between the horror of knowing and the fear of not knowing whether or not her blood tests were negative or positive for HIV antibodies (see Table 6–3). Obviously, these options are neither mutually exclusive nor exhaustive. The blood test results at this time may not indicate the presence of a recent infection because the blood values are not changed as yet. Therefore, sex with a casual partner is not safe as intercourse involves possible infection from any other previous sexual partners of partners.

The options for safe sex are mutually exclusive and exhaustive as Table 6–4 demonstrates. In this example, the value that the individual decision maker places on freedom of choice and sexual liberation is antithetical to

TABLE 6-2. MUTUALLY EXCLUSIVE AND EXHAUSTIVE OPTIONS IN RELATION TO EDUCATION OF A PATIENT WITH A COLOSTOMY

Mutually Exclusive Choices	Exhaustive Options	
Teach Mr. Green colostomy care.	Teach by demonstration and by return demonstration.	Teach through the use of audiovisual aids.
Do not teach Mr. Green.	Discharge without instruction.	Refer to a clinical nurse specialist, the visiting nurse association, home care, or to the cancer society.

TABLE 6-3. OPTIONS IN RELATION TO BLOOD TESTING FOR HIV FACTORS

Mutually Exclusive Choices	Exhaustive Options	
	Positive Test	*Negative Test*
Blood test for HIV antibodies.	Can inform potential sex partners before intercourse to avoid spread of infection.	Can document negative test outcomes and demand similar documentation from potential sex partners.
No blood test for HIV antibodies.	May infect others unknowingly through sexual intercourse.	May be infected through sexual intercourse with infected others who are also untested.

the values of documented safe, monogamous relationships with persons free of risk factors. The identification of values is an important part of any decision. A choice is or ought to be a reflection of individual values.[19] The place of values in controversies is considered to be of sufficient importance to merit further attention in Chapter 7.

Once the outcomes of a decision have been specified, as in Table 6–4, the outcomes can be ranked in order of personal values and preference. Thus the individual ranking safety and security as foremost will clearly

TABLE 6-4. OPTIONS FOR SEXUAL PRACTICES IN RELATION TO AIDS

1. Safer sex/no sex	A completely faithful, monogomous relationship without risk factors of transfusion or intravenous drug use for 10 or more years duration.	Relationship between individuals who are virgins with documented negative blood and free of risk factors.
2. "Safer sex"	Sexual intercourse with the use of condoms and other protective measures.	
3. Unsafe sex	Casual sex	Sex with members of high-risk groups such as bisexual or homosexual persons, persons who have been transfused, intravenous drug users, their spouses, children, or sexual partners.

choose a monogamous relationship documented to be safe and without risk factors or abstain from sex. The individual ranking complete freedom of choice and sexual expression as the foremost value may elect spontaneous, casual, or even anonymous sexual encounters. The individual who values both sexual freedom and safety equally will choose "safe sex" through the use of condoms and all other protective measures.

In any decision, ranking the possible outcomes according to one's own scale of values is a useful device. Given the action options and relevant states of the world, the value rankings placed on possible outcomes help define differences between one choice and another.[20]

Clearly, a decision that has an outcome that is valued more highly is better than an outcome less valued. In making decisions, however, consideration must also be given to the state of the world, and that brings us full circle to the need for knowledge about the state of the world.

Giere proposes a general value matrix for ranking possible outcomes on the individual's scale of values. Should the decision be a corporate one, then the corporation chooses the value matrix—presumably in terms of financial profits and loss.[21] One of the difficulties that professional nurses face, along with physicians, is the change in the primary value of many hospitals from values of charity, compassion, and unconditional acceptance to business and profit centers. Thus, the phrase "the health care industry" characterizes the way many hospitals are administered. There are obvious conditions, such as reduced federal subsidies to health care, that explain but do not justify the change in values of traditional humanitarian institutions devoted to the care and welfare of sick and suffering human beings. Giere contends that, nevertheless, the strategies for making decisions apply, whatever value ranking is given.[22]

Giere's value matrix is based on "a set of possible actions, a set of possible states of the world, and a corresponding set of outcomes (or 'results') of the decision—that is, action–state pairs."[23] Thus, if there are three actions and four possible states of the world, 12 (3×4) different outcomes are possible. In turn, each of these possible outcomes is either assigned an arbitrary number on a value ranking scale or the value is measured in some actual scale, such as money.

An example in nursing follows:

	S_1	S_2	S_3	S_4
A_1	Value	Value	Value	Value
A_2	Value	Value	Value	Value
A_3	Value	Value	Value	Value

- A_1 stands for health protecting behaviors: medical care, avoidance of harmful substances and environment, goal-directed control of nutrition, exercise.

- A_2 stands for health promoting behaviors: control of stress, activity, environment, and preventive medical care.

- A_3 stands for health indifferent behaviors: random sporadic attention to diet, physical, rest, and health activities and practices.

- S_1 stands for a sedentary stressful occupation oriented toward high achievement and goals.

- S_2 stands for a routinized occupation offering complete security, tenure, and predictability.

- S_3 stands for an uncertain, highly demanding, stressful occupation with immediate high financial returns.

- S_4 stands for a fulfilling, stimulating occupation with high demands, rewards, and recognition.

The 12 possibilities are the combination of the action–state pairs, that is, the three A's times the fours states of affairs, S's. An arbitrary scale of values is then used by the individual to rank the outcomes of these combined states of the world and actions. Thus, the value placed on these outcomes is the direct expression of the individual's values. If the decision maker prefers high financial rewards, a health promoting life-style with control of stress seems an impossible or difficult outcome to achieve. The value preference is clear. A higher-valued outcome is preferable to a lower-valued outcome. Typically, the choice of action leading to the best outcome depends on the state of the world at that time. If that knowledge is readily available, the decision process is easy. The choice would simply be the action with that outcome valued as the highest.

Giere defines three categories of decision strategies as dependent on the availability of information. The first category is that in which the state of the world is definitely known. He calls it "decision making with CERTAINTY."[24] Predictably, when nothing is known about the occurrence of the state of the world, that category is called "decision making with UNCERTAINTY."[25] The middle case is knowing the probability of each state's occurrence. This information may be statistical. Giere calls this category "decision making with RISK."[26]

The use of an inductive form of argument in science can never deliver absolute truth, as the possibility of using true premises to reach a false conclusion is always present. When the evidence for a particular state is especially strong, however, the small chance of error is ignored in favor of decision making with certainty.

In some situations, the actions and states are independent. In the previous problem, action in the form of health protecting, health promoting, or health indifferent behaviors can be independent of the state of the world through the individual's occupational choice. Much of nursing, however, involves problems in which action and states of the world are not independent. For example, a nurse may act to meet the perceived nursing needs of the patient. In fact, the nurse's demonstrated competence, intelligence, and kindness evokes the expression of many more patients' needs. A serious difficulty in the practice of nursing, as the above example illustrates, is the allocation of a finite amount of nursing time among patients with nearly unlimited nursing needs and desires. In such circumstances, the nurse's action is never independent of the state of affairs, even though the nurse is practicing in the category of decision making with certainty. The nurse knows enough about the situation to be able to tell what outcome goes with each possible action. In such cases, choosing the action with the outcome most valued in relation to knowledge of the states is the preferred decision. Nurses, then, place their highest value on actions that save the lives of patients with good prognoses rather than on those with prognoses that are poor, such as long-term comatose and Alzheimer victims.

To make a decision with complete uncertainty about states is in effect to make a decision based only on the value matrix. To be completely uncertain about states is to recognize that actions and states are completely independent of each other. The use of a new experimental drug on AIDS patients—purportedly effective against the virus, but never given to humans—may be one example of a decision with complete uncertainty. The outcome of possibly saving lives doomed by AIDS is most valued even though knowledge of the states, such as the desired effects and the unwanted side effects on humans with this infection, are completely unknown.

As Table 6–5 illustrates, actions can be better or worse. The value choices in this simple diagram are explicit. Because probabilities cannot be assigned to the chances of cure, remission, drug effect, death, or harmful side effects, the decision must be made solely on the basis of values. If the AIDS victim prizes the chance for a cure or remission above the unknown length and quality of life left for him or her, then that value is highest. If the subject places the highest value on continuing whatever life is left for him or her, then that value assumes priority over the possibility of death or harmful effects from the drug.

TABLE 6–5. VALUE MATRIX FOR A DECISION WITH COMPLETE UNCERTAINTY

Action	Desired Effects	Undesired Effects
Administer the experimental drug to volunteers	Cure or remission of the disease	Death Serious harmful side effects Ineffective
Do not administer the drug	None	None

One could argue that it would be foolish for an individual with a fatal case of AIDS to refuse a possibly life-saving drug. It appears to be the worst action and it should be eliminated, as these options are exclusive and exhaustive alternatives. The actions and the states are independent and the better option, taking the experimental drug, is the only one available. Therefore, it becomes the BEST action available.[27] That action then becomes a belief shared by other AIDS victims who also clamor for a possibly limited supply of the experimental drug.

In some decision problems with options for actions, the individual ranks the outcomes on a value scale to determine the lowest value regarded as satisfactory or acceptable outcome. If there were no possible action granting a higher value, the choice would be the action ranked as satisfactory or acceptable.[28] Even if this outcome is the only acceptable action in the ranking, it should be chosen.[29] A gambler, in contrast, chooses the highest valued outcome, "all the marbles," regardless of risk.[30] The persistent heavy smoker may be regarded as a gambler. The cautious person, the health protecting person, plays it safe by avoiding bad consequences even if some good ones might happen. For example, such a person might avoid prophylactic doses of a drug, such as aspirin or penicillin, because of possible harmful side effects, even though such a drug might prevent a heart attack or a recurrence of bacterial endocarditis. Such a person tends to "choose the action with the greatest security level . . . to maximize . . . minimum possible value payoff."[31] In comparison, the gambler or the health indifferent person, assigns the highest values to the pleasures of smoking or to eating foods high in calories, fat, cholesterol, and salt (such as thick steaks, hamburgers, whole milk, and rich pastries) or to risking all on the chance of winning.

Another perspective from which to view decision problems is either *from the top* or *from the bottom.*[32] In a simplified version, only two actions and two states are possible. A nursing analogy is the comparison of two states: the best possible hospital system of nursing service or the real state of a given hospital system of nursing service. The two actions can be either increasing the number of professional nurses or maintaining the current number of professional nurses (difficult in current conditions of nursing shortage). The value matrix viewed from the top, meaning administration, trustees, and financial managers, may be quite different from the value matrix from the bottom, meaning staff nurses, patients, and possibly auxillary services such as pharmacy and dietary.

Compare the highest value ranking on the "top" people for maintaining the current number of professional nurses with the hypothetical value matrix for an "Ideal World" decision viewed from the bottom (Tables 6–6 and 6–7). Values placed on the outcomes are dramatically different because of the values nurses and patients place on staffing patterns that will result in the most effective, safe patient care with standards acceptable to professional nurses.

TABLE 6-6. VALUE MATRIX FOR AN "IDEAL WORLD" DECISION VIEWED *FROM THE TOP*

	States of the World	
Action	*Ideal World of Expanded Resources*	*Real World of Limited Resources*
Increase number of professional nurses	2	4
Maintain current number of professional nurses	3	1

Giere's third category is decision making with risk; risk then is known or controlled by probabilities.[33] This is an intermediate level of decision making based on knowledge of the probabilities of possible states.[34] For example, the probabilities of mortality and morbidity from routinized procedures, such as childbirth (normal and cesarian section), abortions, herniorrhaphy, tonsillectomy, cardiac catherization, and coronary bypass surgery, are readily available to persons making operative decisions. The success rate of individual surgeons and institutions may also be available. The obvious choice then for the individual contemplating such procedures is to seek knowledge of the probabilities, consider the costs, and then "choose the action with the greatest expected value . . . It is the product of the probability and the value that matters, not just the magnitude of either separately."[35] For example, the statistical evidence is very strong and complete enough to accept cigarette smoking as the cause of lung cancer with support from a worthy biological model. The statistics show that the risk of lung cancer rises with increasing amounts smoked.[36] The product here is the value of life times the probability of the risk of lung cancer as the basis for the choice of the greatest expected value. Thus, anyone who continues to smoke may be regarded as a gambler, because the causal connection with lung cancer has been so well established. The

TABLE 6-7. VALUE MATRIX FOR AN "IDEAL WORLD" DECISION VIEWED *FROM THE BOTTOM*

	States of the World	
Action	*Ideal World of Expanded Resources*	*Real World of Limited Resources*
Increase number of professional nurses	3	1
Maintain current number of professional nurses	4	2

gambler, however, may value smoking to the extent that the probabilities of developing lung cancer are regarded as complete uncertainty and a not known risk of dying prematurely. The issue becomes one of confronting the probabilities and the values we place on outcomes to determine our choice of action.[37]

For an action to be a causal factor for a harmful effect does not negate the benefits of the agent, as the history of oral contraceptives demonstrates. When the frequency of blood clots in women of childbearing age taking oral contraceptives is quoted as 7.5 times greater than all women of childbearing age, the actual numbers are 15 in a million (taking oral contraceptives) compared to 2 in a million. Fifteen in a million is still a small number.[38]

A new issue is the association of drinking alcoholic beverages with an increased risk of developing breast cancer. According to two new studies, drinking alcohol is connected to a 50 percent increase in the risk of developing breast cancer.[39] This is alarming to women who drink moderate amounts! The standard estimate is that about 9 percent of American women (1 in 11) will develop breast cancer. The reaction to the new studies was that women who drink have an additional 50 percent risk, or a 14 percent risk of developing cancer of the breast. The figures are misleading as the 9 percent estimate includes both women who drink and who do not.[40] The 50 percent extra risk was based on a comparison of drinkers and nondrinkers. The 9 percent figure is doubly misleading because it is based on women at birth. With the passage of time, however, the risk declines as there are fewer years in which breast cancer can develop. A woman has about a 3.3 percent chance of developing breast cancer between ages 40 and 60, whereas the risk to a moderate drinker is about 4.3 percent.[41] "Drinking might be responsible for about 1 to 2 percent of all breast cancer in the United States . . . the strongest 'effect' of alcohol is observed among women below the age of 50, an age at which few breast cancers appear. A proportionately large increase in a very small number is still a very small number."[42] Women with other risk factors (close relatives with breast cancer, early menstruation, advancing age, childlessness, first pregnancy after age 35, and obesity)—states of the world—might wish to take action such as reassessing their drinking patterns if they value the outcome of reducing the risk of breast cancer.

CONCLUSION

A six-step procedure for decision making is offered as a general guideline (this method is but one possibility among others that are similar): (1) uncover unstated, hidden, or suppressed premises that underly what appears to be the real problem; (2) gather information that is relevant, sufficient, and accurate; (3) move from data to inferences as the basis for generating possible conclusions; (4) test possible conclusions for their validity, soundness, and usefulness. True and relevant premises as the basis for true conclusions help to fulfill these conditions; (5) evaluate conclusions to determine what solutions among those tested are workable; and (6) base a decision both on careful evaluation of the previous steps and the frame of reference, including values, in which the decision will be implemented.

Thinking critically about decisions is to choose a course of action and to eliminate others. Freedom from attitudes of "all or nothing at all" or "black and white" thinking are helpful to openness. Options need organization in terms of their exclusivity and exhaustiveness, freedom from repetition and omission. Ranking the possible outcomes according to one's own scale of values is useful in making decisions that must also consider the state of the world and action options. This can be done with a matrix that multiplies action with a state of the world resulting in outcomes that are ranked according to the decision maker's values. Decision making with certainty occurs when the state of the world is definitely known. Conversely, when nothing is known about the world, decisions are made with uncertainty. Decision making with risk is based on the probabilities of each state's occurrence. An inductive form of scientific argument is never absolute truth, because the possibility of reaching a false conclusion from true premises is ever present. Moreover, some premises thought to be true may turn out to be false.

Actions and states of the world can be independent. Much of nursing practice, however, occurs in a context in which actions and states are not independent. A professional quality of nursing care, for example, usually evokes more nursing needs from a patient than was originally perceived by either nurse or patient.

Making a decision with complete uncertainty, as in the use of experimental drugs or in casual, spontaneous sex, is to make a decision based on the value matrix. Action and the state of the world are independent, and the outcome is completely unknown. The decision then must be made on the basis of the decision maker's values. Critical thinking about each phase and dimension of decision making is useful in arriving at decisions that are valid, sound, and useful and that reflect one's most cherished values.

REFERENCES

1. Giere, R.N. Understanding Scientific Reasoning (2nd ed.). New York: Holt, Rinehart and Winston, 1984, p. 332.
2. Ibid. p. 337.
3. Ibid.
4. Ibid.
5. Moore, W.E., McCann, H., & McCann, J. Creative and Critical Thinking (2nd ed.). Boston: Houghton Mifflin Company, 1985, pp. 6–10.

6. Moore, W.E., McCann, H., & McCann, J. Creative and Critical Thinking, p. 7.
7. Ibid.
8. Ibid, pp. 6–7.
9. Bandman, E.L., & Bandman, B. Nursing Ethics in the Life Span. Norwalk, Conn.: Appleton-Century-Crofts, 1985, p. 93.
10. Ibid, p. 86.
11. Mendelsohn, R. L., & Schwartz, L. M. Basic Logic. Englewood Cliffs, N.J.: Prentice-Hall, 1987, p. 223.
12. Moore, W.E., McCann, H., & McCann, J. Creative and Critical Thinking, p. 9.
13. Ibid, p. 10.
14. Ibid.
15. Ibid.
16. Ibid.
17. Ibid, p. 11.
18. Giere, R.N. Understanding Scientific Reasoning, p. 321.
19. Ibid, p. 325.
20. Ibid, p. 332.
21. Ibid, p. 331.
22. Ibid.
23. Ibid, p. 332.
24. Ibid, p. 337.
25. Ibid.
26. Ibid.
27. Ibid, p. 344.
28. Ibid, p. 345.
29. Ibid.
30. Ibid, p. 346
31. Ibid, p. 348.
32. Ibid, p. 349.
33. Ibid, p. 352.
34. Ibid.
35. Ibid, pp. 353–354.
36. *Harvard Medical School Health Letter* 1987; 12(9): July.
37. Giere, R. N. Understanding Scientific Reasoning, p. 360.
38. Ibid, p. 362.
39. *Harvard Medical School Health Letter* 1987; 12(9): July.
40. Ibid.
41. Ibid, p. 2.
42. Ibid.

Chapter 7

The Role of Critical Thinking in Resolving Controversial Issues

The aims of this chapter are to enable the learner to:

1. Apply principles of critical thinking to a rational consideration of controversial issues in nursing.
2. Develop skills of intellectual criticism that help clarify controversial issues in health care.
3. Discriminate between good and bad reasons on behalf of a controversial conclusion.
4. Recognize the scope and limits of rational debate over fundamental disagreements.

INTRODUCTION

There is no shortage of controversial issues in nursing. Should a nurse fail to call a code on an irreversibly comatose patient? Is abortion murder or a woman's prerogative? May Jehovah's Witness parents refuse a blood transfusion for their child? Does an individual have a right to refuse to be tube fed, if not being fed results in death? May a parent of a seriously defective newborn refuse life-saving surgery? May a health professional, including a nurse, kill a hopelessly ill patient in intractable pain? The list of controversies seems endless. There is, however a very short list of processes and procedures for rationally resolving controversies. We will try to show how the use of critical thinking helps to clarify and resolve issues. An important reason for the nurse to know how to help resolve controversial issues is that the nurse is an important moral agent at the patient's bedside. The nurse is often in a position to recognize and advocate on behalf of a patient's best health care needs.

Another reason for applying processes and procedures of critical thinking is to examine controversial ideas by appealing to rational standards. A related reason is to examine conflicts without resorting to the irrational and arbitrary use of physical or political power to settle controversies.

The nursing supervisor who tells staff nurses, "If you go on strike, you'll be fired," is committing an *either–or* fallacy. If the nursing supervisor and the staff nurses know and understand this, they can invoke the fallacy as a rational argument stopper of such a threat. Preferably, they both understand that threats have no place in the rational discussion of issues. The issues that lead to the strike call for discussion, examination, and mutually beneficial negotiation and resolution, not the unreasoning exercise of authority of one side over another.

A third reason for applying critical thinking to rationally resolve controversies is to be an effective advocate on behalf of vulnerable clients or nurses, who are treated irrationally.

A fourth reason for using critical thinking to help settle controversies is to achieve a form of standing conducive to rational respect within the health professions and in the public perception.

DEFINITION OF A CONTROVERSIAL ISSUE

A controversial issue is a contentious, contestable, debatable issue about which available evidence and reasoning may not provide an acceptable resolution. A controversial issue may result in a dilemma, which is an issue or problem neither of whose solutions is satisfactory; or a stalemate, which is an issue in which both sides are in a rational deadlock, or draw or tie. The sides to a controversial issue need not be rational. Each side considers the other unreasonable. A controversial issue arouses opposition; its premises and conclusion are debatable, disputable, and likely to generate a conflict.

A controversial issue is a conflict of principles and policies rather than a disagreement of particular practices. Two nurses may disagree about a patient's condition. But neither of these disagreements is necessarily controversial. What makes an issue controversial is that it is about principles or policies, such as abortion, euthanasia, and the just allocation of scarce health care resources. A nurse may refuse to participate in sex education, family planning for teenagers; and disagree with another person who finds that not participating in these activities to be morally objectionable. A nurse may believe in terminating the life of an irreversibly ill, suffering patient; and another person may disagree, arguing that life is a gift, no matter what quality.

One response to controversy is to shun, deny, avoid, or eliminate differences of position. Some people prefer peace at any price. But the cost of peace is sometimes too high. Some issues are worth fighting for, or preferably debating or arguing over, or negotiating about.

Another appraoch is that of Socratic questioning. To use this approach is to analyze and dissect the assumptions, evidence, and implications of each position, and consider the broad, underlying questions. The nursing issue of entry into practice, for example, is controversial. There are several possible positions to take with regard to the educational preparation of the practitioner: continuation of the current license, titles, roles and educational programs; change to a professional nurse title for the graduate of the baccalaureate degree program and an associate nurse title for the graduate of an associate degree program with changes in licensing, role, expectations and rewards; or change to a masters' degree level of basic preparation for the first professional degree, as do programs of social work, occupational and physical therapy.

The analysis, dissection, and questioning of the assumptions, reasons, evidence, and implications of each position stimulate and illuminate critical and creative thought processes in nursing education.

FIVE KINDS OF CONTROVERSIAL ISSUES IN NURSING

We may single out five kinds of controversial issues in nursing. The first of these issues concerns quantity versus quality of life. A parent asks a nurse to "pull the plug" on her 14-year-old boy who has been comatose for 8 months. The question at issue is: What shall the nurse rationally do? Nurses are in a position to influence questions concerning the quality of life versus the quantity of life. Families ask nurses whether suffering patients with tubes and needles in nearly every bodily orifice should be kept alive.

A second issue concerns freedom versus control and prevention of harm. One example of individual freedom versus control and prevention of harm is that of a frail, elderly patient who wishes not to have a locking waistbelt, but to walk about freely. This freedom is in conflict with the health care team's effort to prevent harm to this patient. Another example is forced feeding of a patient who refuses to eat on grounds of individual rights and freedom. The film "Whose Life Is It Anyway?" further illustrates the issue of freedom versus prevention of harm. Harrison, the paraplegic patient, argues for the right to die and the health professional argues for the conflicting principle of trying to prevent harm to him. A further example is a nurse's freedom to strike for better working conditions and quality care versus the hospital's efforts to prevent harm to patients.

A third issue that critical thinking illuminates is truth-telling versus deception or lying. Reasons for deception and lying are to get one's way, to avoid harm by withholding bad news, or to conceal an abuse pattern, such as alcoholism or narcotic addiction. A further dilemma occurs for a colleague who discovers the abuse, and has to decide whether to join in the concealment effort or "blow the whistle" by telling the truth. A third dilemma occurs if the substance abuser theatens to reveal something that is of a vital professional or personal interest to the would-be whistle blower. An implication of these dilemmas is this final dilemma of what to do about a health professional, who is a substance abuser and in a position to cause serious harm to patients. Another example of the issue of truth-telling versus deception is the proverbial "sink test" for certain urine specimens. Here a laboratory technician takes a specimen to be analyzed, and pours it down the sink and lies about the findings.

A fourth issue is the desire for knowledge in opposition to religious, political, economic, and ideological interests. Faith healing may be preferred over scientific medicine. Research is poorly rewarded by society as investigation often raises disturbing questions about the status quo. Research about cigarettes or a sugar substitute may provide evidence that conflicts with economic interests. Commercial and military interests in research are supported far more extensively than research related to health care or environmental safety. A recent example of knowledge versus opposing interests, religious in nature, is the decision of some states to teach Creationism in preference to traditional biological theories of evolution.

A fifth issue is that of conventional, scientifically based therapy versus alternative, nonscientific therapies. A classic case of nursing is that of a nurse who advocated Laetrile as an alternative to chemotherapy for treating a patient with cancer. Further examples of controversial nonscientific alternative therapies include faith healing and Christian science.

Nursing conflicts generally occur within these five kinds of issues. There are overlaps between these types of issues, and still other issues that may arise.

Exercises

(a) Identify the following examples as controversial by placing a "C" after them. (b) Classify these examples into one or more of five groups: (1) quantity versus quality of life; (2) freedom versus control and prevention of harm; (3) truth-telling versus deception; (4) knowledge versus other social, economic and religious issues; (5) scientific versus nonscientific therapies. (c) Cite the fallacy, if there is one.

1. Shall a nurse keep a 14-year-old boy alive who has been comatose for 8 months by calling the fourth code on this nurse's shift? *Answer:* C, quantity versus quality.
2. A nurse counsels a couple, both of whom are blind from retinoblastoma, "I can't recommend that you have children, since you're at high risk, more than 50 percent, for transmitting this disease to your offspring."

Answer: C, freedom versus control on behalf of prevention of harm.

3. A nurse decides to cheat on a competitor to get a good job.
   Answer: C, truth-telling versus lying.
4. Shall one spend resources on a mentally handicapped child to surgically repair his heart?
   Answer: C, quantity versus quality.
5. Does a pregnant woman have a right to an abortion?
   Answer: C, could be quantity versus quality, freedom versus control, or freedom versus prevention of harm issue.
6. Physician J.H. to Adolescent Nurse Practitioner, "We have to force-feed Dorothy, 14, who has anorexia, otherwise, she'll starve to death." Physician L.K., "But Dorothy specifically wants to die." Both physicians turn to Ms. Jones, a nurse, "What do you advise?"
   Answer: C, freedom versus control.
7. Ms. B. Jazelick, an antiabortion nurse, refuses to participate in abortions.
   Answer: C, quantity versus quality and freedom versus control.

HOW CAN CRITICAL THINKING HELP RESOLVE CONTROVERSIAL ISSUES?

How may the use of procedures, processes, and criteria of critical thinking help resolve controversial issues in nursing? Critical thinking can help resolve controversial issues by the application of formal, inductive, and informal criteria to evaluate arguments made in support of one side or the other of these issues.

With particular reference to the five nursing issues, one can clarify meanings of key terms, make relevant distinctions, expose fallacies, such as the either–or fallacy, appeal to force, abuse of the person, and false cause.

There is, for example, the New Hampshire license plate, which has the slogan, "Live free or die." This slogan commits the complex question of the either–or fallacy. In Monserrat, Spain, there is a sign of a bygone age, which holds that one is either a Christian or one doesn't exist. We can easily expose this either–or fallacy by pointing to non-Christians who exist. An example of the either–or fallacy in health care is this question to a patient, "Do you want to try this experimental drug and live, or not and die?" One can point to the patients who still live without the experimental drug and those who died taking it, to refute the necessity of doing the one or the other. The exposure of faulty logic is a function of critical thinking. Do away with fallacies and we undercut the opportunity to provide a rational demonstration of critical thinking. An example of critical thinking applied to a controversial issue is: If a nursing supervisor tells a staff nurse "You provide care to AIDS patients on this unit or you'll be fired." This supervisor is committing the either–or fallacy. Or, using an example of formal logic, argue that:

Major premise: All diabetics are sick. (True)
Minor premise: All homosexuals are sick. (False or debatable)
Conclusion: All homosexuals are diabetics. (False)

This is to argue fallaciously. This argument contains a controversial proposition, the minor premise. But whether the premises are true or false, the conslusion does not follow logically, because the middle term is undistributed. Moreover, the conclusion is false. Therefore, this is an unsound argument in addition to being invalid. (For further elaboration of formal arguments, see Chapters 8, 9, and 10.) Consider another example:

All RNs are nurses. (True)
All LPNs are nurses. (True or debatable)
∴ All LPNs are RNs.

Here again, the argument is invalid. The conclusion does not follow as the argument has an undistributed middle term. The argument is, in addition, unsound. Although each premise may be interpreted as true, the conclusion is false. Or let us consider this argument:

All assertive nurses are feminists.
All assertive nurses are critics of physicians.
∴ All critics of physicians are feminists.

This argument is invalid through the illicit minor fallacy. Both premises and the conclusion are false.

Exercises

(a) Identify the following examples as controversial by placing a "C" after them. (b) Identify them as informal, deductive, or inductive. (c) Cite the fallacy, if there is one.

1. Nurse L. takes drugs; Dr. W. finds out and Nurse L. tells Dr. W. "If you tell on me, I'll tell your wife which woman I often see you with."
   Answer: C, truth-telling versus lying (tu quouque fallacy).
2. Ms. Gree, LPN, to Nurse White, RN, "We should all get the same salary. After all, we're all nurses and do the same work."
   Answer: C, quantity versus quality. Variation on heap fallacy. The nurse believes that little differences are too small to make a difference. See Chapter 3 on Fallacies.

3. Nurse Lapotina used the new syringe on Mr. Torey, and it works better than the old syringe. Supervising Nurse Boschwitz, "How many times have you used it, and on how many other patients?" Ms. Lapotino, "This is the first time and Mr. Torey is the only patient."
Answer: Not C, inductive fallacy of hasty generalization.

4. Nurse Harman, "A law should be passed prohibiting the growing of tobacco." Nurse Freemon, "That would stifle free enterprise. It's not tobacco availability. The fault lies with people who decide to smoke."
Answer: C, freedom versus prevention of harm.

5. Nurse Peko, midwife, "We've had no newborn males in a week. Twenty-three births, all female last week. I bet the next birth is a male."
Answer: Not C, inductive, Monte Carlo fallacy.

6. Hospital administrator Enson to nursing director Pauley, RN, "This hospital should fire any nurse who refuses to work double shifts." Ms. Pauley, "But a double shift lowers the quality of nursing care." Hospital administrator, "We can't afford more nurses. Besides the nurses here need to know who's boss."
Answer: C, freedom versus control, informal fallacy of appeal to force.

CLARIFYING CONFLICTS: FACTUAL VERSUS VERBAL DISPUTES

A distinction between verbal and factual disputes may help resolve health care controversies. If two nurses, A and B, argue over whether a certain medication is appropriate for a particular patient, with a specific medical diagnosis, the specifications of that medication make that dispute a factual matter. If, however, two nurses, C and D, have a dispute as to whether a 34-year-old, curly haired single male patient is "cute," their dispute may well be verbal. Or if two nurses, E and F, argue about their patient's level of physical, mental, and emotional health, their dispute may be verbal, unless they resort to specific tools of assessment upon which to agree.

If two nurses disagree about the presence of observable blood in a patient's stool, careful observation and testing for the presence of blood can settle their disagreement. But if two nurses disagree about the meaning of *nursing act,* one insisting that it requires knowledge, cognitive skills, and appropriate values and attitudes, and the other that a nursing act requires hands-on-care, this is a verbal dispute. As such, it is not easily resolvable. We may clarify a concept by distinguishing several senses to which the concept applies, clarifying the points of difference. But there are still, what Gallie terms "essentially contested concepts," or intractable disputes, that remain, such as whether a fetus is an unborn person.[1] A result of a clarification of the meaning of terms is either a stalemate or some practical compromise.

A reason some verbal disputes in nursing are more resistant to resolution than others is that some nursing concepts are based on tacit or latent political, ideological, economic, and moral views or assumptions about human nature or social justice. If these disputes are made explicit, the verbal and factual assumptions embedded in them can be disentangled and discussed. In nursing, a systems theory approach is different from a more discrete view of nurse–patient relationships. A result of such clarification is to focus the argument.

Additional terms may be used in various ways in different nursing theories. These terms include *evidence, beliefs, knowledge, truth, necessity, scientific method, inquiry,* and *freedom.* One nurse may define evidence as sense data, whereas another identifies evidence as a public collection of relevant, verifiable data. Two nurses may disagree about abortion, as these definitions show.

- $Abortion_1$: The removal of a parasitic tissue from the uterine wall of a human female.
- $Abortion_2$: The murder of an innocent child for the selfish convenience of his or her mother.[2]

We cannot appeal to facts alone to resolve the abortion issue. Although nursing theories do not exhibit a similar type of divergence, they, too, cannot be rationally resolved as easily as straightforward factual disputes. Nevertheless, a function of critical thinking is to attempt to rationally resolve or dissolve verbal and factual disputes. One way is to make the meanings of disputed terms clearer. Another way of resolving disputes is to appeal to relevant evidence. Some issues, however, spill over into deep attitudinal and value disputes, such as the issue of assessing the meaning of sexual and racial differences. Serious psychological or ideological difficulties may stand in the way of clearly thinking through such differences.

BELIEF AND ATTITUDE DISAGREEMENTS

A further way to use critical thinking is to distinguish between two kinds of disagreements, disagreements in belief and disagreements in attitude. If two parties agree about an event, such as a cardiac patient lighting up a cigar, then they agree in belief. If two parties do not agree that a particular event occurred, then they disagree in belief. If, however, two pediatric nurse practitioners agree that Baby X, born with multiple congenital handicaps was not treated, but have strongly different attitudes about it, one nurse approving and the second disapproving, then they disagree in attitude.[3] The collective bargaining unit of the state nurses' association and the hospital management may agree in attitude that nurses should receive fair wages. But they may disagree in belief about what counts as a fair wage. A nurse and a cardiac patient may both agree in attitude about the value of healthy living, but disagree in belief about the effect of cigarettes on living healthfully. The nurse can use the nurse's and patient's agreement in attitude to help resolve the disagreement in belief. The nurse can also provide authoritative documentation regarding the destructive effects of smoking on health.

Another type of disagreement is that of two parties who disagree in attitude, but agree in belief. For example, Nurse Rogers and Nurse Delaney disagree about Ms. Wyman's being healthy. Rogers says "She's seriously sick," Delaney says, "She's pretty healthy, considering her age and diagnoses." Both nurses may agree, however, on what nursing plan works best for Ms. Wyman. Two nurses may disagree about abortion. Their agreement in belief may help resolve the disagreement in attitude. If Nurse A opposes abortion, but recognizes that uncontrolled growth in population implies a level of worldwide conflict and violence that is intolerable, her acquired factual belief about the consequences of uncontrolled population growth may lead her to change her attitude.

The most difficult disagreement to resolve rationally by using critical thinking seems to be a disagreement in attitude together with a disagreement in belief. If a nurse wants a chronically despondent patient to live, but he wishes to die, and if they disagree as to what will be helpful, then the nurse and the patient have a disagreement in attitude and a disagreement in belief. If there is both a disagreement in attitude and of belief, there may be a breakdown of reasoning. A patient, for example, will not take medication unless there is an interest in getting better; and unless the patient believes that what the nurse says about the medication is true.

If two people disagree in attitude about cigarette smoking in the workplace, one prohibiting it and the other permitting it, there may be no rational way to resolve this disagreement. However, if they agree in belief that cigarettes are causally linked to lung cancer and if they both agree on the value of life, then they may be in a position to use this agreement to resolve their disagreement about the desirability of smoking in the workplace.

Resolution of differences of attitude in problem situations can be facilitated if there is clarity on whether the basis of agreement and disagreement is related to the facts of the case, identified with belief, or to differences in attitude. If the disagreements concern belief, then the usual processes of data collection, inferences, and verification are appropriate. The evidence provides justification for deciding on what to believe. If, however, the source of the disagreement is in differences of attitudes, then issues of values, ethics, motives, and intentions are central. Concepts of *right, wrong, good,* and *bad* have strong emotional significance as moral judgments. Esthetic, political, or economic values may also play a role in shaping attitudes. Clarity concerning the kinds of disagreements and the ways language is used can help to resolve these arguments.

Exercises

Identify the type of disagreement in each pair of statements.

1. Nurse A: "Mr. Gram, in 308, is a troublemaker." Nurse B: "Mr. Gram is meticulous."
   Answer: Disagreement in attitude, because there is no factual belief they agree or disagree about.
2. "Nurse A has a mind of her own." "Nurse A is a nonconformist."
   Answer: Disagreement in attitude, because again there is no factual belief about which these speakers agree or disagree.
3. Nurse A: "Patient C is too sick to make it through the week." Nurse B: "Patient C is sick but has remarkable recovery powers."
   Answer: Disagreement in belief. Both nurses are not disagreeing about the desirability of this patient surviving.
4. "Nurse Doar generously worked overtime." "Nurse Doar only worked for the money."
   Answer: Disagreement in attitude, because there is no factual dispute about Nurse Doar working overtime.
5. "Nurse A almost saved her patient." "Nurse A didn't work hard enough to save her patient."
   Answer: Disagreement in attitude. Both speakers perceive Nurse A differently. The first is laudatory, whereas the second is derogatory.
6. "Mr. L had lots of blood in his stool." "Mr. L had very little blood in his stool."
   Answer: Disagreement in belief about the amount of blood in Mr. L's stool.
7. "Nurse A talked incessantly at the staff meeting." "Nurse A was stupidly silent."
   Answer: Disagreement in belief as to whether Nurse A talked or not. But there is no disagreement in attitude.
8. "Nurse Liz has a great imagination." "Nurse Liz lacks respect for data."
   Answer: Disagreement in belief that not all her statments are true. Also disagreement in attitude. A approves. B disapproves.
9. "This bottle is half full." "This bottle is half empty."
   Answer: Disagreement in attitude.
10. "Life is in front of that young 50-year-old man." "Life is over for that old 50-year-old man."
    Answer: Disagreement in attitude. There is no disagreement about the facts.

11. "Never mind having college-educated nurses. Nurses need to be at the bedside." "Today's complex health care needs require that nurses be optimally educated with at least a Master's degree. Never mind the patient's bedside."
Answer: Disagreement in attitude about the role of nursing.

SOME MEANINGS OF RESOLVABILITY

We may find it helpful to clarify the meaning of an issue being resolvable. At one time, some people thought the earth was flat. That was controversial. They were proved wrong. That issue was resolvable, but apparently not at that time. At one time, slavery was condoned, as were racism, sexism, elitism, and indecent treatment to working people and children. Using condoms was at one time unacceptable to certain groups. But in time, with education and rational persuasion, it became acceptable. The AIDS epidemic gave reasons for using condoms. Prostitution, still accepted in some cultures, is unacceptable in others. The issue whether to condone or oppose prostitution is controversial, and is currently regarded as unresolvable. But in time, we may show how this issue is rationally resolvable.

One method for resolving controversial issues has traditionally been the use of *argument* in the task or try sense. We present an argument. This may be followed by a counter-argument, and so on. Another method for resolving conflicts has been to compromise differences. If nurses want a higher salary and the hospital initially refuses, and if both sides agree to talk, they may come up with a compromise, one that partially satisfies one or both parties.

In talking, we negotiate; and in negotiating, the parties come to agree as to what is or is not negotiable. In negotiating, both parties confine themselves to negotiable items, which usually include salary and time. In the process of negotiating, both parties present arguments, which consist of claims or conclusions and reasons. One party or the other appeals to some reasons to come to an agreement.

Although both sides disagree, they agree to the principle that agreements are desirable, that rational methods of arriving at agreements are also desirable. Such methods include the principle that coercion without rational persuasion by either side is undesirable.

LOGICALLY AND TEMPORALLY UNRESOLVABLE ARGUMENTS

We may distinguish between logically unresolvable issues and temporally unresolvable ones. Most, if not all controversial issues, where we can find agreement, are logically, if not temporally, resolvable. The claim that there are logically unresolvable arguments is premature.

There are several pitfalls to avoid. One is begging the question, or arguing in a circle. This is done if we define a rational argument as one that is resolvable. A second pitfall rests with the qualifier *rationally.* One or both parties to a dispute may use irrational arguments. If they do, that does not make an argument rationally unresolvable. For those who use irrational arguments may be falling into one or more fallacies, such as slothful induction, the refusal to consider any alternative. To argue irrationally is the fault of the arguers, not the fault of an argument.

VALUE ARGUMENTS

Despite clarifications of meanings, distinctions, analogies, and arguments expressed on either side, some issues are said to resist rational resolution, such as whether abortion is murder or a woman's right. These are sometimes referred to as "deep disagreements."[4] According to one view, there is no way the parties can rationally agree. Whether deep disagreements are resolvable is itself a controversy.[5] There are arguments, however, showing that some value arguments break down.

In a valid, deductive argument, the conclusion is certain. In an inductive argument, the conclusion is likely or probable. In a value inference, the values one person or group of persons favors may collide with the values held by another person or group. In such an event, there may be a moral stalemate. This is illustrated in the value of conserving all life in collision with the Jehovah's Witness's right to refuse a life-saving blood transfusion.

In addition to moral stalemates, there are unresolvable moral dilemmas, some of which result in human tragedy. One illustration is the scarcity of health care resources. Thousands of eligible patients apply for the artificial heart to save their lives. Only a few persons, such as Barney Clark, were chosen to receive it, because only a few artificial hearts are available. This is the quantity versus quality issue. This example shows that in applying critical reasoning to ethics, even if we could overcome stalemates, there is a feature that is not always rationally resolvable, namely tragedy.

CAN A WAY OF LIFE BE JUDGED RIGHT OR WRONG?

The five health care issues presented are controversial. People debate about abortion, forced feeding, truth telling, value of knowledge, and scientific versus nonscientific medicine. One argument is that these issues stem from differences in ways of life and that there is no sense in disputing ways of life. According to one claim, we cannot argue with a Muslim, a segregationist, a Jehovah's Witness, an Amish, a Nazi, a Buddhist, a fundamentalist, a snake worshipper, a head hunter, a faith healer, a creationist, an evolutionist, a sexist, an antisexist, or a proponent or opponent of homosexuality or suicide. Each goes his or her way, and there is no rational way to reconcile differences or change the other's outlook. Fundamental commitments remain unchangeable, according to this view.

But there is a way out of this impasse between the claim that all controversies are rationally resolvable and that none are; namely that some controversies are rationally resolvable. To begin with, a way of life, like anything else, is made up of parts. If we find that crucial parts of a way of life are irrational or clearly wrong and filled with fallacious reasoning, then we can judge at least those parts of a way of life to be defective. We can also judge a way of life by finding characteristics that make it rationally defensible and worthwhile. We can generate arguments showing that one part of a way of life is better than another. Then someone else will produce an argument countering a previous argument.[6] But there will be ways to judge who has the better argument. How?

PRACTICAL REASONING IN DECIDING CONTROVERSIAL ISSUES

One way to justify a decision to believe or to act is to construct a practical argument. We can build our own practical arguments, as well as evaluate other people's arguments. To that end, Aristotle's practical syllogism is useful. If, for example, patients should be helped not to smoke and Mr. L is a patient, then Mr. L should be encouraged not to smoke. This conclusion is based on a practical syllogism, which states: All patients should not smoke. Mr. L is a patient. So, Mr. L should not smoke. Or patients with lobar pneumococcus pneumonia ought to be given appropriate antibiotics. Mrs. R has this infection. So, Mrs. R ought to be given appropriate antibiotics.

We use the general statement of ends along with a statement of means to an end to imply a practical conclusion. A nurse applies means–ends reasoning to a controversial issue with this example: Abortion is a procedure that is morally impermissible. Nurse Jones is assisting in an abortion. Therefore, Nurse Jones is assisting in a procedure that is morally impermissible.

UMBRELLA STATEMENTS

One method for rationally resolving a controversy is to take some statement about which disputants agree and use it to settle their disagreement.

We identify the statement about which the disputants agree as an *umbrella statement.*

We use the umbrella statement to justify a particular conclusion. Applied to the five controversial nursing issues, we cite an umbrella statement to which both sides of a dispute agree. These may include:

1. The quality of life is more important than the quantity of life.
2. Individual freedom is better than prevention of harm.
3. Truth telling is better than deception.
4. Knowledge is better than ignorance.
5. Science is better than nonscientific alternatives.

Or we may take the opposite views. We then house intermediate means–ends statements under the umbrella statement, and then draw a conclusion as follows:

1. Modern health care contributes to a life with quality. Therefore, support modern health care.
2. Freedom in health care means a patient consents to or refuses various therapies. Therefore, support the freedom to choose.
3. Telling what Jenkins actually did in taking drugs promotes truth telling. Therefore, tell what Jenkins did.
4. Modern medicine applies science to health care problems. Therefore, use modern medicine.

Agreement on the umbrella statement and the means–ends statement implies agreement with the conclusion. If, two disputants agree with an umbrella statement, but disagree about a means–ends statement, then the burden is on both disputants to show that their means–ends statement is consistent with the umbrella statement. Two nurses in a dispute may, however, agree that preventing harm is more important than a patient's individual freedom. They may also agree that a locking waistbelt protects a patient, but diminishes the patient's freedom. Therefore, they are justified in using a locking waistbelt on a patient.

> Preventing harm is more important than the patient's individual freedom.
> Using a locking waistbelt prevents harm to patients who may fall without it.
>
> ∴ Using a locking waistbelt is more helpful in preventing harm than letting the patient go without it.

If individual life is more important than death, and if saving a spina bifida infant gives it life, then one tries to save the infant's life. But if both sides agree that a quality of life is to serve as an umbrella value, then they use it as a criterion to help resolve the controversy about saving a particular baby's life. The argument would look like this:

Umbrella statement:	Do not save infants who show evidence of having a poor quality of life.
Intermediate statement:	Infants with spina bifida show evidence of a poor quality of life.
Conclusion:	Do not save infants with spina bifida.

If saving a life is all important, and a Jehovah's Witness refuses a life-saving blood transfusion, then we use the umbrella statement to decide to give the Jehovah's Witness patient a blood transfusion. It all depends on agreement with an umbrella statement. Some health care disputes are intractable; the disputants are impervious to rational dispute settling. They cannot agree on an umbrella statement. Their mutual interests are served if they can find one.

We begin with certain U (Umbrella) statements, which are generally accepted on rational grounds, such as the U statement that treating people decently is better than treating people indecently. We place the umbrella statement together with the intermediate statement, and generate a conclusion, as the example below demonstrates:

Umbrella statement:	Organizations and ideas that advocate treating people decently are good.
Intermediate statement:	Feminism advocates treating people decently.
Conclusion:	Feminism is good.

Exercises

Identify the umbrella statement or rephrase the statement into an umbrella statement. Tell whether the controversy is resolvable or not. Using critical thinking procedures, try to show how it is resolvable.

1. Nurse Adler: "I refuse to take care of AIDS patients. It's their own fault. And my life is more valuable to me than theirs." Nurse Sanches: "We're all God's children, and we must take risks to help the sick and weak among us. That's what nursing is about."
   Answer: U_1, each person's life is more important to that person than any other person's. Too difficult to resolve without intermediate statements that show more reasons and evidence toward tipping the moral scale, assuming it can be tipped.
2. Nurse Solares: "I told Katy B., 14, that she should use condoms to avoid pregnancy. But we have to get her out of this mess. Her mother will crucify her if she comes home with a baby." Nurse Styles: "But Katy loves children, even though she's one herself. Let her have her child. It's God's will. We'll be punished if we commit murder."

Answer: Although the word *abortion* is not used, the controversial issue between them is whether abortion is morally permissible. Nurse Solares's U statement is "Abortion is morally permissible" and Nurse Styles's U statement is "Abortion is morally impermissible." Not easily resolvable.

3. Nurse Blue: "I tried to tell Stokes to stop smoking. He looks awful with a lung missing. But I feel sorry for him." Nurse Green: "Let him kill himself. He's just a freeloader, anyway."
   Answer: U_1 "One should care for everyone, even for smokers." U_2, "Each person is responsible for his or her own life-style, including indolent smokers." Too difficult to resolve without more data to strengthen the intermediate statement.

A LINK ARGUMENT: THE FIVE ISSUES CONNECTED

We will try to show that these five controversial nursing issues (quantity versus quality, freedom versus prevention of harm, truth-telling versus deception, knowledge versus other interests, conventional versus nonconventional therapy) are partially resolvable on rational grounds. One argument is: These issues are linked together, and they imply fundamentally important common values. A position on one side of the truth telling versus the deception issue affects the knowledge versus the competing values issue. A position favoring or opposing knowledge, in turn, affects our view regarding conventional, scientifically based therapies versus alternative nonscientific therapies. Our position on scientific medicine affects our position on the quantity versus quality debate. Our position on the quantity versus quality debate, in turn, affects the value we place on freedom. The values of truth, knowledge, science, quality of life, and freedom radiate in many directions. Valuing truth implies a preference for knowledge; and knowledge, in turn, implies a preference for scientifically based therapy. If truth, knowledge, and scientifically based therapy have value, these, in turn, point to the value of quality in human life.

Regard for truth, knowledge, science, and quality of human life, in turn, implies the value of freedom, the freedom to think. The freedom to think leads us to decide what to accept as true or false independently of any coercive efforts. But what if someone denies the value of truth, knowledge, science, quality of life, or freedom? One kind of opponent of truth is a Relativist, who claims that there is no rational basis for preferring one value over any other; and that there are no truths.

If a Relativist argues that no values are better than any others, there is a counter-argument, that the Relativist's values are no better than anyone else's either, in which case the Relativist cannot prove that this position is better than the non-Relativist's position. Moreover, there are, at least, some values that are clearly better than others. Or, if one argues that there are no true statements, then all statements are false, or neither true nor false. But then the statement that "All statements are false, or neither true nor false," is also false, or neither true nor false. This application of the *Reductio ad absurdum* argument logically contradicts the Relativist's argument. At least, some statements have to be true, otherwise *true* has no meaning, and is also of no use. Also, to place a value on statements means some statements have more value than others. To value any statements is to assess some statements as having more value than others.

A FURTHER USE OF A CHAIN ARGUMENT: FEMINISM

We can use a Chain-linked argument or further amplification as follows: Nursing is largely a woman's profession: and one which is deservedly in need of substantial social, political, and economic upgrading. Feminism advocates social, political, and economic benefits for women's professions. Women's professions include nursing. Therefore, feminism advocates social, political, and economic benefits for nursing.

We can continue building the Chain. (In technical terms, a *sorite* is a chain argument with more than two premises.) We make this value assumption: Feminism advocates principles and practices that socially, politically, and economically benefit women's professions and society at large. Feminist advocacy of the baccalaureate degree as a professional entry requirement benefits women's professions. Women's professions include nursing. Therefore, feminist advocacy of the baccalaureate degree as an entry requirement benefits the nursing profession. Therefore, it clearly benefits nurses to prefer entry into the profession with, at least, a baccalaureate degree. For this argument, feminist advocacy provides the umbrella principle; and with a description of nursing, the umbrella statement together with the intermediate, means–ends statements, implies the conclusion for nursing, consistent with the principles of feminism.

But if one rejects feminism, then one rejects the chain leading to the conclusion that advocates the upgrading of nursing. As some sexists have said, "The nurse belongs at the patient's bedside at the behest of the physician, hopping at his or her every command."

However, what if people disagree about umbrella statements, such as "Treat all people decently"? A sexist might argue that only men are real people. Or an elitist might argue that only certain types of people deserve to be treated decently. At any rate, a conflict between umbrella-type statements results in a deadlock. One strategy is for both sides to work to find umbrella statements of greater generality on which both sides can agree, and then determine which intermediate statement of values is more conducive, compatible, or consistent with achieving the newly agreed upon umbrella statement.

Is the issue between feminism and sexism resolvable in the long run? It probably is, if one recognizes the moral and rational preferability of feminism over sexism.

WHAT MAKES A WAY OF LIFE WORTHWHILE?

A way of life that denies the importance of truth, knowledge, freedom, quality of human life, and science is irrational at crucial points; and is not in accord with the precepts of critical thinking. Such a view does not make a life as worthwhile as one that accepts these values.

The resolvability of controversial issues does not eliminate difficult issues, deadlocks, or dilemmas. Moreover, some issues, such as freedom versus control, or freedom versus prevention of harm, call for clarification as a preliminary condition for resolving conflicts.

Moreover, freedom and control need not necessarily be antagonistic. Freedom is sometimes closely correlated with control. Freedom may also overlap with prevention of harm. John Dewey is cited by Nagel as saying: "All intelligent thinking means an increment of freedom of action, an emancipation from chance and fatality."[7] Quantity and quality are not always antithetical either. The quality of life in a community may be enhanced by having an increased population.

What makes a way of life humanly worthwhile is the ability and opportunity to reason about all things, including the final ends of life. The ends may collide. Humans who prefer civilization to chaos, however, make assumptions that even the deepest controversies are rationally resolvable, at least in part. Civilized human beings also assume that those who disagree agree not to kill each other over deep differences. They agree, furthermore, to use reason to settle their differences. One form of reasoning is to have a short list of values that they and their proponents hold in common. One of those values is the commitment to use rational means to persuade those who disagree.

But when that short list of fundamentally important values is threatened, as it is with some forms of evil, such as Nazism, apartheid, slavery, racism, sexism, and arbitrary tyranny of any kind, we can no longer harken to the ordinary forms of dialogue and uses of argument. We then recognize the breakdown of argument and rationality and prepare "to fight in the hills" against those who would exterminate what is of value in human life.

BASIC ASSUMPTIONS IN DEALING RATIONALLY WITH HEALTH CARE CONTROVERSIES

Freedom is one assumption basic to the values for which we argue. With freedom, we can describe events, make judgments, or take actions on the basis of discriminating among options. If a nurse is not free to make decisions as an autonomous professional, he or she cannot exercise independent judgments that are designed to show appropriate care for patients. In a decisive argument, Noam Chomsky refuted B. F. Skinner's contention that human beings are not free.[8] Chomsky argued that even to choose between the values of true and false, or any two values, p and not p, or p and q, requires the freedom to think.

Freedom is important to critical thinking in nursing. We can build a chain argument and explicate the case for freedom as a basic value. To engage in critical thinking in nursing makes the fundamental assumption:

1. The freedom to think and to express ideas is a highly important value in this society.
2. The freedom to think in nursing implies the freedom to inquire, no matter where the inquiry leads. C. Peirce's maxim aptly applies to critical thinking, "Do not block the way of inquiry."[9]
3. The freedom to inquire implies the freedom to make or draw inferences, analogies, guesses, conjectures, speculations, hypotheses, and metaphors that lead to truth and knowledge.
4. The freedom to make inferences implies the freedom to investigate, check, inspect, examine, verify, confirm, test, and attempt to justify one's inferences.
5. The freedom to attempt the justification of one's inferences implies the freedom to try to form sound, reasonable, rational, warranted, justifiable, and credible judgments.

A result of engaging in these conditions is for nurses to adopt methodological guidelines that imply credible health care conclusions, including those that involve controversial issues in nursing.

I. Scheffler makes a similar point regarding the concept of teaching. To teach, according to Scheffler, unlike some other ways of forming beliefs, rules out brainwashing. The student's freedom to think includes "the student's right to ask for reasons" and the student's "right to exercise independent judgment on the merits of the case."[10] A nurse can only make independent and worthwhile judgments if a nurse has the freedom to think and to inquire on the merits of the case before her.

SOME PROCEDURES FOR RATIONALLY RESOLVING CONTROVERSIAL ISSUES IN NURSING: APPEAL TO THE PARADIGM CASE ARGUMENT

A study of selected aspects of critical thinking provides rational procedures for helping to resolve some conflicts. An important basis of appeal for rationally settling controversial issues in nursing is to consider a standard example of a commonly accepted set of values. Such values will not, as matters stand, be accepted by everyone. Moreover, there are people for whom irrationality serves a purpose, however self-defeating.

What are commonly accepted human values? J. Rawls refers to these as "primary goods." Rawls identifies primary goods as those anyone wants "whatever else a person wants."[11] One example is health. Whatever else a person wants, she or he wants health. Because we cannot always have health, we want a related value, namely health care. A list of commonly accepted values, CAVs, will be short, but it will include adequate income, literacy, opportunity, freedom, life, protection from harm, security, love, human companionship, trust, devotion, sexual fulfillment, and appropriate forms of physical, social, and emotional well-being.

We think a list of CAVs will include the means to human happiness, including health care with decency, dignity, and respect, and relevant forms of human fulfillment, such as artistic and aesthetic enjoyment. These commonly accepted values, in turn, imply other values, such as autonomy, truth telling, knowledge, and regard for a high quality of human life. These expanded values, in turn, help us decide controversies that occur in everyday nursing practice.

We appeal to commonly accepted values to help resolve controversies, analogous to the way we appeal to an umpire or referee to decide the score in a sports event. We also appeal to a dominant example of commonly accepted values, their linchpin, without which they would topple down.

There are two pitfalls to avoid. If there is a role for critical thinking in helping to resolve controversial issues, we want to avoid absolute and inflexible values, about which there is no debate, no discussion, no change. According to this view, values are fixed forever. An opposite pitfall is the appeal to subjective relativism, where no value is better than any other. There is no rationality. All opinions are equally good.

There is a passageway between these unacceptable alternatives of absolute objectivity and relativistic subjectivity in rationally settling controversial issues in nursing. A promising lead consists in appealing to standard examples or paradigms of commonly accepted values. A paradigm is a touchstone, a model, an outstanding example of some principle. A paradigm is also used in critical thinking to refute counter-arguments.

In the case before us, a paradigm is an example of one or more of our commonly accepted values, one that appeals to rational values, whatever else that person accepts. Paradigms or standard examples are partway between subjectivity and objectivity. In metaphysics, F. H. Bradley, a philosopher of this century, once argued that "Time . . . has most evidently proved not to be real."[12] Another philosopher, G. E. Moore, then offered this refuting paradigm with the example, "I had breakfast before lunch."[13]

In ethics, Moore offered a classic refutation of Mill's argument that whatever is desired is, therefore, desirable. To refute Mill's argument, Moore cited examples of bad desires.[14]

A nursing example of how the paradigm case argument works in settling controversial issues in nursing is the view held that patients and nurses have no rights. To refute this, appeal is made to standard examples that show now important rights in health care function for both patients and nurses. The exposure of the Tuskeegee experiment showed decisively that if there are any justified values at all, they include the human rights of patients, subjects, and health professionals to informed consent.[15] Citing the Tuskeegee experiment provides a paradigm, a standard example that refutes the contention that patients, subjects, and nurses have no rights to informed consent.

A second standard example or paradigm case argument on behalf of human rights consists in the account of Nazi medical experiments. The unfolding of these horrors in health care emphasizes the appeal to commonly held values designed to prevent the reoccurrence of such evils. A standard example or paradigm of such values is found in *The Universal Declaration of Human Rights, 1948,* and a standard example of the right to informed consent of subjects and patients is found in *The Declaration of Helsinki, 1975.*

A third illustrative paradigm case argument for human rights and women's rights, in particular, is the Supreme Court 1973 decision in the case of Roe vs. Wade, which states that first trimester abortion is a private decision made by an affected woman. An earlier argument is by J. J. Thomson, *In Defense of Abortion,* showing that for anyone to have any rights at all is to have rights in and to one's body.

In nursing, H. Peplau and C. Fagin refuted the idea that patients and nurses have no rights by arguing that nurses have a right to refuse to assist in administering electroconvulsive therapy.[16]

Another refuting paradigm in nursing is the argument against the "Captain of the ship" doctrine that the physician always knows best. In D. K. Darling versus Charleston Community Memorial Hospital, physicians were held responsible for neglecting Kenneth Darling.[17] One nurse was also charged with neglecting to report her observations, which, according to the court, could have saved Darling's leg. After 14 days in a poorly prepared cast, Darling's leg turned gangrenous and was amputated. The Darling case was a paradigm illustrating that nurses are also responsible. With responsibility, training, and ability come decision-making rights. As a result of this case in 1965, rights and responsibilities legally apply to nurses, both to exercise rights and responsible judgment.

The appeal to human rights encompasses such values as decency, dignity, respect, an attitude of "live and let live," and an environment for helping resolve conflicts rationally. One fundamentally important basis for helping to resolve controversial issues in nursing is to appeal to human rights, to patients' bills of rights, and to rights provisions in the *Nurses' Code.* Generally, rights defenders point to five conditions for having a useful set of rights. These are: (1) freedom to do as one wishes, with appropriate constraints against harming others; (2) correlative duties against other relevant persons, parties, corporations, and states; (3) appeal to rationally defensible principles of justice; (4) enforceability; (5) compensation if one's rights cannot be enforced.[18]

Rights defenders point to several kinds of rights: (1) civil and political liberty rights, such as the right to physical security, the right to equal political participation; (2) rights to be cared for socially and economically, such as rights to food, clothing, shelter, health care, and education; and (3) the right to try to develop and flourish throughout one's life. Respect for liberty rights and rights to be cared for helps orient our judgments of complex cases that arise with the five controversial issues. The appeal to human rights implies that rights are steadfast, not absolute, but not mere negotiable interests either. Rights provide appeal to entrenched values, not easily discarded.

FIRST-ORDER AND SECOND-ORDER CHANGE: APPEAL TO HUMAN RIGHTS AS A SECOND-ORDER CHANGE

Adapting P. Watzlawick's distinction between first- and second-order change, [19] we may regard a position taken within a controversial issue as a proposed first-order argument, either favoring or opposing one side of an issue. The appeal to human rights to settle such an issue may be regarded as a second-order argument. We appeal to the second-order argument to settle the first.

In the case of abortion, however, we may agree to appeal to rights, such as a woman's right in and to her body; but then an argument opposing abortion may appeal to the right of a fetus to be born. At this point the controversy gets waged as to who has, or can have, rights. We may then have what W. B. Gallie calls "an essentially contestable concept."[20] That route may lead us to a stalemate. There is another route, however. In a stalemate or toss up, who has the stronger case for a more entrenched, deeper level right, a pregnant woman or a fetus?

One effort to make the case for a fetus is to call it an "unborn child," a fairly obvious effort at a persuasive definition. Does it work? Its use is a tip-off that the case for including a fetus in the category of persons is weaker than the case for including an actual child. Moreover, on linguistic grounds, rights belong primarily to those who can protect their own interests. On these grounds, a woman has a stronger, linguistic basis for asserting a right than does a fetus.

TASK AND ACHIEVEMENT SENSES OF CRITICAL THINKING APPLIED TOWARD RESOLVING CONTROVERSIAL ISSUES

We may apply the task or try sense of rationally resolving a controversial issue to those controversies before us. Who defends slavery today? Who rationally even defends segregation by race or sex? As the evolution/creationist controversy shows, it is not true that the abortion debate is a tie. The weight of argument tilts more and more heavily in the direction of a woman's right to an abortion. All values, whether liberal, radical, or conservative, are not always equal. On some issues, one side or the other emerges as the winner. But it is somewhat like the process that occurs in a sports contest, the winners and losers are not immediately evident.

There is no formula for gaining immediate successes when using critical thinking to resolve controversial conflicts. The methods presented and illustrated help; but critical thinking cannot guarantee absolute results. Critical thinking does not provide a priori assurances. Critical thinking is a process with procedures that are for the most part inductive and empirical.

An upshot of studying the role of critical thinking in controversies and in rational conflict resolution is to recognize a predicament. We cannot escape the *try* or *task* sense of critical thinking, analogous to developing "habits of workmanship" in the sciences. In these models, the parties submit their disputes to impartial criteria, procedures, and rules for testing the suggestions made on the feeling and vision levels. Still, we cannot be sure that mistrials will not occur. We have no choice but to try to apply critical thinking to rational conflict resolution.

THREE MODELS ORIENT CRITICAL THINKING IN RESOLVING CONTROVERSIAL ISSUES

Three models help orient the role of critical thinking in the process of rationally resolving controversies. These are influenced by I. Scheffler's philosophical models of teaching.[21] These are feelings, impressions, and data. In health care, appeal to *feelings* calls for attention to signs, symptoms, and clues, such as skin pallor, pulse, weight changes, body sounds and smells, and attention to patient's expressed feelings. There is no health care or nursing without attention to patients' feelings, such as pain, discomfort, relief, and joy in recovering.

A second model with which to interpret feelings and a patient's data is to consider hypotheses, vision, insights, ideas, and inferences. This may be called the *vision model.* An example of a visionary idea governing social and political institutions is *The Declaration of Independence.* Another is the *Universal Declaration of Human Rights,* and its application to patients' rights. Appeal to rights as due process values helps resolve health care controversies.

Feelings and ideas, however, are not a sufficient basis for forming sound and wise judgments in health care without checking, corroborating, testing the feelings and ideas of the earlier models; therefore, there is a third model. We act reasonably on an idea, insight, or vision by reflecting on it with the help of relevant criteria. We may call this the *examination model,* the search for appropriate rules of inference, along with rational principles of investigation, testing, inspecting, verification, confirmation, corroboration, and justification. One basis for this model is Socrates' statement that "an unexamined life is not worth living." So, too, an unjustified feeling, datum, idea, act, belief, or decision is not worth having. The idea that one can use rights to justify a health care decision or action, or appeal to rights to resolve health care conflicts, calls for appropriate justifying arguments. In some instances, appeal to rights passes the examination model, in others it does not.

CONCLUSION

Critical thinking in both the narrow and broad sense helps rationally to resolve health care controversies. In the narrow sense, we appeal to relevant rules of inference or to the relevant fallacies as tie breakers to resolve disagreements, conflicts, and dilemmas. In the broad sense of critical thinking, we appeal to more informal rules or criteria of argument. These include (1) the testing of analogies and metaphors, (2) *reductio ad absurdum,* (3) the process of elimination, (4) the exposure of fallacies and category mistakes, (5) the use of "inference tickets" or inference warrants, (6) the paradigm case argument or the appeal to standard examples, and (7) the use of umbrella statements as rational tie breakers in otherwise intractable disputes.

Cogent arguments are a rational basis for justifying our verdicts, decisions, and actions. Such health care judgments are designed rationally to resolve health care conflicts. The judgment that antibiotics and the germ theory are acceptable, for example, refutes belief in the Navajo medicine man. The appeal to scientific standards of reasoning refutes the claims of Laetrile and various kinds of faith healing. All five steps involved in the freedom to reason complement the medical reasoning process, the nursing process, and scientific problem solving.

In these steps toward conflict resolution, we may move inferentially from step 1, the freedom to think to step 2, the freedom to inquire, to step 3, the freedom to draw inferences, to step 4, the freedom to try to justify one's inferences, and to step 5, the freedom to try to form credible and justifiable judgments. Such judgments are the grounds for nursing decisions and actions. The credible and justified judgments in step 5 are the major premises of arguments, the umbrella statements. These provide the principles or mainsprings of action, tie breakers, due process dispute settlers. The principles in steps 1 through 5 constitute justifying values designed to help resolve controversial issues.

The role of critical thinking in resolving health care conflicts means that we move from the freedom to think and to express ideas and feelings, to an enriched freedom, freedom with reasoned restraints, such as the formal, inductive, and informal rules of inference. Critical thinking applied to conflict resolution, in effect, says, "If you want to get this right and reason correctly, follow such and such procedures, techniques, and rules." A role for critical thinking is to help resolve health care conflicts. The attempt to resolve health care conflicts consists in rationally examining contestable health care concepts, policies, and practices. The attempt to resolve controversies is an ongoing process.

But even when all the strategies of critical thinking are cited, there are still difficult questions that go unanswered, such as the questions of which patient to treat first, or what a health professional might tell a patient facing a mastectomy. We often do not know what to do or say to a patient. Nor do we know how to resolve a health care conflict between the dying patient's wishes, close family members, and various health professionals. We would really like to know, but we sometimes really do not know, whether a patient in a locking waistbelt needs it all the time or whether a breast cancer patient really needs a mastectomy instead of radiation or chemotherapy. We seek conceptual and practical methods to get access to the inner dynamics that are the causes of conflicts. Perhaps, as an ancient Greek philosopher said, "we know nothing . . . For the truth is hidden in the deep;" or as a contemporary of his said, "everything is but a woven web of guesses."[22] So, too, with some intractable value controversies, we may not be able to resolve them.

All is not lost. If we are puzzled, we may be guided by Wittgenstein's remark that "an inner process is in need of outer criteria."[23] A map, as an *outer criterion,* helps a traveler to find the way. A conflict has an inner process of causes and effects, and the role of formal, inductive, and informal, outer criteria of logic is to assess these inner processes. The *outer criteria,* as with a detective, diagnostician, scientist, or nurse, help orient an investigator to understand and evaluate an inner process. The inner process may include the factors that account for a controversy.

Against this often unknown inner process, we can use critical thinking in the task sense to try to resolve controversies. This critical thinking process consists in assessing the data that surrounds disputes, examining assumptions, generating and testing inferences, and in forming and continuously revising our judgments of what we may reasonably regard as credible and justifiable. Deep and nearly intractable controversies are resolvable through the steady development of insights and inferences, in the hope and assumption that we can, by degrees, penetrate "the woven web of guesses."

There are some guidelines for the use of critical thinking in the rational resolution of health care controversies. One is the continuing use off inference through controlled inquiry, leading to better and better founded nursing decisions. A result of the process of controlled inquiry is that justifiable arguments form the basis for justifiably resolving health care conflicts. Critical thinking is not only critical; it is also creative, and may help to resolve controversial issues in nursing, step by step, rather than all at once. Critical thinking helps generate ideas, inferences, and arguments to deal rationally with health care controversies.

REFERENCES

1. Gallie, W. B. Philosophy and the Historical Understanding (2nd ed.). New York: Schocken Books, 1968, p. 157.
2. Fogelin, R. The Logic of Deep Disagreements. *Informal Logic* 1985; VII(1): 1–8, Winter.
3. Copi, I. Introduction to Logic (7th ed.). New York: Macmillan, 1986, pp. 78–82.
4. Fogelin, R. The Logic of Deep Disagreements, pp. 5–7.
5. Lugg, A. Deep Disagreement, and Informal Logic: No Cause For Alarm. *Informal Logic* 1986; VIII(1): 47–53, Winter.
6. Ibid, pp. 47–52.
7. Nagel, E. (Ed.), Sovereign Reason. Glencoe, Ill.: Free Press, 1954, p. 140.
8. Machan, T. The Pseudo Science of B. F. Skinner. New Rochelle: Arlington House Publishers, 1974.
9. Hartshorne, C., & Weiss, P. (Eds.). Collected Papers of C. S. Peirce. Cambridge, Mass.: Belknap Press of Harvard University Press, 1960, p. 56.
10. Scheffler, I. Reason and Teaching. Indianapolis: Bobbs Merrill, 1973, p 62.
11. Rawls, J. A Theory of Justice. Cambridge: Harvard University Press, 1971, pp. 90–95.
12. Bradley, F. H. Appearance and Reality (2nd ed.). Oxford: At The Clarendon Press, 1897, pp. 31–36.
13. Moore, G. E. In Defense of Common Sense, in Philosophical Papers. London: George Allen & Unwin, 1954, pp. 32–59.
14. Moore, G. E. The Concept of Reality, in Philosophical Studies. London: Routledge & Kegan Paul, 1922, pp. 207–219.
15. Final Report of the Tuskeegee Syphilis Study Ad Hoc Advisory Panel. *Report.* Washington, D.C.: U.S. Public Health Service, 1973, pp. 5–15.
16. Fagin, C. Nurses' Rights. *American Journal of Nursing* 1975; 75(1):82.
17. Charleston Community Memorial Hospital v. Dorrence K. Darling. 33, Ill. 326, 211 NE, 2nd 253, 1965.
18. Becker, L. Individual Rights, in Regan, T., Van de Veer, D. (Eds.), And Justice For All. Totowa, N.J.: Roman & Littlefield, 1982, p. 203.
19. Watzlawick, P. The Language of Change. New York: Basic Books, 1978, p. 119.
20. Gallie, W.B. Philosophy and the Historical Understanding (2nd ed.). New York: Schocken Books, 1968, pp. 157–191.
21. Scheffler, I. Philosophical Models of Teaching, in Scheffler, I. (Ed.), Reason and Teaching, pp. 67–81.
22. Popper, K. Back to the Pre-Socratics. *Proceedings of the Aristotelian Society* 1958–59; 59:1–24.
23. Wittgenstein, L. Philosophical Investigations. Oxford: Blackwell, 1953, p. 153.

Part III
STRUCTURES OF ARGUMENT IN NURSING

Chapter 8

Deductive Reasoning

The purpose of this chapter is to enable the learner to:

1. Apply logical procedures in the process of reasoning.
2. Discriminate between general and particular arguments, and between deductive and inductive arguments.
3. Distinguish between valid and invalid arguments.
4. Distinguish between valid and sound arguments.
5. Analyze the relationship of logic to the scope of critical thinking.
6. Apply the above procedures and distinctions to thinking critically in nursing.

INTRODUCTION

Logic is the study of criteria of appraisal for judging arguments. Arguments are at the core of logic. In logic, an argument is a claim that one statement or proposition follows from or is implied by another. For example, John is wearing a green scrub suit in a hospital. Nurse A infers that John is a staff member. At the outer scope of critical thinking is the analysis of controversial issues in science, religion, politics, economics, ideology, and philosophy. Analysis of controversial issues includes abortion, euthanasia, freedom, consent, democracy, terrorism, slavery, racism, and sexism. Figure 8–1 represents the relation between the core and the scope of logic and of critical thinking.

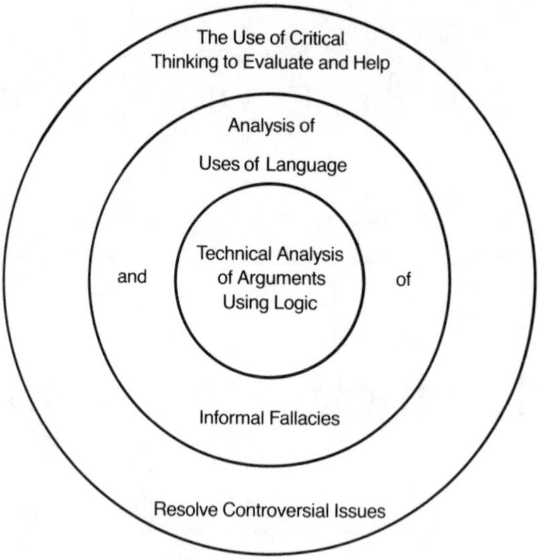

Figure 8-1. Aspects of the Scope of Critical Thinking

WHY DEDUCE?

Deduction, as distinct from induction, consists in drawing conclusions of which we can be certain. Certainty about our conclusions is a natural desire. Knowing which types of inferences lead to certainty and those that do not helps us to avoid useless inferences and to look for useful inferences.

We deduce to draw unmistakable conclusions. We want to know if Patient Y will recover if given treatment X. By identifying types or patterns of inference that imply certain conclusions, we can use these patterns to generate innumerable conclusions that are also certain. The more we can do with deductive reasoning, the less we have to rely on the vagueries and uncertainties of inductive reasoning. The use of deductive reasoning reduces our dependence on forces of unreason to settle the deepest issues of life.

The significance of studying any forms, types, or patterns is that all instances that fit these patterns will have identical values of being either valid or invalid.

Deduction is useful to place values, facts, expressions, and propositions into formulas that generate inferences from initial premises. If a supervisor knows that all professional nurses work no more than a single 12-hour shift, and Mr. Henry is a professional nurse, then Mr. Henry works no more than a single 12-hour shift.

PATTERNS OF REASONING IN NURSING: DEDUCTIVE AND INDUCTIVE

There are two major forms of argument, deductive and inductive. The difference between deduction and induction is itself controversial.

Some people mistakenly believe that deduction consists of going from the general to the particular; and that induction consists in moving from the particular to the general.[1] This is wrong. Valid deductive arguments make use of universal propositions in the premises and the conclusion.

Example:
All nurses are health professionals.
All psychiatric nurses are nurses.
∴ All psychiatric nurses are health professionals.

A deductive argument may also have particular propositions both for the premises and the conclusion.

Example:
If nurse Kelly gave Smith acetaminophen, then she gave Smith a pain reliever.
Kelly gave Smith acetaminophen.
∴ Kelly gave Smith a pain reliever.

An inductive argument may have universal propositions among its premises and its conclusion.

Example:
All psychiatric nurses are health professionals and work with patients.
All surgical nurses are health professionals and work with patients.
All pediatric nurses are health professionals and work with patients.
∴ All health professionals probably work with patients.

Inductive arguments may conclude with particular propositions.

Example:
Nurse White, a Hunter College graduate, is competent.
Nurse Brown, a Hunter College graduate, is competent.
Nurse Clark, a Hunter College graduate, is competent.
Nurse Davis, a Hunter College graduate, is competent.
∴ Nurse Emerson, a Hunter College graduate, is probably competent.

An inductive argument with a general premise may be followed by a particular conclusion.

Example:
Most nurses are women.
Reilly is a nurse.
∴ Reilly is probably a woman.

Consequently, deductive arguments do not necessarily generate particular conclusions from general or universal premises; nor do inductive arguments necessarily generate universal conclusions from particular premises.

A more effective way to perceive the difference between deduction and induction is this: In a valid deductive argument, its premises imply its conclusion. So we have:

All nurses are health providers, and
All health providers are persons.
∴ All nurses are persons.

The conclusion follows by absolute necessity. Therefore a more useful distinction between a deductive and an inductive argument is this: The premises of a deductive argument provide complete evidence for the conclusion, whereas an inductive argument provides only some evidence for its conclusion. Deductive arguments are certain; inductive arguments are uncertain.

A useful basis for distinguishing deduction from induction is that a deductive argument is one in which the premises, if assumed to be true, are sufficient to establish the truth of the conclusion. In an inductive argument, on the other hand, the premises provide some reason for accepting the conclusion. But the premises of an inductive argument are not sufficient to assure, insure, or guarantee the truth of the conclusion. In an inductive argument, even if the premises at a given time are believed to be true, the conclusion may still be false.

Reasons in the premises for drawing a conclusion that is certain, as distinct from a conclusion that is probable or possible, distinguishes a deductive from an inductive argument. A deductive argument, which is valid, is one that, if the premises are true, the conclusion is likewise true.

A second basis for distinguishing a deductive argument from an inductive argument is that a deductive argument contains all of its reasons within its premises. In contrast, an inductive argument makes or implies reference to data that call for further, external verification. A deductive argument is self-enclosed. An inductive argument depends on facts in the external world for further corroboration. If, for example, Jane is sitting next to Mary, then Mary has to be next to Jane. We cannot say, however, that Mary has to sit next to Jane, because Mary could be standing or lying down. Or, if Jane is Mary's aunt, then Mary has to be Jane's niece. If Buenos Aires is south of New York, then New York has to be north of

Buenos Aires. A deductive argument is airtight. There is no room in a valid, deductive argument for exceptions. The conclusion is absolutely certain, and necessarily follows from the premises beyond any rational doubt. A valid, deductive argument is decisive, and it is what every decision maker needs and wants. It is, however, often inappropriately used. Too many arguments look certain, but are uncertain, such as the supposition that "the patient in the next bed will die today." People seek certainty. They often claim to have it without sufficient rational authority. The possibility that an argument could have a different conclusion shows that such an argument is either invalid or inductive.

A clue to distinguishing between a deductive and an inductive argument is the appropriateness of using the term *probably* in the conclusion.

Example:
All members of the CIO voted for the Democratic party.
Smith is a member of the CIO.
∴ Smith voted for the Democratic party.

Contrast this with:

The *majority* of the CIO members voted for the Democratic party.
Smith is a member of the CIO.
∴ Smith probably voted for the Democratic party.

In the first argument, it makes no sense to conclude that Smith probably voted for the Democratic party. In the second example, however, it does make sense to say that Smith *probably* voted for the Democratic party.

THE DIFFERENCE BETWEEN CERTAINTY AND UNCERTAINTY

Knowing the difference between certainty and uncertainty of conclusions is a useful tool of critical thinking. Training in the difference between certain and uncertain conclusions is an important part of nursing education. Such training consists in doing frequent exercises, so as to gain experience in knowing how to distinguish between certain and uncertain conclusions.

Exercises

Determine if the argument is deductive or inductive and explain why.

1. Either John Adams or George Washington was the first president of the United States. John Adams was not the first president. Therefore, George Washington was the first president.
Answer: Deductive, because if the premises are true, then the con-

clusion has to be true. All of the information in the conclusion is found in the premises. Therefore, the conclusion follows.

2. Mary has lobar pneumonia. Antibiotics are usually given to patients with lobar pneumonia. Therefore, Mary should be given an antibiotic.

   Answer: Inductive, because the conclusion is not certain and it is implied solely by the information cited in the premises.

3. The largest city is generally the capital of a country. New York is the largest city of the United States. Therefore, New York is the capital of the United States.

   Answer: Inductive, because we cannot tell for sure from the phrase "is generally," whether the conclusion is implied from what is given in the premises.

4. All nurses are women. Kimberly is a nurse. Therefore, Kimberly is a woman.

   Answer: Deductive, because if the premises are true, the conclusion would have to be true in a valid argument.

5. Ninety-six percent of nurses are women. Tiffiny is a nurse. Therefore, Tiffiny is probably a woman.

   Answer: Inductive, because we cannot tell from the premise that 96 percent are X, whether the next one referred to, namely Tiffiny, is a woman, even though there is a 96 percent probability that Tiffiny is a woman.

6. Nora is a premature infant who weighs 1 pound. Nora has myelomeningocele with mental retardation. Nora cannot suck. Infants with such anomalies usually die within 2 weeks. Therefore, Nora will die within the next 2 weeks.

   Answer: Inductive, as no certainty is implied from the premises to the conclusion. The odds are against Nora surviving beyond 2 weeks, but she may defy the odds.

7. Tony is a prisoner performing hard labor. Therefore, Tony is a criminal.

   Answer: Inductive, for two reasons. First, Tony could be a prisoner due to an unfair trial, from which he is later vindicated. Second, Tony could be a prisoner of war. In either case, the conclusion, that Tony is a criminal, does not necessarily follow.

8. Nick was at the scene of the crime. His fingerprints were on the gun. Therefore, Nick must have committed the crime.

   Answer: Inductive, because fingerprints alone do not prove conclusively that Nick is the one who committed the crime.

9. Mary is wobbling around. Mary is attending a cocktail party. Therefore, she drank too much.

   Answer: Mary could be suffering from muscular dystrophy, multiple sclerosis, or some other condition. Therefore, the conclusion is uncertain and the argument is inductive.

10. Almost every known carcinogen causes cancer in animals. Therefore, compounds that cause cancer in animals are also potential human carcinogens.[2]
Answer: Inductive, as the premises do not state that all carcinogens cause cancer in animals.

11. Wall Street brokers are customarily members of the New York Stock Exchange. O'Leary is a Wall Street broker. Therefore, O'Leary is a member of the New York Stock Exchange.
Answer: Inductive, as the clue word "customarily" in one premise does not guarantee the truth of the conclusion.

12. "In a certain flight crew, the . . . pilot, copilot and flight engineer are Allen, Brown, and Carr, though not necessarily in that order. The copilot, who was an only child, earns the least. Carr, who married Brown's sister, earns more than the pilot. What position does each person hold?"[3]
Answer: Deductive, because if one explicates the meaning of the premises, the conclusion is necessarily implied by the premises. The following argument shows how one may arrive at the conclusion deductively.

Given	Reasons
1. Allen, Brown, Carr are pilot, copilot, and flight engineer.	Given
2. Copilot, only child, earns least of the three.	Given
3. Carr married Brown's sister.	Given
4. Carr earns more than the pilot.	Given
Inferences	
5. Carr is not the pilot.	(4) Because Carr earns more than the pilot, Carr cannot be the pilot.
6. Carr is not the copilot.	(2 and 4) Carr earns more than the pilot.
7. Hence Carr must be the flight engineer.	Process of elimination (5 and 6).
8. Brown has a sister.	(3) If Carr married Brown's sister, then Brown has a sister.
9. Brown is not the copilot.	(2 and 3) If Brown has a sister, Brown is not an only child.
10. Brown is not the flight engineer.	(7) Because Carr is the flight engineer, Brown cannot be.
11. Therefore, Brown is the pilot.	Process of elimination (9 and 10).
12. Allen must be the copilot.	Process of elimination (7 and 11).

The nursing example that follows also illustrates the distinction between a deductive and an inductive argument.

13. (1) Ada, Betty, and Clara are staff nurse, head nurse, and supervisor, though not necessarily in that order. (2) Ada was beaten by the head nurse in a bridge game. (3) Betty is the supervisor's neighbor and (4) is unbeatable at bridge, having played the other nurses. (5) Clara wants to become a head nurse or supervisor. Match up the nurses with their positions. *Answer:* Deductive argument and it is solvable. Number the relevant data or *givens,* as in the previous example and use a similar format.

Given	Reasons
1. Ada, Betty, Clara are staff nurse, head nurse, and supervisor.	Given
2. Ada was beaten in bridge by the head nurse.	Given
3. Betty is the supervisor's neighbor.	Given
4. Betty is unbeatable at bridge.	Given
5. Clara wants to become a head nurse or supervisor.	Given
Inferences	
6. Ada is not the head nurse.	(2) Because Ada was beaten by the head nurse, she cannot be the head nurse.
7. Betty is not the supervisor.	(3) The supervisor's neighbor is presumably not the supervisor.
8. Betty, the bridge winner, is the head nurse.	(2 and 4).
9. Clara is not the head nurse or supervisor.	(5).
10. Therefore, Clara is the staff nurse.	(9) Process of elimination.
11. Ada is the supervisor	(6 and 10) Process of elimination.

Another way to solve the above problem, influenced by Copi, is as follows:

	Supervisor	Head Nurse	Staff Nurse
Ada	✓ Step 7 (6 and 10).	× Step 1 (2).	
Betty	× Step 2 (3 and 7).	✓ Step 3. Process of elimination.	
Clara	× Step 4 (5 and 9).	× Step 5 (5 and 9).	✓ Step 6 (9 and 10). Process of elimination.

We begin with Step 1: × in Step 1 means Ada is eliminated as the head nurse. In Step 2, × means Betty is eliminated as the supervisor. The check ✓ in Step 3 means that Betty is the head nurse by the process of elimination. In Step 4, × means Clara is not the supervisor. The reasons are 5 and 9, based on the preceding format using a given, reasons, and inferences. In Step 5, Clara is eliminated as the head nurse, again for reasons 5 and 9. Therefore, in Step 6, Clara is the staff nurse, and this by reason 9. In Step 7 (because of reasons 6 and 10), Ada is the supervisor.

These *brain teasers,* as they are sometimes called, illustrate deductive arguments. They are solved by extrapolating what is given.

14. Green has chest pain, a cough, sputum, elevated temperature, and questionable chest x-ray. These symptoms are typical of pneumonia. Therefore, Green has pneumonia. *Answer:* Inductive, because the premises alone do not provide conclusive evidence of the truth of the conclusion.

15. 93 percent of a random sample of newborns weigh more than 5.5 pounds. Baby Jones is a (full-term) newborn American. Therefore, Jones weighs more than 5.5 pounds.[4]
Answer: Inductive argument, we do not know conclusively from the premises whether the conclusion has to follow.

THE RELATION OF TRUTH AND FALSITY TO VALIDITY AND INVALIDITY

Validity characterizes the relation between premises and conclusions. In logic, arguments are valid or invalid. Statements or propositions that make up the premises and conclusions of arguments are either true or false. Arguments themselves are not true or false; nor are statements or propositions valid or invalid.

The word *valid* means *valor,* meaning value. One could argue that words, such as valid, could mean whatever their speakers and writers wish them to mean. But the terms *valid, invalid, true,* and *false* have taken on precise, technical meanings. Terms communicate more effectively when limited by technical rules.

An argument is valid if, when the premises are true, the conclusion of that argument is likewise true. But premises and conclusion of a valid argument need not be true for the argument to be valid. All that is claimed for an argument to be valid is that if the premises are true, the conclusion is also true. The point of validity and invalidity in deductive arguments is that a certain form or structure is exhibited in the relation between premises and conclusion. For example, "if only women are permitted to use the Ladies Room and Jane is a woman, then Jane is permitted use of the Ladies Room" is a valid argument. Similarly, if all islands are surrounded by water, and Greenland is an island, then Greenland is surrounded by water.

Valid arguments may contain both true premises and true conclusions. In the English alphabet, A precedes B and B precedes C; therefore, in the English alphabet, A precedes C. An argument, however, may still be valid if it has a false conclusion, providing that the premises are likewise false.

Example:
In the English alphabet, B precedes A, and
C precedes B in the English alphabet.
∴ C precedes A in the English alphabet.

This argument has obvious false premises and a false conclusion, but it is nevertheless a valid argument. What matters is the relation of the premises to the conclusion.

The above argument, however, would be invalid if after the premises were asserted, the conclusion was instead that A precedes C in the English alphabet. That conclusion would not be implied by the premises, which precede the conclusion. Another example of an invalid argument is that if Nurse Jones works at Presbyterian Hospital and Presbyterian Hospital is in Manhattan, then Nurse Jones does not work in Manhattan. In deductive logic, we assume that if the premises are or can be true, the conclusion will follow as true in the same sense. We also assume that in a deductive argument if the premises are false, then a false conclusion follows.

The following example may help make the relation between truth and validity clearer. We will mark each component premise and conclusion with a T to stand for true.

T. If I were Bob Hope, I'd be a great comedian.
T. I am not Bob Hope.
T. ∴ I'm not a great comedian.

Most people who conceded that the premises of this argument were true would also agree that the conclusion, as applied to them, was true as well. Even though the premises and conclusion of this argument are all true, the argument is invalid, because the premises although true, could still result in a false conclusion. If, for example, the speaker were Victor Borge or George Burns, he'd still be a great comedian. For either of them, it is not true that "Therefore, I'm not a great comedian." The premises could be true, as they are in the above example, but the conclusion could still be false.

Example:

T. If I were Florence Nightingale, I'd be a great nurse.
T. I am not Florence Nightingale.
T. ∴ I'm not a great nurse.

This example again contains true premises and the possibility of a false conclusion. Although some nurses might concur with the conclusion, there are some nurses about whom the conclusion would be false. For example, Lillian Wald was also a great nurse. It all depends who we substitute for *I* in the conclusion. For most cases, the conclusion might well be true. But if the conclusion could be false in the presence of true premises, the argument would be invalid. A deductive argument is invalid, then, if the premises are true and the conclusion could be false. Although we will discuss criteria of soundness in later chapters, it may be helpful to distinguish validity from soundness. An argument, in addition to being valid, is sound, if, in fact all the premises and the conclusion are true. The validity of an argument concerns the relation between premises and conclusion, and is sometimes identified as the structure of an argument. The soundness of an argument characterizes the truth of the component propositions or statements that comprise the content of the argument. One reason for studying validity before soundness is that if an argument is invalid, it cannot be sound.

We, therefore, resume with attention to validity. Another rule of valid arguments is that the conclusion cannot contain more terms than there are in the premises. For example, if A precedes B and B precedes C, then A precedes C. It would be an invalid argument to say that if A precedes B and B precedes C, that, therefore, A precedes D. D was not cited in the premises, and therefore, cannot appear in the conclusion of a valid argument.

An argument may be valid, even though it consists of false premises and a false conclusion.

Example:

F. All five-legged beings can fly.
F. All horses have five legs.
F. ∴ All horses can fly.

This is a valid argument because the conclusion logically follows from the premises.

The following type of argument is valid even though it consists of nonsensical or obviously false sentences.

F. All skyscrapers are over 8 miles tall.
F. All undergraduates are skyscrapers.
F. ∴ All undergraduates are over 8 miles tall.

This argument, however absurd in appearance, is valid, because of the relation of the premises to the conclusion. The conclusion logically follows from the premises.

Two steps may help to appreciate the relation of premises to conclusions in determining whether an argument is valid or invalid. The first step is to translate the terms into symbols representing abstract forms. For example, in place of "All skyscrapers are over 8 miles tall," we say "All S's are T's," and in place of "All undergraduates are skyscrapers," we say "All U's are S's." In place of "Therefore, all undergraduates are over eight miles tall," we say, "All U's are T's." Schematically, the example is:

All S's are T's.
All U's are S's.
∴ All U's are T's.

In schematizing, symbolizing, or formalizing, we divest the structure of its content as well as its factual and emotional associations. In deductive logic, we refer to a different sense of truth from truth in science. The essential difference is that in a deductive argument, the conclusion is contingent or dependent on the premises. The conclusion is a formal abstraction that follows from and is implied by the first part of the form, that is the premises.

To determine the validity of the argument:

All S's are T's.
All U's are S's.
∴ All U's are T's.

the question is, if all S's are T's and if all U's are S's, then are all U's therefore T's?

To appreciate the point about structure, in place of letters, we may find pictures easier to follow.

If all △'s are ▭'s.	If all triangles are rectangles.
And if all ○'s are △'s.	And if all circles are triangles.
∴ All ○'s are ▭'s.	∴ All circles are rectangles.

Or

If all dentists earn more than nurses.
And if all physicians earn more than dentists.
∴ All physicians earn more than nurses.

The validity or invalidity of some arguments is intuitively more obvious than others. To extend our intuitive powers, we look to forms and rules. Some rules of inference are like rules of crossword puzzles; other rules of inference are like cookbook rules, rules of the road, rules of a sport or social activity, or like microscopes and telescopes, all of which are used to check and extend our intuitively obvious inferences.

CONCLUSION

If there is even a logical possibility of the antecedent being true with the possibility of the consequent being false, then an argument is invalid. If the premises are false and the conclusion of an argument is either true or false, then the argument is valid, but not sound. An argument is valid if the conclusion follows from or is implied by the premises.

REFERENCES

1. Copi, I. Introduction To Logic (7th ed.). New York: Macmillan, 1986, pp. 547–550.
2. Salsburg, D., & Heath, A. When Science Progresses and Bureaucracies Lag—The Case of Cancer Research. *The Public Interest* 1981; 65:34, Fall.
3. Copi, I. Informal Logic. New York: Macmillan, 1986, pp. 57–58.
4. Gordon, M. Nursing Diagnosis: Process and Application. New York: McGraw-Hill, 1982, p. 14.

Chapter 9

Syllogistic Reasoning

The study of this chapter enables the learner to:

1. Distinguish among syllogisms, enthymemes, and sorites arguments.
2. Discriminate between immediate and mediate inferences.
3. Differentiate the quantity and quality of categorical propositions.
4. Use the square of opposition as it applies to nursing.
5. Distinguish between contraries, contradictories, and subcontraries.
6. Apply the doctrine of distribution to syllogistic reasoning.
7. Show how the rules of the syllogism distinguish a valid from an invalid classical argument.
8. Illustrate the test for validity of classical argument through the use of Venn diagrams.

INTRODUCTION

Deductive logic is divisible into classical syllogistic logic and symbolic logic. Syllogistic logic or classical reasoning then divides into (1) immediate inference or enthymeme, using one premise followed by a conclusion; and (2) mediate inference, using two or more premises. An enthymeme is an argument that uses one premise, whereas an argument using two premises is a syllogism. An argument with more than two premises is a sorites. For example, in the premise: A is bigger than B, an immediate inference is that B is smaller than A. Another inference or conclusion is that A and B are not the same size.

An enthymeme is an argument consisting either of a single premise or a suppressed, missing, or unstated assumption. In ordinary conversation, an argument with a suppressed premise is frequently appropriate, as everyone in a given context knows the missing premise. For example, when a health professional tells a colleague that Mr. Smith, a patient, is in Room 204 of St. Barnaby's Hospital, the health professional need not add that Mr. Smith has a serious enough illness to justify hospitalization. We omit missing premises hundreds of times a day, partly to economize on communication and also to avoid excessive boredom. When mother asks Johnny to go to the store, it's often understood that he is to get milk. When someone says, "Ms. Jones is a member of the ANA," we can assume that Ms. Jones is a nurse, as only nurses are members of the ANA. One could formalize this into a standard argument form by saying: All members of the ANA are nurses. (Missing premise.)

Ms. Jones is a member of the ANA.

∴ Ms. Jones is a nurse.

A second type of example is:

A is bigger than B.
B is bigger than C.

∴ A is bigger than C.

In this example, there are two premises. An argument with two premises and a conclusion is a syllogism.

One could extend this process of A's and B's further.

Example:
A is bigger than B.
B is bigger than C.
C is bigger than D.
D is bigger than E.

∴ A is bigger than E.

This sort of argument, with three or more premises, is called a *sorites.*

Immediate Inference

To Aristotle (384–322 BC), who was probably the major originator of classical logic, there were four kinds of propositions, A, E, I, and O. An A proposition is a universal affirmative. It asserts that all the members of a class are to do something. A proposition is defined as a sentence with a subject and a predicate. Each of these types of propositions is about the relation between subject and predicate. An A proposition makes a complete assertion about its subject in relation to its predicate. This is sometimes called class inclusion. An E proposition completely denies that one class, the subject of the sentence, is included in the predicate. This is called class exclusion. An I proposition asserts that some members of a class, expressed in the subject of the sentence, have an affirmative relation with another class, represented by the predicate. Finally, an O proposition denies that some members, expressed in the subject, have a relation to another class, represented by the predicate of the sentence or proposition.

Example:
A. All women are nurses.
E. No women are nurses.
I. Some women are nurses.
O. Some women are not nurses.

Or

A. All nurses are intelligent and caring persons.
E. No nurses are intelligent and caring persons.
I. Some nurses are intelligent and caring persons.
O. Some nurses are not intelligent and caring persons.

A glance at these four propositions suggests that the first and second of these propositions, the A and E, are clearly false. We know some nurses who are not intelligent and caring, and we also know some who are. So, the bottom propositions, I and O may, in fact, both be true. In the first example, *women* is the subject and *nurses* is the predicate. A categorical proposition asserts or denies something about its subject. What each of these propositions asserts about its subject is its predicate. In the second example, *nurses* is the subject and *being intelligent and caring persons* is the predicate. We typically abbreviate the subject and the predicate of a categorical proposition with S and P, respectively.

An A proposition asserts that all members of the class belong to another class. For example, all pediatric nursing practitioners are nurses. This is a clear illustration of class inclusion. We cannot rationally deny that a pediatric nurse practitioner is a nurse, anymore than we can rationally deny that a puppy is a dog or a kitten is a cat, or that a left-sided shoe is a shoe. An A proposition asserts that some entity referred to as S, the subject, cannot be an S without also being included in another category referred to as P, the predicate. By abbreviating these relations into symbols, such as S and P, we symbolize their relation as follows:

A. All S is P.
E. No S is P.
I. Some S is P.
O. Some S is not P

VENN DIAGRAMS FOR CATEGORICAL PROPOSITIONS

We may represent A, E, I, and O propositions with the help of Venn diagrams (Figs. 9–1 through 9–4), named after the logician John Venn (1834–1923). In all S is P, we number the regions and shade region 1, meaning that it is made empty and relocated into regions 2 and 3 of the P cir-

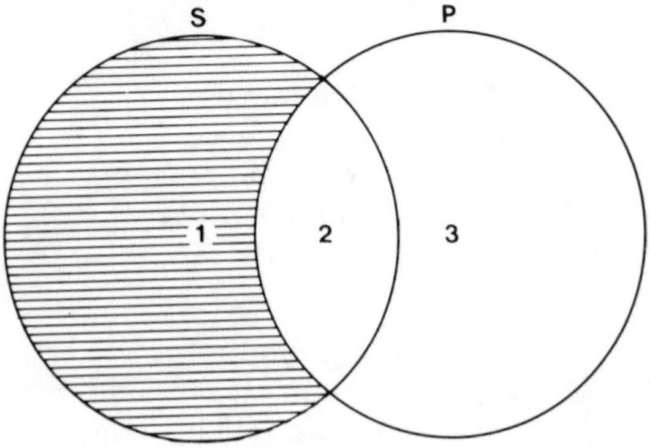

Figure 9-1. An A Proposition.
1 = Nurses;
2 and 3 = women
(E.g.: All nurses are women. All N is W.)

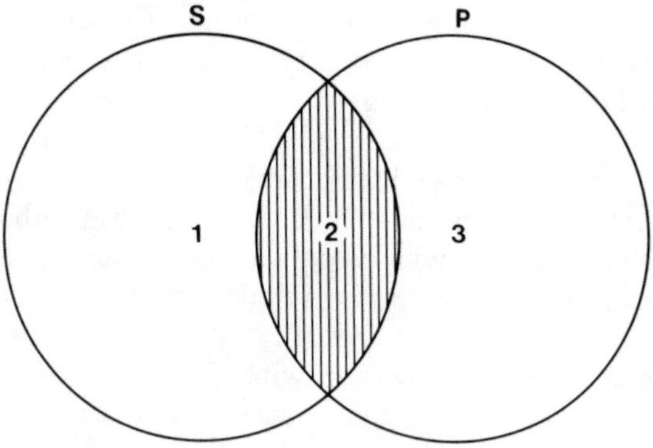

Figure 9-2. An E Proposition.
1 = Nurses;
3 = Women;
2 = Nurses who are not women.
(E.g.: No nurses are women. No N is W.)

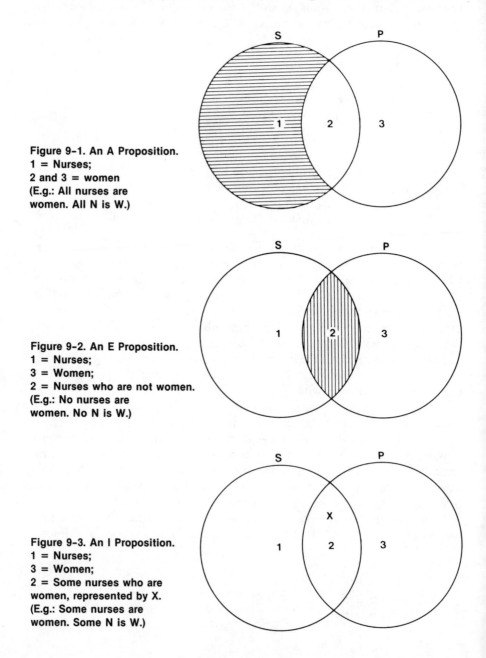

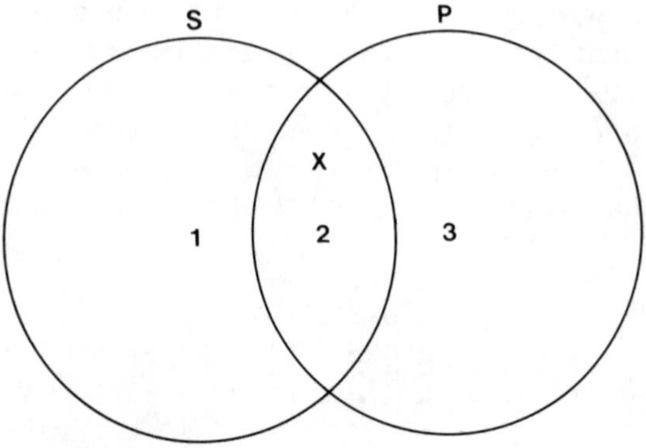

Figure 9-3. An I Proposition.
1 = Nurses;
3 = Women;
2 = Some nurses who are women, represented by X.
(E.g.: Some nurses are women. Some N is W.)

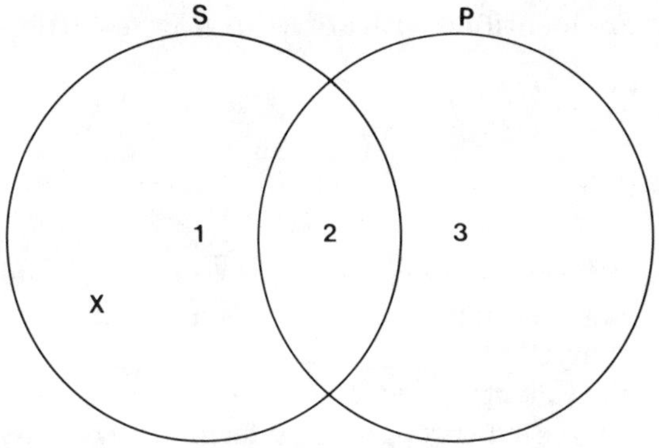

Figure 9-4. An O Proposition. 1 = Nurses; 3 = Women; X = Some nurses. (E.g.: Some nurses are not women. Some N is not W. Some nurses, X in 1, are outside 2 and 3, the class of women.)

cle. If all pediatric nurses are nurses, then there are no pediatric nurses left over who are not also nurses. In effect, we herd all members of S in region 1 into regions 2 and 3. In an E proposition, region 2 is shaded, showing complete exclusion of both classes from one another. In an I proposition, region 2, the intersection between circles S and P contains at least one member. Finally, in the O proposition, region 1 in the circle S contains at least one member, meaning that there is at least one X in S that is not a member of the class represented by P.

THE MEANING OF "SOME" AND OF SINGLE INDIVIDUALS IN CLASSICAL LOGIC

In ordinary language, the term *some* refers to one or more, but not all, in relation to what is being asserted. Another usage of some in classical logic confines some, not to one or more, but to two or more. A reason for this use of some is that single individuals are identified with classes rather than with parts of classes. For example, in the classical argument,

1 All humans are mortal.
2 Socrates is human.
3 ∴ Socrates is mortal.

Lines 2 and 3 refer to all of Socrates rather than to part of him. The preferred convention is to render line 2 as follows: "All individuals identical to Socrates are human," and line 3 is rendered or interpreted to mean, "All individuals identical to Socrates are mortal." Because there is only one individual identical to the original Socrates, the above syllogism is interpreted as one with three universal, affirmative propositions. Assertions about single individuals are identified with affirmative or negative, universal propositions.

QUANTITY AND QUALITY

To preface a proposition with *all, none,* or *some* specifies a quantity, and is called the *quantifier.* Every categorical proposition has a quantifier and answers the question, "How many?"

The quality of a proposition is identified with its assertion or denial; and this quality is generally expressed through some form of *yes* or *no,* or a positive or a negative. Every categorical proposition has both a quantity and a quality. An A proposition is universal affirmative; an E proposition is universal negative; an I proposition is particular affirmative; and an O proposition is particular negative.

Quantity, which refers to how many entities, is a huge topic in logic, philosophy, science, nursing, and the history of critical thinking. Some modern thinkers, such as A. Whitehead[1] and A. Kaplan,[2] have pointed out that a science advances in proportion to the level and degree of mathematical quantity it refers to. These thinkers have this thought in common: Advances in science and technology depend on substituting exact quantities for inexact qualities. Instead of saying, "The patient is feverish," or "The patient is not drinking enough," we use precise measurements, such as thermometers, liquid and weight measures, and highly sophisticated laboratory tests, that achieve the required quantification. We could say that human knowledge advances to the extent that initial estimates are replaced with precise measurements.

To think critically is to use some form of either *yes* or *no* to states of affairs in the world. One form of yes or no is green and red lights. Another important form of yes or no is *true* or *false.* These are two fundamental words in logic, critical thinking, science, nursing, the arts, the humanities, ethics, and in all practical action.

True and false discriminations are important to the sciences and the measuring of precise quantities. A researcher's initial assumptions and findings in health care depend on the clear use of true and false judgments.

If one conclusion is true, its denial is false. The analysis of falsehoods, sometimes identified with negation, is no less important than the analysis of truth or affirmation. To assert one statement is to deny another. If Supervisor S says, "Nurse Brown can handle some primary care problems," the supervisor denies that nurses cannot handle primary care problems.

In nursing, and health care generally, we expect people to tell the truth, and abjure people against lying and deceiving others. In all our social institutions, especially in the family, we place a value on truth and falsity as forms of affirmation or assertion and negation. Without some form of assertion and denial, it is doubtful that we could think critically about anything.

THE DOCTRINE OF DISTRIBUTION

The doctrine of distribution is fundamental to classical logic. Any term S or P in a categorical proposition is distributed if definite reference is made to each and every entity referred to in the proposition. For example, in the proposition, "All pediatric and geriatric nurse practitioners are nurses," definite reference is made to each and every pediatric and geriatric nurse practitioner. There are no exceptions. The quantifier *all* makes definite reference to each and every pediatric and geriatric nurse, referred to in the subject of this A proposition. An A proposition distributes its subject.

The word *all* has a prominent role in laws of science, which have the form, "All A's are B's.[3] The form "All A's are B's" characterizes a lawlike relation, as in Newton's law of gravitation. According to Newton's law, all particles or any two particles attract one another proportionately to the product of their masses and inversely to the square of the distance between them. Although Newton's formula is written as: $F = G\,M_1\,M_2/D^2$, the unstated but critical term in front of F is *all*. We may test the law by looking for exceptions. One exception disproves the generalization or rule. Also, universal propositions, which withstand the test, provide inference–warrants[4] for drawing particular conclusions.

Example:
All roses are red, and
Here is a rose.
∴ It is red.

This conclusion follows deductively. For a second illustration, if "No practicing nurses are practicing physicians," we may then use this exclusionary proposition to rule out a practicing nurse from being a practicing physician. Or if "No vegetarians are meat eaters," is true, it provides a basis for reliably inferring the behavior of vegetarians regarding the consumption of meat. To say "No nurses are drug addicts" or "No nurses are cigarette smokers," if true, provides a warrantable basis for future nurses' behavior.

Some inclusions and exclusions may be implicit, but they have force in civil law and custom. For example, a rest room may explicitly say "Ladies" but the implied directive is "Ladies only." The implied message is "All who are ladies and none who are not ladies may enter." Clear and unambiguous exclusions and inclusions are important inference–tickets for guiding people's behavior, as the above rest room examples illustrate.

Such inclusions and exclusions presuppose a doctrine of distribution, in which we make definite reference to all the members of the class. The ladies room makes definite reference to all ladies; and by exclusion, makes definite reference to all men.

In I type propositions, neither the subject nor the predicate is distributed. In "Some nurses are researchers," indefinite reference is made to both the subject *nurses* and the predicate *researchers.* We do not know from this example of an I proposition which nurses are referred to and which researchers. On the other hand, in "All nurse directors are administrators," the subject, but not the predicate is distributed.

The predicate of an A type proposition, however, is undistributed. In "All pediatric nurse practitioners are nurses," we do not know anything definite about nurses. In an E type proposition, definite reference is made both to subjects and predicates, as in "No practicing nurses are practicing physicians." Here definite reference is made to all practicing nurses and to all practicing physicians. There is a mutual class exclusion. The members of either class cannot belong to the other class.

In I propositions, both subject and predicate are undistributed, as no definite reference is made to either the subject or the predicate regarding class inclusion or exclusion. For example, "Some nurses are hard workers" does not tell us which nurses are referred to, or which nurses are hard workers and which ones are not.

Similarly, the O type proposition is without a definite reference in the subject. For example, "Some students are on the Dean's list," leaves indefinite which students are referred to. However, the predicate of an O type proposition is distributed, because it holds that the entire predicate class excludes some entities, which ones we do not know. In this example, the entire Dean's list excludes some students. Or, in "Some dogs are not Great Danes," the term *dogs* is undistributed, meaning that we cannot refer to the entire class of dogs. However, the entire class of Great Danes excludes some dogs.

In summary form, the doctrine of distribution, then looks like this:

	Subject	Predicate
A	D	U
E	D	D
I	U	U
O	U	D

where D = distribution and U = absence of distribution.

As we will see shortly, the doctrine of distribution is vitally important to determine the difference between a valid and an invalid syllogistic argument. This doctrine also enables us to make some immediate inferences.

CONVERSION

A further immediate inference we may make is to reverse an A proposition and notice if the reverse is valid, that is, if switching subject and predicate implies the same meaning as we had in the initial statement. If, for example, "All nurses are health professionals," does it follow that all health professionals are nurses? Clearly not, as some health professionals include physicians, x-ray technicians, and respiratory therapists. Therefore, an A type proposition does not validly convert. By conversion, we mean that the subject and the predicate may be switched and that we may validly infer the same truth value by reversing the subject and the predicate of the original proposition. This is clearly impossible in an A proposition.

In an E proposition, however, such as "No practicing nurses are practicing physicians," we can reverse the subject and the predicate of this proposition and validly infer that, therefore, "No practicing physicians are practicing nurses." Or, if we say "No left-sided shoes are right-sided shoes," this validly implies that, therefore, "No right-sided shoes are left-sided shoes."

If we next consider an I proposition, such as "Some nurses are scholars," we can reverse the subject and predicate of this proposition and validly infer that "Some scholars are nurses."

Finally, the O proposition, "Some S is not P" also does not convert validly. To say "Some nurses are not pediatric nurses," it would be absurd to reverse the subject and the predicate and conclude that "Some pediatric nurses are not nurses."

Another look at the doctrine of distribution shows that where there is symmetry between distributed or undistributed terms, as in E and I, we may validly convert; otherwise we cannot.

THE SQUARE OF OPPOSITION: CONTRARIES, CONTRADICTORIES, AND OTHER IMMEDIATE INFERENCES

There are several kinds of immediate inferences we may validly make. If "All nurses are health professionals," "All patients have health problems," or "All books have pages" are true, then we know that their opposites or contraries "No nurses are health professionals," "No patients have health problems," and "No books have pages" are false. A proposition is the contrary of another if it has the same universal quantifier, but has a different quality; that is, if the second proposition denies what the first asserts, or vice versa.

If, however, "All nurses are women" is false, as it is, that does not imply that "No nurses are women" is true, which it is not in fact. Or, if

"All doors are made of wood" is false, then its contrary, "No doors are made of wood" is not necessarily true. In fact, both statements are false. Both pairs of statements, prefaced by "All" or "No" are contraries of one another. Although both have a different quality, one asserting what the other denies, they have the same quantity, namely the universal affirmative or universal negative *all* or *none*.

Two propositions are contraries, then, if either they cannot both be true or if they can both be false. Clearly, "All nurses are women" and "No nurses are women" are both false. Two contraries cannot both be true, but they can both be false. For example, the contrary of "Nurse Jones is rich" is "Nurse Jones is not rich." Both statements may be false, but they cannot both be true. Nurse Jones may be neither rich or not rich, but if she is either rich or not rich, she cannot also be the other at the same time or "in the same respect," to cite a useful phrase of Aristotle's.

A different relation between propositions, a contradictory one, occurs if both of two such propositions have a different quality. One asserts what the other denies, using a different quantifier. If one of two contradictory statements is universal, affirmative, the second proposition is a particular negative. If "All nurses are women" is false, as it is in fact, then "Some nurses are not women" is true, which happens to be the case. On the other hand, if "All nurses are health professionals" is true, its contradictory, "Some nurses are not health professionals" is false, which, again happens to be the case.

Accordingly, a contradictory relation is one in which if the first of two propositions is true or false, the contradictory proposition has the opposite truth value of the first proposition. Two contradictories cannot both be true; nor can they both be false. If either of two contradictories is true or false, the other has the opposite truth value. If, for example, "Some women are nurses" is true, then "No women are nurses" is false. Contradictories differ in both quantity and quality; and cannot both be either true or false.

A way to remember a contradictory is that it takes back what it asserts. The contradictory of "Ms. Rose is a good nurse" is "Ms. Rose is not a good nurse." The contrary of the first statement, "Ms. Rose is a good nurse," is "Ms. Rose is a bad nurse." With contradictories, as in "Mary has a tall patient" and "Mary does not have any tall patients," there is no way for both statements to be both true and false. If it is true that Mary has a tall patient, then it is not true that she has no tall patients. If Mary does not have a tall patient, then it is not true that she has any tall patients. Contradictories both exclude and exhaust all other truth values.[5] The case is different for contraries. If "Mary's only pneumonia patient is tall" is true, then "Mary's only pneumonia patient is short" is false. But both statements may be false, such as "Mary's only pneumonia patient is middle sized." being true.

People who do not think critically may confuse a contrary with a contradictory. For example, the New Hampshire license plate slogan "Live free or die," makes sense if it expresses a contrary relation. However, if someone lives in a despotic regime, corporation, or family, that person may not accept either alternative, and work for reforms instead. For a contrary relation, we can avoid either alternative. A patient may not be tall or short, but middle sized. A nurse may be neither rich nor poor. But in a contrary relation, the assertion is made that if one is true, the contrary cannot be true; and both may be false, as Mary's pneumonia patient example illustrates. A useful way to understand a contradiction is that it is the complete cancellation of one's assertion. Smith utters a contradiction if he says "Patient Jones is alive and patient Jones is not alive." If either is true, the other is false, and vice versa.

Two propositions, I and O, are subcontraries, if they can both be true, but not both be false. For example, "Some nurses are highly conscientious" and "Some nurses are not highly conscientious" may both be true, but they cannot both be false. Moreover, if one of two subcontraries is false, the other is true. To reiterate a point about I and O propositions, they both have the same quantifier, namely *some,* but differ in quality, the one asserting what the other denies.

We may schematize the relation of these four categorical propositions in what is called the *square of opposition.* We may refer to this as a "Lazy Susan," a turnaround table, useful for making valid inferences. For example, if "All nurses are women" is true, then we may validly infer that "Some nurses are women" is true as well. Or, if "All aspirin tablets have a pain relieving property" is true, then we can validly infer that "Some aspirin tablets have a pain relieving property" is also true.

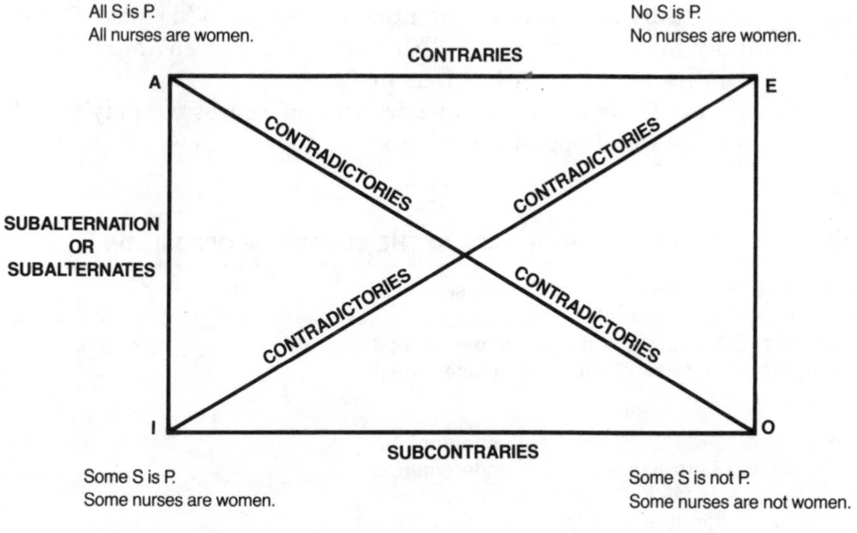

Figure 9-5. The square of opposition.

By being given the truth value of one proposition, and by knowing the meanings of *contradictory, contrary, subalternate,* and *subcontrary,* we can validly infer the truth values of the other propositions. If, for example, "All nurses are health care providers" is true, then we can move to the O proposition and immediately infer that "Some nurses are not health care providers" is false. If an A type proposition is true, we can next move to an E proposition and knowingly infer that E has to be false. If E is false, we can cross the square of opposition and conclude that I, the contradictory of E, has to be true. Or, again, if we know that A is true, we can infer that I, which is covered by A, is likewise true. If all S's and P's is true, then some S's and P's is likewise true. To return to our brief discussions of the values of laws of science, a law that functions like an A proposition provides a cover or umbrella for an I proposition. If all X's are Y's is true, then the next X will be Y is also true.

Also, if the E, "No vegetarians are meat eaters" is true, then we can go to I and infer validly that "Some vegetarians are meat eaters" is false. We may also lateral across to A, "All vegetarians are meat eaters" and infer validly that it is false. We can then go from A to O and infer validly that "Some vegetarians are not meat eaters" is also true.

A virtue of these types of inferences in the square of opposition is that they are not only true, but absolutely true. They cannot be false. Deductive reasoning, if valid, implies certainty. Becoming familiar with rules of deduction provides a nurse with training in certainty. This sort of training helps us also to develop training in uncertainty, which may be as important. But to know either requires knowing the differences between them.

In the square of opposition, however, there are three values, true, false, and undetermined. If I is true, for example, "Some nurses are women" is true, we can validly infer that E "No nurses are women" is false. But we cannot validly infer that either A, "All nurses are women" or O, "Some nurses are not women," is either true or false.

We can use Table 9–1 to summarize the inferences we may validly make in the square of opposition.

TABLE 9-1. VALID INFERENCES MADE IN THE SQUARE OF OPPOSITION

If A is true, E is false, I is true, O is false.
If E is true, A and I are false, O is true.
If I is true, E is false, A and O are undetermined.
If O is true, A is false, E and I are undetermined.

and

If A is false, O is true, E and I are undetermined.
If E is false, I is true, A and O are undetermined.
If I is false, A is false, E is true, and O is true.
If O is false, A is true, E is false, and I is true.

Exercises

Assume the propositions below to be true, then false, and use the procedures of the square of opposition to validly infer other propositions.

1. a. All successful nurses are college graduates. (A statement)
b. No successful nurses are college graduates. (E)
c. Some successful nurses are college graduates. (I)
d. Some successful nurses are not college graduates. (O)
Answer: If A is true, E is false, I is true, O is false (Table 9–1). If A is false, then O is true, E and I are undetermined.

2. a. All patients improve after their first hospital stay. (A)
b. No patients improve after their first hospital stay. (E)
c. Some patients improve after their first hospital stay. (I)
d. Some patients do not improve after their first hospital stay. (O)
Answer: If A is false, O is true, E and I are undetermined.

3. a. All professors bore their students to death. (A)
b. No professors bore their students to death. (E)
c. Some professors bore their students to death. (I)
d. Some professors do not bore their students to death. (O)

4. a. All nurses like competent, considerate physicians. (A)
b. No nurses like competent, considerate physicians. (E)
c. Some nurses like competent, considerate physicians. (I)
d. Some nurses do not like competent, considerate physicians. (O)

5. If O is false, what can we validly infer about A, I, and E?
Answer: A is true, E is false, I is true.

6. If E is true, what can we validly infer about A, I, and O?
Answer: A and I are false, and O is true (Table 9–1).

7. If A is false, what can we validly infer about I, E, and O?
Answer: O is true, I and E are undetermined (Table 9–1).

THE CATEGORICAL SYLLOGISM

We next provide rules and procedures to explain and test arguments using two premises. These arguments are called syllogisms. Let's consider:

No anemic persons are blood donors. (E)
Some nurses are blood donors. (I)
∴ Some nurses are not anemic. (O)

We may symbolize this argument as follows:

AP e BD		P e M
N i BD	or	S i M
∴ N o AP		∴ S o P

AP stands for anemic persons, BD stands for blood donors, N stands for nurses, e stands for an e proposition or a negative universal, i stands for an i proposition or a particular affirmative, and o stands for a particular negative proposition. The small letters e, i, and o, at S. Barker's suggestion, stand for the quantity and quality of the propositions in the argument.[6] Next, the S, P, M arrangement is as follows: S stands for the subject of the conclusion of a syllogism; P stands for the predicate of the conclusion; and M stands for the middle term. S, the subject of the conclusion, is also called the minor term, and P, the predicate of the conclusion, is called the major term. The major term, along with the middle term appears in the top line of a syllogism. The minor term, S, appears along with the middle term in the next line of the premises. The conclusion contains the major and minor terms, but never the middle term.

The structure of a syllogism is determined by noting the position of the middle term. In the example before us, M is on the right in both premises. There are four possible arrangements for the position of M, one being that it is in the predicate position in both premises. Another possible arrangement is that the middle term is in the subject position in the major premise and that the middle term is in the predicate position in the second or minor premise. For example, in the argument:

All health professionals work in, or are oriented by, hospitals.
All nurses are health professionals.
∴ All nurses work in, or are oriented by, hospitals.

The middle term is health professionals. It appears first in the subject position in the major premise, and second, the middle term, health professionals, appears in the predicate position in the minor premise. The above argument may be schematized as follows:

Major premise:	HP a H		M a P
Minor premise:	N a HP	or	S a M
Conclusion:	N a H		S a P

The above is called a first figure syllogism. The first example was a second-figure syllogism.

Two other possible arrangements for the middle term are that the middle term is in the subject position in both premises; and that the middle term is in the predicate position in the major premise and in the subject position in the minor premise. If the middle term is in the subject position in both premises, we call this a third-figure syllogism. For example, in the syllogism:

> All underpaid and overworked persons include nurses.
> Some underpaid and overworked persons are altruists.
> ∴ Some nurses are altruists.

The middle term *underpaid and overworked persons* appears in the subject position in both premises. This argument may be schematized as follows:

P a N
P i A
∴ N i A

P = underpaid and overworked persons; N = nurses; and A = altruists

or

M a S
M i P
∴ S i P

M = middle term; S = subject of conclusion; and P = predicate of the conclusion

Finally, in the fourth arrangement, the middle term appears in the predicate position in the major premise and in the subject position in the minor premise. That is:

> All nursing is a form of interaction.
> All interaction is a form of communication.
> ∴ All nursing is a form of communication.[7]

Interaction is the middle term, and appears in both premises. This argument may be schematized as follows:

N a I		P a M
I a C	or	M a S
∴ N a C		∴ S a P

If we look at all four arrangements, we can draw a diagonal from left to right in the first example, and a diagonal from right to left in the fourth example. In the second example, the middle term is in predicate position, and in the third example, the middle term is in the subject position. Schematizing these four examples, we have:

$$
\begin{array}{cc}
\text{M} \quad \text{P} & \text{P} \quad \text{M} \\
\quad \diagdown & \mid \\
\text{S} \quad \text{M} & \text{S} \quad \text{M} \\
\hline
\text{S} \quad \text{P} & \text{S} \quad \text{P}
\end{array}
\qquad
\begin{array}{cc}
\text{M} \quad \text{P} & \text{P} \quad \text{M} \\
\mid & \diagup \\
\text{M} \quad \text{P} & \text{M} \quad \text{S} \\
\hline
\text{S} \quad \text{P} & \text{S} \quad \text{P}
\end{array}
$$

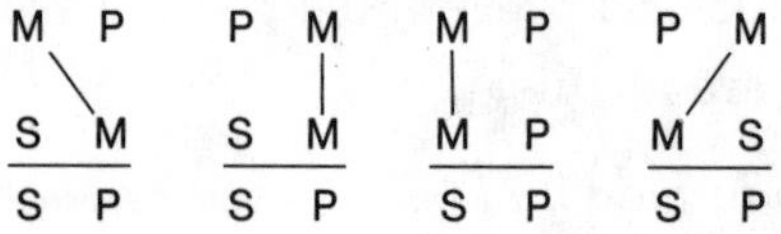

The first and fourth arrangements are relatively easy to remember. A device for remembering the second and third arrangements is to say to yourself, MP-2, meaning that the middle term is in the predicate position in the second arrangement; and MS-3 for the third position, meaning that the middle term is in the subject position in the third arrangement.

We may ask, "Why do we need to learn all these abstractions?" The answer is that to determine the validity of a syllogism, we need to know the figure and the mood of the syllogism, along with rules of validity. Some of these rules depend on the doctrine of distribution.

We want to know if these examples of arguments and numerous others that are used in nursing are valid or invalid. An advantage of looking for valid arguments, and also for schematizing arguments, is that valid arguments are valid for any substituted instances. Thus, one could replace these examples with any others and if they were valid, other examples with the same structure and mood would also be valid. But let us now determine if these examples of syllogisms are valid. First, we need to identify the rules of syllogism.

RULES OF A VALID SYLLOGISM

Rule 1. The middle term is distributed at least once.
Rule 2. Any term distributed in the conclusion is distributed in the corresponding premise.
Rule 3. If any syllogism has a negative premise, the conclusion is negative.
Rule 4. If any syllogism has two negative premises, there is no conclusion.
Rule 5. If the premises are universal, the conclusion is universal.

A device may help remember these rules. Rule 1 is that the middle term is distributed at least once (MT1). Rule 2 is that any term distributed in the conclusion is distributed in the premise (TDCDP). Rule 3 is that two negative premises cannot imply a conclusion (NPNC). Rule 4 is that if there is one negative premise, it is followed by a negative conclusion

(1NPNC). Last, rule 5 is that if a syllogism contains two universal premises, then the conclusion is universal (2UPUC).

We now consider, the first syllogism with the rules as a checklist.

	AP e BD	No anemic persons are blood donors.
	N i BD	Some nurses are blood donors.
∴	N o AP	∴ Some nurses are not anemic persons.

Rule 1, is the middle term distributed? BD is the middle term. An E proposition distributes both subject and predicate, therefore, this syllogism passes rule 1. As for rule 2, AP is distributed in the conclusion. AP also appears in the major premise as an E proposition. An E proposition distributes both subject and predicate, therefore, the syllogism passes rule 2. We can readily see that premise 1 is negative, as is the conclusion; and the second premise is particular, as is the conclusion. Hence, the argument is valid.

We consider the next syllogism symbolized.

	HP a H	All health professionals work in, or are oriented by, hospitals.
	N a HP	All nurses are health professionals.
∴	N a H	∴ So, nurses work in, or are oriented by, hospitals.

Because this syllogism passes all the rules, it, too, is valid. A comparison of the next two syllogisms with the rules also shows that these syllogisms, beginning N a A and N a I, are also valid.

But how about this syllogism?

All cardiologists are health professionals.
All nurses are health professionals.
∴ All nurses are cardiologists.

Schematically, we have

	C a H	or		P a M
	N a H			S a M
∴	N a C		∴	S a P

Here, the middle term is in the predicate position both in the major and minor premises. Is the middle term distributed? No. Therefore, this syllogism does not pass the test. To pass the test, all rules of the syllogism must be satisfied. We may recall that an A proposition does not distribute its predicate term. The middle term, H, therefore, is not distributed. Hence, the syllogism is invalid.

Let's consider this syllogism:

All nurses are health professionals.
Some health professionals favor national health insurance.
∴ Some nurses favor national health insurance.

This syllogism may be schematized as:

	N	a	HP		S	a	M
	HP	i	NAI	or	M	i	P
∴	N	i	NAI		∴ S	i	P

Because the I proposition distributes no terms and the A proposition only distributes its subject, with HP, the middle term, undistributed, this syllogism is likewise invalid.

Rule 2 states that any term distributed in the conclusion is distributed in the premise. The following syllogism illustrates this rule.

All nurses are health professionals.	(A)
No physicians are nurses.	(E)
∴ No physicians are health professionals.	(E)

The conclusion is obviously absurd. But we may wish to know why this argument is valid or invalid. The conclusion is an E proposition. An E proposition distributes both its subject and its predicate. If we look at the premise in which *physicians* appears, we find another E proposition, which means that *physicians* is distributed in the minor premise. But if we look at the major term *health professionals* in the conclusion, and then traces it to its role in the major premise, we find that, as with any other A proposition, the predicate *health professionals* is undistributed. Therefore, we have a term *health professionals* distributed in the conclusion but not in the premise. This is called *illicit major* and violates rule 2. The syllogism is, therefore, invalid. If the minor term is distributed in the conclusion, is undistributed in the premise, then we have the illicit minor fallacy.

Rule 4 states that we cannot have two negative premises, as the following syllogism illustrates.

No Muslims are Christians.	M e C
Some Muslims are not women.	M o W
∴ Some women are not Christians.	∴ W o C

An advantage in looking for the mood in a syllogism is that we can tell right away that a set of premises that are negative, such as e and o, imply no conclusion. The next rule is that if one premise is negative, the conclusion must be negative. Such a syllogism is likewise easy to spot in terms of its being either valid or invalid.

Finally, rule 5 says that we cannot have two universal premises followed by a particular conclusion.

All pets are tame animals.
No wild animals are tame animals.
∴ Some wild animals are not pets.

Schematically, this syllogism has this form:

P a T		P a M
W e T	or	S e M
∴ W o P		∴ S o P

This syllogism passes the first four rules, but not the fifth, because it contains two universal premises followed by a particular premise, called the Existential Fallacy. This syllogism is, therefore, invalid.

VENN DIAGRAMS FOR THE SYLLOGISM

A Venn diagram is not a proof, but illustrates a proof. To diagram a syllogism (see Fig. 9–6), we will use our earlier syllogisms:

Example:
No anemic persons are blood donors.
Some nurses are blood donors.
∴ Some nurses are not anemic.

Schematized, this takes the form:

AP e BD
N i BD
∴ N o AP

We diagram the conclusion, like eyeglasses, on top, with the middle term on the bottom.

We want to determine if the premises represent no more than the conclusion. So, we first take the top line, the major premise, AP e BD (making sure it is the premise that contains the major term plus the middle

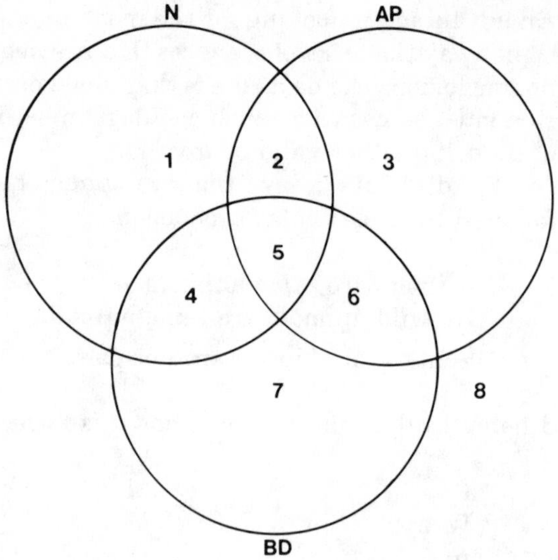

Figure 9-6. Schematic representation of syllogism.

AP = Anemic persons;
BD = Blood donor;
N = Nurses.

term), using circles AP and BD or regions 2, 3, 4, 5, 6, and 7; and covering part of circle N, as follows, and shade in regions 5 and 6 (see Fig. 9–7).

Proceeding to the next premise, the minor, N i BD, we put our hand over region 3 of circle AP, assuming for the moment that we are only dealing with circles N and BD.

The reason that our asterisk (see Fig. 9–8) is in region 4 rather than in regions 4 and 5 is that the major premise, first to be spoken for, calls

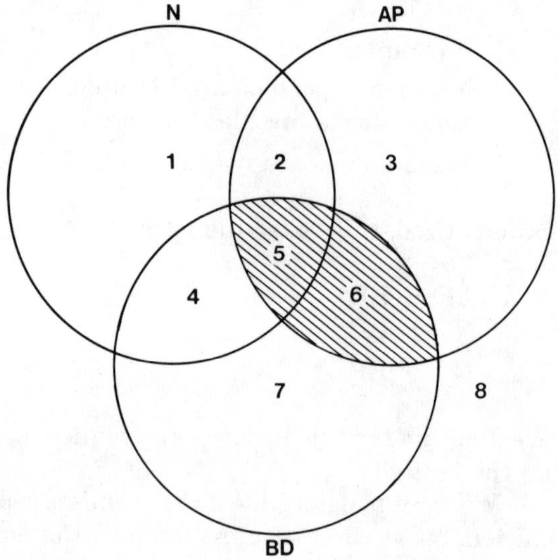

Figure 9-7. Venn diagram of major premise. AP e BD.

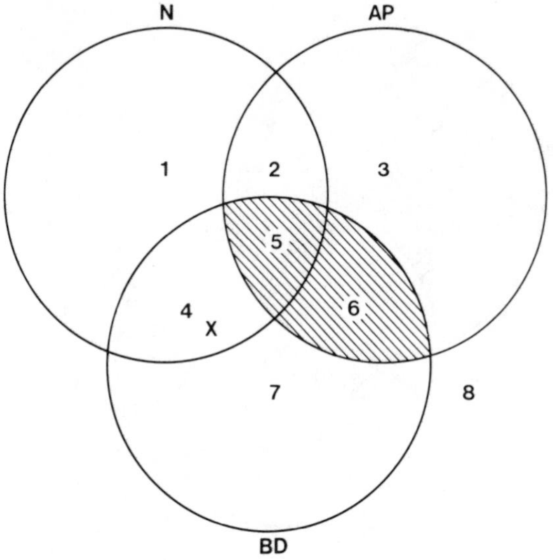

Figure 9-8. Test for conclusion. N o AP.

for regions 5 and 6 to be empty. For Venn diagrams, we add the rule that "emptiness wins." This means that if a region is empty and another Venn part conflicts with it by placing an asterisk in part of the empty region, the emptiness pushes the asterisk into the next region. Because the asterisk was originally in regions 4 and 5, it is pushed into region 4. Now we put the pen down and ask "Does the conclusion, N o AP, represent what I marked up in the premises?" In the conclusion, some N is represented as being outside AP. Therefore, this syllogism, as illustrated, appears valid.

We consider next the syllogism.

Example:
All nursing is intervention.
No intervention is passive.
∴ No nursing is passive.

Schematized, this takes the form:

N a I
I e P
∴ N e P

To analyze this syllogism, we use the checklist of rules. The middle term *intervention* is distributed in the minor premise. The predicate of the conclusion, *passive*, is distributed in the conclusion, an E proposition. But it is also distributed in the minor premise. The subject of the conclusion,

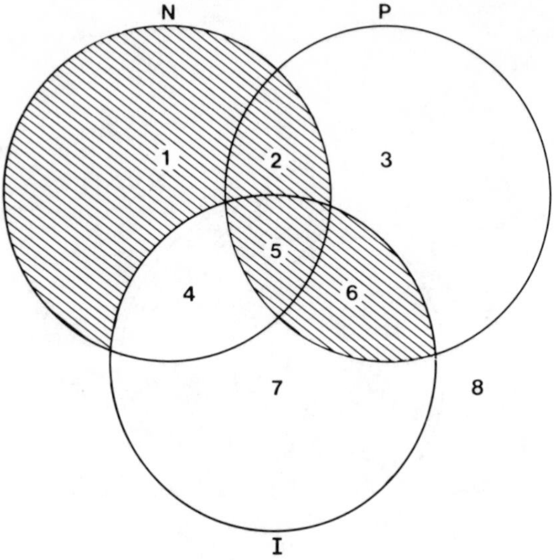

Figure 9–9. Test for validity of conclusion. N e P.
N = Nursing;
I = Intervention;
P = Passive.

nursing, is also distributed. But it is also distributed in the major premise, "All nursing is intervention." The conclusion, following a negative premise, is negative. Therefore, the syllogism is valid. We may check this with a Venn diagram (see Fig. 9–9). To be valid, regions 2 and 5 need to be shaded. They are.

Example:
All nursing is intervention.
All intervention is active.
∴ All nursing is active.

Schematized, this takes the form:

N a I
I a A
∴ N a A

Again *intervention* is the middle term; and it is distributed, this time in the minor premise or second line. The term *nursing*, the subject of the conclusion, the minor term, is distributed in the conclusion. But it is also distributed in the major premise or the top line. Using our checklist, this syllogism passes all five rules. We may note that there are no negative premises; therefore, the conclusion is, quite correctly, affirmative. As for the fifth rule, the premises are universal, and so is the conclusion. Therefore, this syllogism is valid.

The Venn diagram for this example is shown in Figure 9–10. For this

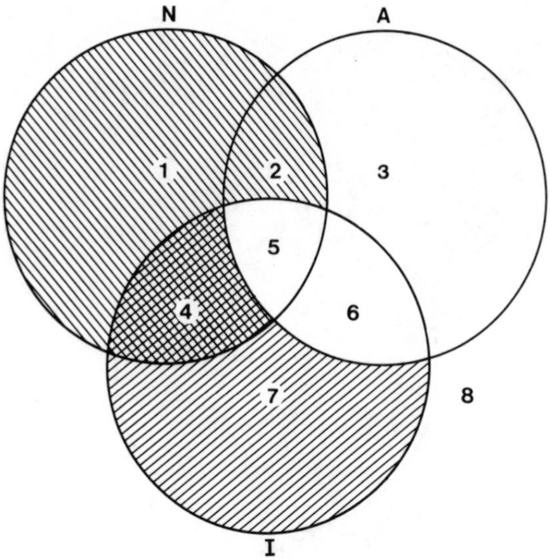

Figure 9–10. Test for conclusion. N a A.
N = Nursing;
I = Intervention;
A = Active.

syllogism to be valid, regions 1 and 4 need to be shaded, meaning that they are empty. They are. Here is how it works: We take circles N and I, and say, as the major premise states it, "All nursing is intervention," or "All N's are I's." "All N's are inside I," involving regions 4, 5, 6, and 7, where all the N's of regions 1, 2, 4, and 5 are put. Next, we take the minor premise, "All I's are A," and place all the I's of regions 4 and 7 into circle A. For the syllogism to be valid, the conclusion, "All N's are A's" should be represented accurately. If "All N's are A's," regions 1 and 4 should be empty. They are. Therefore, the syllogism is valid.

Let's consider the next syllogism:

Example:
All psychotherapists are health professionals.
All nurses are health professionals.
∴ All nurses are psychotherapists.

We schematize this to read:

P a H	or	P a HP
N a H		N a HP
∴ N a P		∴ N a P

The checklist of syllogistic rules shows that, because an A proposition does not distribute its predicate, the middle term H is undistributed. Therefore, the syllogism is invalid.

A Venn diagram is shown in Figure 9–11. Region 4 is unshaded

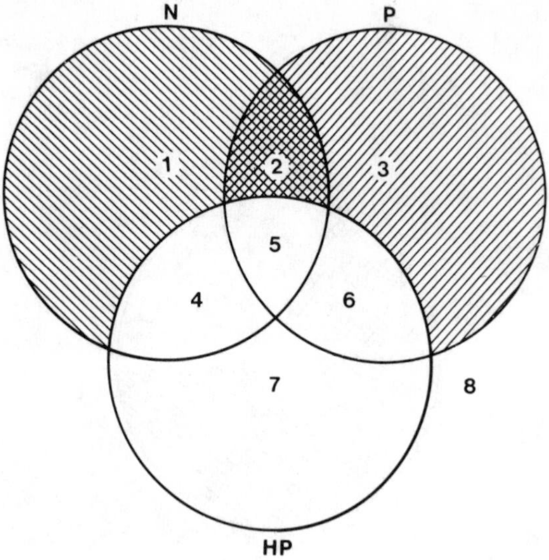

Figure 9-11. Test for validity of conclusion. N e P.
N = Nursing;
P = Psychotherapists;
HP = Health professionals.

according to the indications of the two premises; therefore, the syllogism is invalid.

Exercises

Schematize the following syllogisms, then determine by the rules whether they are valid or not; and then apply Venn diagrams to illustrate their validity or invalidity.

1. All mismanaged enterprises are unprofitable ventures.
No hospitals are unprofitable ventures.

∴ No hospitals are mismanaged enterprises.

Answer: M a V
H e V
∴ H e M (Second figure, a e e, valid.)

2. No nursing is ever restful.
All restful activities are pleasurable.

Answer: N e R
R a P
N e P (Fourth figure, illicit major, invalid.)

3. No persons who burn out make good leaders.
Some nurses make good leaders.

∴ Some nurses are not persons who burn out.

Answer: P e L
N i L
∴ N o p (Second figure, e i o, valid.)

4. All communication is a form of interaction.
All nursing is a form of interaction.

∴ All nursing is a form of communication.[8]

Answer: C a I
N a I
N a C (Second figure, a a a, undistributed middle, invalid.)

5. All protective body responses work to establish homeostasis.
Some pain is a protective body response.

∴ Some pain works to establish homeostasis.[9]

Answer: B a H
P i B
∴ P i H (First figure, a i i, valid.)

6. Nursing is indispensable to health care.
The nursing process is indispensable to nursing.

∴ The nursing process is indispensable to health care.

Answer: N a H
P a N
∴ P a H (First figure, a a a, valid.)

7. Test the following syllogistic forms by constructing propositions to fill the schemata, and then examine by using the syllogistic rules, and by Venn diagrams.

a. AAE-1
b. AEO-2
c. OAO-3
d. EIO-2
e. IAE-1
f. EAO-4
g. EAE-3
h. EIO-2
i. AOO-4
j. AEE-4

Answers for a to j:

a. M a P
S a M
S e P
(Illicit major)

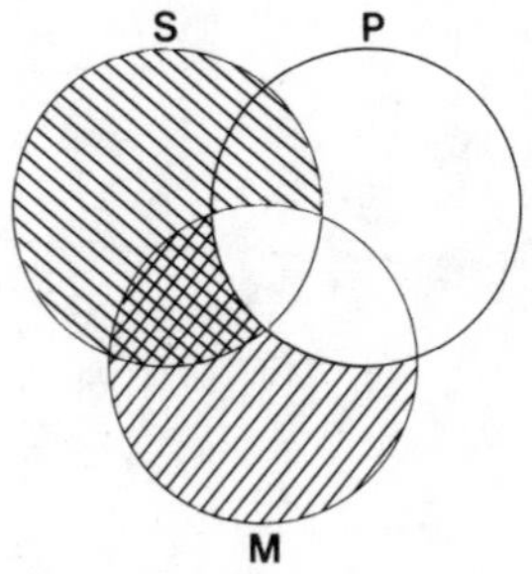

b. P a M
S e M
―――――
S o P
(Existential fallacy)

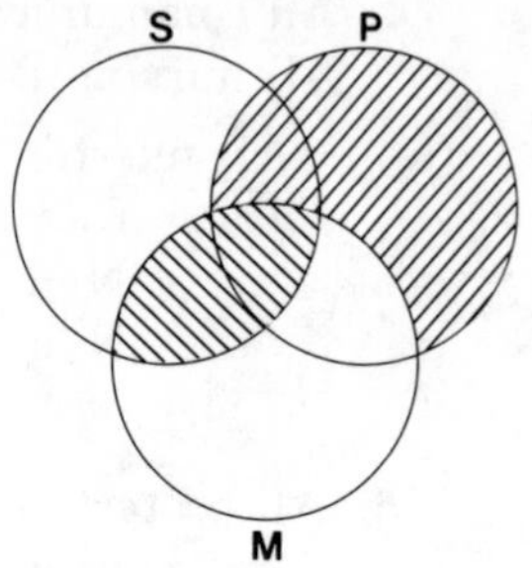

c. M o P
M a S
―――――
S o P
(Passes all syllogistic rules, valid)

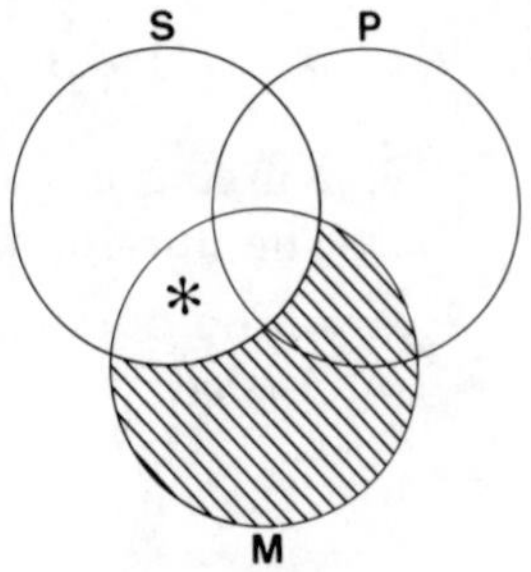

d. P e M
S i M
―――――
S o P
(Passes all syllogistic rules, valid)

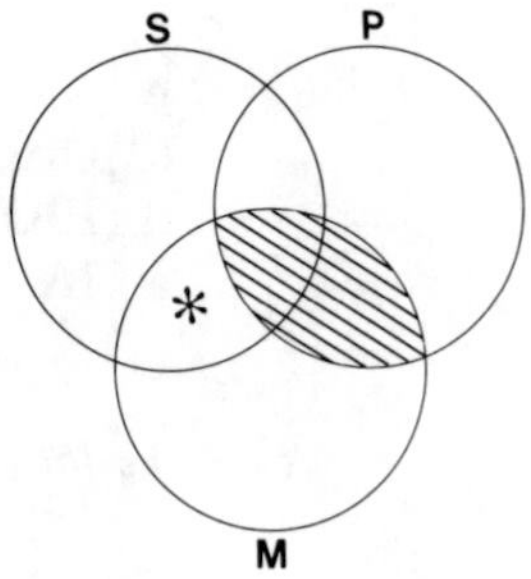

e. M i P
S a M
―――――
S e P
(Undistributed middle, illicit major)

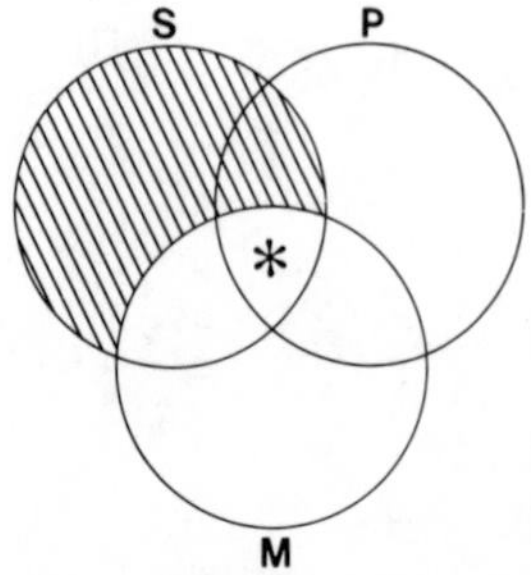

f. P e M
M a S
S o P
(Existential fallacy)

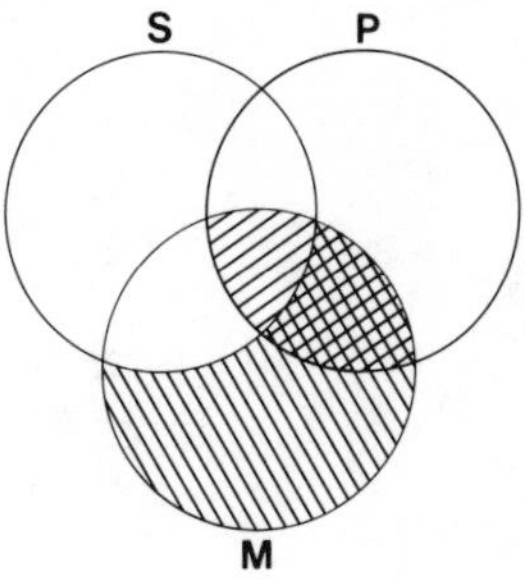

g. M e P
M a S
S e P
(Illicit minor)

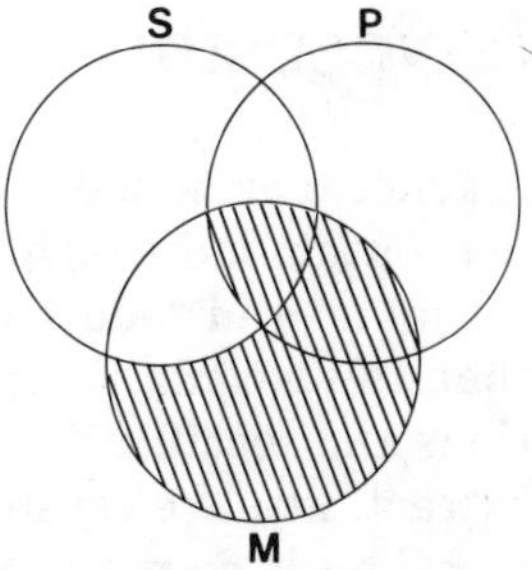

h. P e M
S i M
S o P
(Passes all rules, valid)

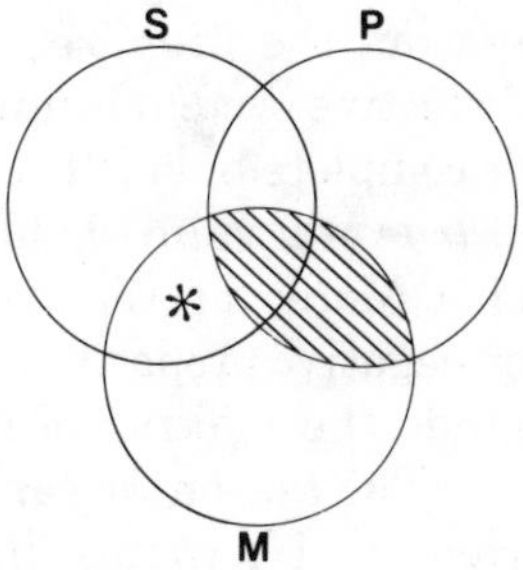

i. P a M
M o S
S o P
(Undistributed middle)

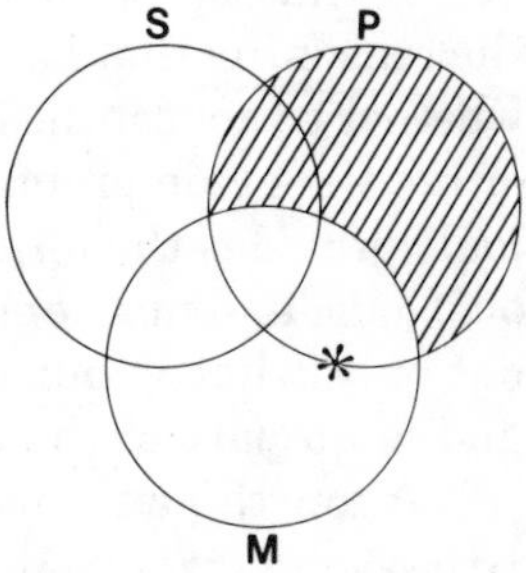

j. P a M
M e s
———
S e P

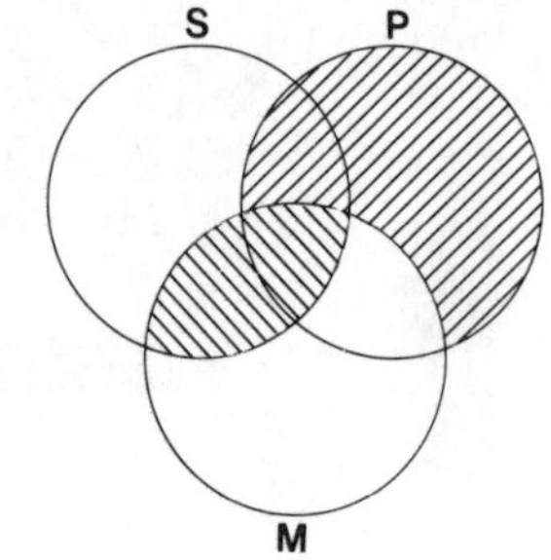

CONCLUSION

A general principle we may draw is that a valid deductive argument does not contain more terms than there are in the premises. A second principle is that a valid deductive argument is certain, due solely to its form rather than to its content. The form of a deductive argument consists in definitions and specifications of terms for specialized purposes of explicating an extract, idealized system, one that guides rational thinking somewhat as a cookbook may guide practice.

A third principle we may draw from a valid, deductive system is that it is self-enclosed. The definitions. specifications, and rules are adequate to generate a system of inferences without external reference. For this reason, the premises, if assumed true, validly imply the conclusion. A deductive system is unlike an inductive system, which is never self-enclosed or complete by itself. The premises, assumed true, in a special logical sense of *true* of a valid, deductive argument, guarantee the truth of the conclusion. Moreover, the major premise in a syllogism or a universal affirmative or negative proposition, A and E, function as covering rule principles, which guide the making of valid inferences.

The reason we can count on a deductive argument is explained by Carl Hempel. He writes that "it is a basic principle of scientific inquiry that no proposition and no theory is to be accepted without adequate grounds."[10] Barbara Stevens points out that "the criterion of logical development requires that every conclusion set forth in a theory logically follows from the reasoning that has preceded it . . . Logical development has to do with whether or not conclusions can be derived from given premises, not whether or not the given premises or conclusions are themselves true.[11] Deductive logic provides the forms into which to insert the facts. As Hempel points out, logic and mathematics are like an orange juice extractor. It squeezes out only what is put into the machine by way of the facts of the world, and is no part of the oranges.[12]

A fourth principle we may draw is that the presentation of a deductive system gives us the opportunity to achieve training in certainty, which is indispensable to training in uncertainty. To achieve training in uncertainty is to have training in the difference between certainty and uncertainty. To reiterate an earlier example, if A is bigger than B and if B is bigger than C, we know that, therefore, A is bigger than C. We cannot validly conclude, however, that A is, therefore, bigger than D. This is what we mean by a system of proof. The conclusion could not be other than what it is; and only because the premises provide sufficient grounds for rationally compelling the acceptance of the conclusion.

Deduction consists in explicating or translating what we already know. There are myriad examples around us, such as that three strikes imply that one is out in baseball, unless the catcher drops the ball; or the king in chess may only move one square at a time; or for X to be a triangle means it has to have three enclosed sides. As Einstein once put this similar insight, "As far as the laws of mathematics refer to reality, they are not certain, and as far as they are certain, they do not refer to reality."[13]

REFERENCES

1. Whitehead, A. Science and the Modern World. New York: Mentor, 1948, pp. 20–39.
2. Kaplan, A. Sociology Learns the Language of Mathematics, in Wiener, P. (Ed.), Readings in Philosophy of Science, New York: Charles Scribner and Sons, 1953, pp. 394–412.
3. Hospers, J. An Introduction to Philosophical Analysis (2nd ed.). Englewood Cliffs, N.J.: Prentice Hall, 1967, pp. 250–252.
4. Toulmin, S. The Philosophy of Science. London: Hutchinson's University Press, 1953, pp. 99–104.
5. Mendelsohn, R., & Schwartz, L. Basic Logic. Englewood Cliffs, N.J.: Prentice Hall, 1987, pp. 20–32.
6. Barker, S. Elements of Logic (4th ed.). New York: McGraw Hill, 1985, pp. 57–60.
7. Stevens, B. Nursing Theory (2nd ed.). Boston: Little Brown, 1984, p. 61.
8. Ibid.
9. Ibid, p. 62.
10. Hempel, C. On The Nature of Mathematical Truth, in Feigl, H., & Sellars, W. (Eds.), Readings in Philosophical Analysis. New York: Appleton-Century-Crofts, 1949, p. 222.
11. Stevens, B. Nursing Theory, pp. 60, 62.
12. Hempel, C. On The Nature of Mathematical Truth, in Feigl, H. & Sellars, W. (Eds.), Readings in Philosophical Analysis, p. 235.
13. Hempel, C. Geometry and Empirical Science (Einstein quoted by Hempel), in Feigl, H. & Sellars, W. (Eds.), Readings in Philosophical Analysis. New York: Appleton-Century-Crofts, 1949, p. 249.

Chapter 10

Symbolic Reasoning

Study of this chapter enables the learner to:

1. Use symbolic logic as a tool of thinking critically about nursing judgments.
2. Use conjunctions, disjunctions, implications, and truth tables in thinking critically about nursing judgments.
3. Justify particular arguments in nursing through the use of rules of inference in symbolic logic, such as hypothetical and disjunctive syllogisms.
4. Analyze and construct dilemmas that arise in nursing practice.
5. Make inferences in nursing with the help of simplification, conjunction, addition, and short-cut methods.
6. Make natural deductions that apply to nursing judgments.
7. Use symbolic logic to distinguish good from bad nursing arguments.

INTRODUCTION

Although AEIO logic (universal affirmative, negative, particular affirmative, and negative) is helpful in characterizing the relation between categorical propositions that apply to nursing, all propositions do not come in AEIO form. Propositions that are used in nursing also come in other forms, such as if–then propositions, propositions prefaced with *unless,* and propositions having the form *either–or*. Although AEIO or syllogistic logic is useful up to a point, there are other sentences, that are better rendered through a more modern logical system, namely symbolic logic.

There are arguments using if–then forms that are not represented by the categorical syllogism. Modern symbolic logic makes use of propositions and logical connectives to represent *or,* a disjunction, *and,* a conjunction, and *not,* a negation. Symbolic logic is a more effective tool for handling some kinds of inferences in modern science and technology, including clinical aspects and even value judgments in nursing.

HOW SYMBOLIC LOGIC IS USEFUL TO NURSING

One reason for studying symbolic deduction is that nurses can extend, strengthen, and deepen their inferential powers. Although classical logic is useful up to a point, it is inflexible in its use of four forms to render propositions. This results in limits imposed on evaluating arguments. Modern symbolic logic provides flexibility in translating propositions into symbolic notation. This offers a distinct advantage over the older, rigid AEIO formulation.

Rendering sentences, using logical connectives, such as implication, if–then, conjunction (two propositions connected by *and*), disjunction (two propositions connected by *or*), negation, using *not,* provides advantages over syllogistic logic. Rendering sentences in these ways, when combined with other sentences in argument form, helps set them up for evaluation as either valid or invalid. The use of propositions with logical connectives to generate arguments enables us to expand our inferential powers beyond our unaided intuitions and beyond the limits imposed by the four-form structure of syllogistic logic.

An analogy may help a nursing student of symbolic logic to appreciate the extent of its conceptual power. The analogy is made to the airline industry. People who fly commercially recognize the value of instrument flying and landing over the use of direct observation. Direct observation is limited as in foggy weather. Even in good weather, direct sighting is limited to our visual perimeter. The use of instruments to guide takeoffs, flights, and landings provides far more accuracy and a broader data base than does a pilot's visual acuity. With the use of symbolic reasoning, therefore, we acquire a conceptual power that frees us from the limits of using direct intuition to determine validity. Syllogistic logic provides some conceptual advantages over direct intuition. Syllogistic logic has the disadvantage, however, of inflexible limits, analogous to primitive instrument landing assistance. In contrast, symbolic logic, with its flexible use of natural language connectives, such as *or, and, if–then,* and *negation* offers a powerful conceptual basis for evaluating the use of arguments.

The usefulness of symbolic reasoning to nursing includes nurses knowing what they may not infer as valid, as well as knowing how to infer what is valid. For once an argument is correctly judged invalid, it is pointless to continue with either premises or conclusions of such arguments, even though they may be true. If an argument is shown to be invalid, its components have no formal or structural value. Without structural value, it is useless to pursue the component parts of a nursing argument. If we know how to use symbolic reasoning, we can evaluate nursing arguments; eliminate bad reasoning in nursing; construct or generate arguments; and strengthen nursing judgments. By improving the quality of nursing judgments, we thereby improve the quality of nursing care. The use of symbolic reasoning helps us to structure arguments, thus organizing and converting isolated fragments into meaningful wholes, which comprise the bases of sound nursing judgments.

Symbolic logic also provides added ways to determine the validity or invalidity of an argument, such as truth tables, the short-cut method, and most ingenious of all, *natural deduction,* a method of generating new and also valid inferences on the basis of a few rules and assumptions that are presented as *given.*

APPLYING INCLUSIVE AND EXCLUSIVE USES OF "OR" TO NURSING JUDGMENTS

There are two uses of the disjunction *or.* The word or may be used inclusively, as in Nurse Smith gave either acetaminophen *or* codeine. In the inclusive use, the nurse could give one or both medications. The sentence would still be true, whether the nurse gave one or both. The word or, however, may also be used in an exclusive sense, as in "Either Smith gave acetaminophen or morphine, but not both." In the exclusive sense, choosing one rules out the other. Restaurant menus give people a choice of main dishes, meaning that we may choose one but not both. In joining a religion, a profession, a spouse, a full-time workplace, the exclusive sense of *or* is appropriate.

Some nursing judgments involve the inclusive use of *or,* whereas others involve the exclusive use. The reader who recalls the distinction between a contradictory and a contrary knows that in a contradiction, one alternative totally excludes the other. For Nurse Jones to give Mr. Andrews, a severe, emergency, hot-water burn victim, "cool, sterile, saline soaks to the burn area" rules out applying "ice packs to the burn area" or applying "vaseline gauze."[1] An indicated intervention excludes one that is contraindicated. But a nurse who does not apply critical thinking may not distinguish a contradictory from a contrary. If a physician tells a patient, "Have this operation or die," or if a nursing supervisor says, "Either work or you'll be fired," both may be ignoring other options, which a contrary does not rule out. A patient may find an alternative in the form of a new medication; and a nurse may go on strike but negotiate, and not be fired.

A contrary use of *or* may mask the exclusive use, as in a mugger's threat, "Your money or your life," whereas it may not be either the one or the other.

Or in the exclusive sense places a more severe limit on our choices. But *or* also facilitates decision making. If it is not our choice, it is the other. Effective decision making may require the narrowing of choices to two, an either–or choice, that may take the form of true or false. Some scientists point to the advantages of converting "What is?" type of questions, such as "What is diabetes?" into "yes or no" questions or conditional questions, such as: "If one has sugar in the urine, does that imply diabetes?" The form of the answer, yes or no, true or false, in the exclusive sense of *or* narrows down the job of decision making.

There are valid exclusive uses of or in nursing. If a patient has a spinal surgery, a nurse may be taught either to keep the patient on a flat surface or raise the head of the bed. This may be symbolized: F ∨ R (F = Flat; ∨ = or; R = raise); F /∴ –R (F = Flat; /∴ = therefore).* Other symbols are: – = not; R = raise. The formula says: Either keep the patient on a flat surface or raise the head of the bed. Place the patient on a flat surface. Therefore, do not raise the head of the bed. The exclusive *or* rule is that if one disjunct is true, the other is false, and vice versa. Or if a patient has a broken neck, a nurse is taught to move the whole patient like a log and is told "not to move the parts of the body." We may restate this: For a patient with a broken neck, move the whole patient like a log or move the parts of the patient. Move the whole patient. Therefore, don't move the parts. Symbolized, it reads: W ∨ P, W /∴ –P. (W = Whole; ∨ = or; /∴ = therefore; – = not; P = parts. According to the exclusive use of *or*, if one disjunct is true, the other is false, and vice versa.

There are also valid inclusive uses of *or* in nursing. For example, a nurse is taught that if a patient is in shock from loss of blood, always lower the patient's head or raise the patient's legs. A nurse could do both. Lowering the head does not rule out raising the legs. Here, the inclusive use of *or* is at work.

There are occasions, however, when the exclusive use of *or* leads one to the black or white thinking fallacy. A supervisor who tells a nurse, "Either you stay an extra shift or don't bother to come back," is an example. A physician who says to a patient, "Either you have a coronary bypass or you'll be dead within two years," may be leaving out medical alternatives that may be as effective as surgery. To avoid the black or white thinking fallacy and confusing a contrary with a contradiction, the inclusive use of *or* is generally adopted, unless we can show that the exclusive sense is appropriate.

To return to the question whether there is medical or nursing diagnosis, we can use *or* in the inclusive or exclusive senses. Some nurs-

---

* A virgule (/) is used if the conclusion and at least one premise are on the same line. Three dots (∴) after the virgule symbolize or are abbreviatory for "therefore."

ing scholars claim that the exclusive model of nursing diagnosis applies. We may, however, recognize an advantage to the inclusive model, applying here. According to this use of or, diagnosis is medical or nursing, or both. A critical thinking skill in nursing is knowing which use of *or* is appropriate.

Exercises

Determine if the inclusive or exclusive use of *or* applies; and if it is exclusive, which fallacy, if any, is committed.

1. a. Better dead than red.
   b. Better red than dead.
   Answer: Exclusive, black or white fallacy.
2. Either you or your husband have to sign the consent to operate form for your 8-year-old child.
   Answer: Inclusive use, one or both.
3. Either take your insulin injection or you are likely to die.
   Answer: Exclusive use seems generally appropriate here.
4. A probable nursing diagnosis of thyroid hormone excess includes (1) Alteration in cardiac output; (2) alteration in nutrition; (3) sleep pattern disturbance; (4) alteration in thought processes; (5) potential impairment of skin integrity; (6) potential for injury; (7) alteration in bowel elimination; (8) diarrhea.[2] Do the above "diagnoses" presuppose *or* in the exclusive or inclusive sense?
   Answer: Inclusive, one or more are tended to be included in the probably nursing diagnoses.
5. For a nurse teaching Eugene to inject himself with insulin, the best method for entering the subcutaneous tissue is: (1) stretch the skin to make it taut. (2) Hold the skin so that it remains relaxed. (3) Compress the skin by pinching. (4) Do not touch the skin after wiping with an alcohol swab.[3] In this question, which use of *or* is the examiner assuming?
   Answer: The exclusive use of *or*. The answer is (3); and the student is expected to rule out (1), (2), and (4). Pinching the skin ensures that the injection will enter the subcutaneous fatty layer beneath the dermis.[4]

RECOGNIZING ARGUMENTS BY FORMS

A function of symbolic reasoning is to extend our intuitive inferences beyond our native powers. In this sense, logic is to critical thinking what the magnifying glass is to the naked eye. Both syllogistic and symbolic logic extend our inferential powers.

One form of reasoning, an extension of disjunction, is called the disjunctive syllogism. For example, Nurse Smith either gives Jones acetaminophen or codeine. She does not give the first. Therefore, she gives Jones the second. Symbolically, this example of the disjunctive syllogism reads as follows: (A v C) & −A /∴ C, where A = acetaminophen, C = codeine, v = or; & = and; − = not; /∴ = then; therefore, or so. Here, A or C are the two disjuncts. What this formula says is that if of two alternatives in the inclusive sense, it is not the first (in this case A), then it must be the second (C). In the inclusive use of or Nurse Smith could give both acetaminophen and codeine. But on the basis of the inclusive use of or, if she does not give Jones, the patient, acetaminophen, then she gives codeine. It is valid to assert C on the basis of −A (not A). But in the inclusive use of or, it is not valid to assert A and then deny C, since it is not one or the other. The inclusive use of or asserts that one or both values is true; and that if one is false or denied, then the remaining disjunct must be true for the argument to be valid.

The generalized form of the disjunctive syllogism reads: P v Q, −P /∴ Q. We can substitute examples, such as A v C, and if used correctly, come out with valid arguments. How do we know this and other logical forms are valid? We know this by the truth tables.

TRUTH TABLES

A truth table is a way to evaluate whether an argument is valid or invalid. We proceed by assigning a truth value of T or F to any proposition (P). As P can be either true or false, and we want to cover all possibilities for P, our truth table for P, one letter, is this:

P
T
F

If we want a truth table for the negation of P, it will have the opposite truth values and look like this:

−P
F
T

P and −P (not P) will look like this:

	P	−P
Line 1	T	F
Line 2	F	T

Line 1 reads: P is true: −P is false. Line 2 reads: P is false; and −P is true. If P is true, −P is false, and if P is false, −P is true. −P is the contradictory of P.

Truth tables depend on how many letters or propositions there are. As most arguments make use of two or more propositions, it is helpful to indicate how many lines of alternative truth values are required. A useful rule to follow is this:

For 1 letter $2^1 = 2$ truth value assignments.
For 2 letters $2^2 = 4$ truth value assignments.
For 3 letters $2^3 = 8$ truth value assignments.
For 4 letters $2^4 = 16$ truth value assignments.[5]

We now illustrate how a truth table works by returning to one of our initial problems. Ms. Smith gives either acetaminophen or codeine. She does not give the first, therefore, she gives the second. We symbolize this as follows: A v C, −A /∴C. We now assign truth values:

	A	C	−A	(A	v	C)	&	−A	/∴	C	(A v C)	&	−A	/∴	C
Line 1	T	T	F	T		T		F		T	T	F	F	T	T
Line 2	F	T	T	F		T		T		T	T	T	T	T	T
Line 3	T	F	F	T		F		F		F	T	F	F	T	F
Line 4	F	F	T	F		F		T		F	F	F	T	T	F
											1	3	2	5	4

An explanation of this truth table may show why this is a valid argument. As there are two different propositions, A and C, with −A as the contradictory of A, there are four lines of truth tables. In the far left, lines 1 through 4, all possible truth value combinations are cited. In the middle is the formulation of the problem, with initial truth values cited, consistent with the truth value assignments of the far left. On the right, the problem is worked out, using rules for disjunction, or, conjunction, and, and implication. To arrive at the conclusion in column 5, we first use columns 1 and 2 to arrive at 3, and then use columns 3 and 4 to arrive at the truth values of 5. Later, as conjunction and implication are explicated, the proof in this sample problem will become clearer. A helpful way to learn how to use a truth table is to understand the definitions of key logical connectives, such as disjunction, conjunction, and implication. A disjunction is true in the inclusive sense, the one used in the above truth table, *if one or both disjuncts are true, and false otherwise,* that is, if both disjuncts are false. In the sample problem, Ms. Smith did not give acetaminophen, but she gave codeine; therefore, one of the disjuncts is true. Next, we explain conjunction.

CONJUNCTION

A conjunction is true only if all of the conjuncts are true together. If any conjunct is false, the entire conjunction is false. For example, in recommending nursing procedures for women in labor, nurses are frequently taught prescriptions intended to be taken in conjunction. To prevent infection nurses are taught to "(1) wash hands scrupulously; (2) wear cover gown, scrub clothes, hair and shoe covers; (3) use sterile gloves for vaginal examinations, inspection of the introitus; (4) take temperature every four hours; (5) . . . if ordered, shave pubic area gently using sterile equipment; (6) place disposable pads under buttocks and remove promptly when soiled; (7) use antiseptic solution to prepare perineal area for delivery."[6] A nurse is expected to follow all of these inclusively; not choose which one or more of these procedures to follow. This is an example of a conjunctive prescription.

In caring for the client with cardiac surgery, a nurse follows a conjunction of procedures. She is told to "(1) inspect suture line(s); (2) observe for bleeding from body orifices; (3) monitor vital signs . . . ; (4) check skin for signs of hemorrhagic areas; (5) assess for abdominal pain; (6) report bright red blood from chest tubes, urinary catheter, and/or nasogastric tube; (7) monitor coagulation profile . . ."[7] A nurse follows all of these procedures. In this example, a nurse also uses a conjunction of propositions in formulating a nursing care plan.

Similarly, a nurse treating a diabetes patient looks for "(1) fluid volume deficit; (2) alteration in nutrition; (3) alteration in tissue perfusion; (4) potential for injury; (5) potential for infection; (6) potential impairment of skin integrity; (7) sensory perceptual alteration . . ."[8] Diseases are also diagnosed by noticing a conjunction of signs and symptoms. A conjunction is true only if all of its parts together are true. A truth table for conjunction looks like this:

	P	&	Q
Line 1	T	T	T
Line 2	F	F	T
Line 3	T	F	F
Line 4	F	F	F

We first put combinations of TFTF under P, and TTFF under Q. Then we look at line 1 under P and under Q. As we note two T's, the conjunction or & sign makes this true. But in line 2, we note that P has an F and Q has a T, therefore, the conjunction under & is false. Line 3 also has one false, namely Q; and line 4 has both P and Q false; therefore, the conjunction is false in line 4.

Now we can return to our initial problem, A v C, −A /∴ C; and notice why there are four F's under column 3. The conjunct propositions from which the conjunction is derived have at least one false proposition; therefore, the conjunction is false. We turn next to an important principle associated with conjunction, the principle of exclusion, and another useful basis for valid decision making in nursing.

EXCLUSION

Conjunction implies an additional rule for decision making that is applicable to nursing called exclusion. Using another example, if a mother brings her 2-year-old daughter, Armanda, into the emergency room with a half-empty bottle of aspirin and says, "Armanda ate the rest," the nurse should immediately do the following: ". . . give her 15 milliters of ipecac syrup and a large glass of water."[9] The nurse should not immediately "prepare her for gastric lavage."[10] We have the propositions: (I) The nurse gives Armanda "15 millileters of ipecac syrup, a large glass of water." (G) "Prepare her for a gastric lavage." (We abbreviate these as I and G to identify key terms in these propositions, where I = giving ipecac syrup, and G = preparing Armanda for gastric lavage.)

We can use the exclusion formula[11] and symbolize this problem as follows: – (I & G), meaning not both I and G. We have I; therefore not G. The exclusion principle applied to this problem reads: [– (I & G), I] / ∴ – G. Exclusion is another valid reasoning type or pattern that says that if two values P and Q, or I and G, "are not both true, and one is true, the other has to be false."[12] This can be proved with a truth table. The exclusion principle, based on conjunction, is an important form of decision making, and provides an alternative to the exclusive use of *or.*

To complete an explanation of our initial problem, A v C, – A /∴ C, we need one more logical operator, the rule for using implication. Now, we turn to implication.

IMPLICATION

We recognize that all roads of reasoning lead to implication. Whether it is the assertion of a proposition, its negation, double negation, disjunction, conjunction, or the principle or exclusion, an argument is only complete with the help of implication. The all important word *therefore, or so, or then* in an if–then relation, refers to the logical passageway between premises and conclusion. To evaluate whether an argument is valid or not, we need to examine the relation between the *if* and the *then,* the antecedent and the consequent or conclusion of an argument. This relation is clearer in symbolic reasoning than in syllogistic reasoning.

There are various ways the word *implication* is used. For convenience, we distinguish six kinds of implications: (1) definitional implication, such as "nursing implies the nursing process;" (2) logical implication,[13] such as, If the nurse gives this patient an effective pain reliever, then this arthritic patient is willing to walk, and if this patient is willing to walk, then his or her circulation and morale will improve. Therefore, if the nurse gives an effective pain reliever, then both the patient's circulation and morale will improve. (3) Causal implication,[14] occurs if one or more actors bring about an effect. If a person has an absence of vitamin C in the diet, low bodily resistance, and poor bodily hygiene, then that person is more apt to catch a cold than otherwise. Or if Nurse Lee successfully teaches Mr. Jones to follow his diet, test his urine, administer insulin accurately, maintain hygiene, exercise, and comply with follow-up care, then Mr. Jones will control his diabetes. (4) A significant meaning in an act, as when Ms. Hackish asks, "What does my involvement with dying patients imply?" or "What is the meaning of keeping these patients alive?" Questions of life and death compel health professionals to consider the implications of human actions.

The distinctions between the idea or implication as a clue or suggestion, as a strong cause–effect relation, as a purpose, intention, or motive, and as a reference to a significance add to the usefulness of referring to implication in nursing.

(5) Practical implication or suggestion is, for example, if a nurse asks a patient, "Would you like me to pull the curtain?" The nurse implies or suggests that the patient might want to void. Or if a patient says, "My pills are on the table," the suggestion is to give them to the patient. Nursing implications are frequently practical, situational, and "here and now." (6) Technical meaning, also called material implication,[15] governs the validity and soundness of implications. Technically, an implication is made up of an antecedent and a consequent. In a technical sense, to use an implication is to assert that if the antecedent is true, the consequent likewise is true. If Mr. Lee, a licensed professional nurse, is on duty at his nursing station, then he is responsible for the nursing care of his assigned patients. If we assert the implication, or even assume it, then the antecedent, "Mr. Lee, a professional nurse is on duty," is assumed to be true. If the antecedent is true, then the conclusion, "He is responsible for the nursing care of his assigned patients," is also true for the implication to be valid.

If Mr. Lee changes the position of Mr. Jay, an immobilized patient, every 30 minutes, then this will prevent Mr. Jay from getting decubiti. If Mr. Lee moves Mr. Jay every 30 minutes and Mr. Jay still gets bed sores, then the antecedent is true, but the consequent is false. We have, then a $T \rightarrow F$ in the antecedent consequent relation, meaning that the antecedent is true, but the consequent is false. This forces us to consider other causes of decubiti. Perhaps, Mr. Lee should secure an alternating pressure mattress for Mr. Jay. A $T \rightarrow F$ relation suggests another cause of action to the one expressed in an implication. What we want in a valid and sound nursing implication relation is a T → T in both the antecedent and the consequent. This is a useful way of testing nursing interventions such as the examples cited.

Holding a nurse responsible in the antecedent is also a way of holding a nurse accountable for the consequences of a nursing action or inaction. In the landmark Illinois case, *Charlestown Community Memorial Hospital v. Dorrence Kenneth Darling*, 1965,[16] the nurse and a physician were held accountable for failing to report the signs and symptoms of leg gangrene from an improperly applied cast. The implication is: if a nurse is responsible for giving competent nursing care, then the nurse is required to report signs and symptoms of dysfunction and alteration of body functions. The antecedent was true, but the nurse failed to fulfil the requirements of the consequent. So, we have here a T → F relation between both parts of an implication. For an antecedent to imply a consequent means that if the antecedent is true, the consequent likewise is true.

Unlike causal, definitional, or practical implications, in a material implication, there needs to be no connection between the antecedent and the consequent. For example, "If 2 + 5 = 8, then nurses are the only health professionals who work around the clock." In material implication, if one or more premises are false, and the conclusion is either true or false, the argument is valid. In a valid material implication, if the premises are true, the conclusion is also true.

We sometimes use a material implication to cast doubt on the truth of the antecedent. For example, a speaker who is skeptical of faith healing or therapeutic touch may say, "If Smith can cure cancer by therapeutic touch, then I'm the Prophet Elijah." The speaker's intention is to deny the truth of the antecedent namely that therapeutic touch cures cancer; and the speaker does so by denying the consequent, that he or she is the Prophet Elijah.

According to the technical definition of material implication, if the antecedent or set of premises is false, the consequent may be either true or false, and the argument will, in either event, be valid. In a valid argument, therefore, the antecedent is either false or the consequent is true. Material implication provides a basic rule in helping us evaluate between valid and invalid deductions. The function of material implication is to provide a criterion to test the validity of any argument. The criterion is that in a valid argument, if the antecedent is true, the conclusion is also true. If an argument has a true premise or premises, followed by a false conclusion, the argument is invalid. If an argument has a false premise, the conclusion may be either true or false for the argument to be valid. For example, in the argument, "If all snakes are poisonous, then rattlesnakes are poisonous,"[17] the antecedent is false, but the consequent is true. This argument is valid. Moreover, the antecedent and consequent have no logical connection to one another. Similarly, "If all nurses have BAs, then college level nursing instructors have BAs" presents another valid use of material implication. Here, the antecedent is false, and the consequent is true; and the argument is valid. We could also say, "If all nurses have BAs, then practical nurses have BAs," which has both a false antecedent and a false consequent, and yet is a valid use of material implication.

Exercises

Distinguish the following types of implication.

1. Nurse Clark is enrolled in a required course, Foundations of Nursing, which is a prerequisite for adult nursing. Adult nursing is a prerequisite for psychiatric nursing. Therefore, foundations of nursing is a prerequisite for psychiatric nursing.
   Answer: Logical implication.
2. If there is diabetes, then there is inadequate insulin secretion.[18]
   Answer: Definition implication.
3. Nurse Stone works with brain-impaired people. The brain impaired are dysfunctional. Therefore, Ms. Stone works with dysfunctional people.
   Answer: Logical implication.
4. If Mundy is a bronchitis patient in a mist tent, to the professional nurse this implies that she has to change Mundy's clothes frequently so that they remain dry.[19]
   Answer: Practical implication.
5. The presence of bradycardia and rising blood pressure implies that intracranial pressure is increasing.[20]
   Answer: Causal implication.
6. Hypertension implies having a persistent elevation of blood pressure at or above 140 mmHg systolic, 90 mmHg diastolic in adults.[21]
   Answer: Definitional implication.
7. A two-year-old child who swallowed six or more tablets of adult aspirin implies that a nurse gives 15 milliliters of ipecac syrup and a large glass of water.
   Answer: Practical implication.

HYPOTHETICAL SYLLOGISM

We turn next to a type of syllogism noted earlier; only it is referred to as a Hypothetical Syllogism, HS, or Chain argument. It is one of the most elegant and powerful arguments in critical thinking. If all humans are animals and if all animals have the same responses to laboratory tests, then we can conclude that humans have the same responses to laboratory tests as do other animals. Or if person A engages in sex with an AIDS patient, then A is at risk for AIDS, which causally implies that A may get AIDS. And if A gets AIDS, then A is at high risk for dying prematurely. Therefore, if A engages in sex with an AIDS patient, then A is at high risk for dying prematurely.

With suitable modification, the chain argument or hypothetical syllogism is pivotal to nursing arguments as well. For example, Florence Nightingale implemented her hypothesis that proper nutrition, sanitation, hygiene, and nursing care of wounded soldiers during the Crimean War would lower the mortality rate. Suppose she first tested this hypothesis, call it NSHNC (nutrition, sanitation, hygiene, and nursing care) among the members of a regiment, we could reason as follows: If NSHNC applies to Regiment 104, and if the soldiers of Regiment 1076 are like those of Regiment 104, then NSHNC applies also to Regiment 1076. Therefore, if NSHNC applies to Regiment 104, then NSHNC applies to Regiment 1076.

The Chain argument also shows the value of generalizing. We use the Chain argument even if we are unsure of the conclusion. For example, if people who smoke two packs of cigarettes a day for 25 years are at risk for getting lung cancer, and Ms. Jones smoked 2 packs of cigarettes a day for 25 years, then she is at risk for getting lung cancer. Or if someone discovered a disease with a known cause that was identical to diseases with unknown causes, we could use the new discovery to illuminate diseases with unknown causes. Deduction is useful in the sense that if the known is identical to the unknown, the known helps us uncover the unknown. The Chain argument is a large part of the process of inferring the unknown from the known.

Another example of a chain argument is that if a patient eats a wide variety of wholesome foods, then the patient will take in a wide variety of vitamins, minerals, proteins, complex carbohydrates, and fats. If the patient takes in vitamins, minerals, proteins, then the patient will have adequate nutrition. Therefore, if a patient eats a wide variety of wholesome foods, then the patient will have adequate nutrition. We may symbolize such arguments by letting certain letters represent sentences in the argument. Let F represent the patient eating a wide variety of foods; let V represent various vitamins; let N represent the patient having adequate nutrition. We may then symbolize the argument as follows:

If F then N.		$F \rightarrow N$	
If V then N.		$V \rightarrow N$	
∴ If F then N.	or shorter	$\therefore F \rightarrow N$	or one may

place this chain argument on a single line: $F \rightarrow V, V \rightarrow N /\therefore F \rightarrow N$.

Several useful generalizations in organizing and symbolizing chain arguments occur. One is that a chain argument gives us a middle term, in this case, V. Second, it eliminates the middle term. Third, we may use the chain argument or hypothetical syllogism rather than the categorical syllogism of classical logic. The use of if–then or implication is closer to our ordinary thinking than is the categorical syllogistic structure.

Exercises

Organize and symbolize:

1. If patient Jones, 68 years old, gets pain relief, from arthritis, then he will be more apt to move out of bed and walk about. If Jones walks about, he will improve his circulation and his cardiac condition. Therefore, if Jones gets relief, he will improve his cardiac condition.
   (*Answer:* R → W, W → C /∴ R → C)
2. If Lacey has a stroke, then the nurse looks for bradycardia and a rising blood pressure. If the nurse looks for bradycardia and a rising blood pressure, then she aims to control intracranial pressure. Therefore, if Lacey had a stroke, then the nurse aims to control intracranial pressure.[22]
   (*Answer:* S → B, B → IP /∴S → IP [S = stroke; B = bradycardia; IP = intracranial pressure.] We could also write the above formula:

   S → B
   B → IP
   ∴ S → IP

3. If Ms. Rooney, a diabetic, is on insulin, then she may get an insulin reaction. If Rooney gets an insulin reaction, the nurse's instruction to her is to "drink a glass of apple juice." Therefore, if Ms. Rooney, a diabetic on insulin, gets an insulin reaction, the nurse's instruction is "to drink a glass of apple juice."
   (*Answer:* D → IR, IR → A /∴D → A).

MODUS PONENS

We now turn to two important principles. The first, used heavily in science, medicine, nursing, and the nursing process, is called *modus ponens.* This is a significant formula for stating and testing if–then, law-like, or regular relationships. First the if–then statement. Second, we include an instance under it. Third, we use the if–then statement and the included instance to affirm a conclusion.

Example:

If I have pneumonia, then I'm sick.
I have pneumonia.
∴ I'm sick.

If the first and second are true, the third follows. Or if I have a cat, I have a pet. I have a cat. Therefore, I have a pet.

There are more complex cases in nursing. If Mr. Lacey had a stroke, then a nurse would look for Bradycardia, a rising blood pressure, and an increase in intracranial pressure. Mr. Lacey had a stroke. Therefore, a nurse looks for Bradycardia, a rising blood pressure, and an increase in intracranial pressure.[23] Symbolizing the above pneumonia example, P → S, P/∴ S. We can also symbolize the more complex nursing example: S → B, S /∴ B (modus ponens).

Or if Ms. Arbiton, a professional nurse, looks for and finds singed nasal hair in a facial and nasal burn victim, then she has evidence of airway obstruction and possible damage to the patient's respiratory tract. Ms. Arbiton finds singed nasal hair in a burn victim. Therefore, there is evidence of airway obstruction and possible damage to the patient's respiratory tract.[24] We may symbolize this:

SNH → AO
SNH /∴ AO

Or consider, if Mr. Temple has rusty sputum, temperature of 38.8C (102F), respiratory rate of 45, and is lethargic, then this confirms a nurse's initial assessment that Mr. Temple has bronchial pneumonia.[25] Mr. Temple has rusty sputum, a temperature of 38C, a respiratory rate of 45, and is lethargic. Therefore, this confirms the initial assessment that Mr. Temple has bronchial pneumonia. We symbolize this argument: R → P, R /∴P (modus ponens).

If Ms. Kishon successfully completes baccalaureate requirements in nursing and passes State Boards, then she will be a professional nurse. Ms. Kishon has successfully completed baccalaureate requirements and has passed the State Boards. Therefore, Ms. Kishon is a professional nurse. We symbolize this: B → P, B /∴P. The assertion and testing of causal laws is oriented structurally by modus ponens.

There is, however, a fallacy that appears valid, but is a misuse of modus ponens. This is the fallacy of affirming the consequent. Suppose someone said, "If I have pneumonia, I'm sick. I'm sick." Would it follow that I have pneumonia? Not at all. Or consider this further example. If Jones has AIDS, then he has an infection. Jones has an infection. Does it follow that he has AIDS? No. It is only true that if Jones has AIDS then he has an infection. Jones has AIDS. Therefore, he has an infection. To say that he has an infection, therefore, he has AIDS, is to commit the fallacy of affirming the consequent. We may not say, using the general formula:

P → Q
Q /∴ P.

For example, if Florence Nightingale was killed in an airplane crash, then Nightingale is dead. Nightingale is dead. Therefore, she was killed in an airplane crash. This example commits the fallacy of affirming the consequent.

Modus ponens is a valid form of argument, but it requires that we first assert the antecedent followed by the consequent, as in

$$P \rightarrow Q$$
$$P \;/\therefore\; Q.$$

Exercises

Distinguish appropriate uses of modus ponens from the fallacy of affirming the consequent and symbolize.

1. If John has spots over his body, then he has measles. John has spots all over his body. Therefore, John has measles.
   (*Answer:* Modus ponens, appropriate. S → M, S /∴M.)
2. If I have a fox terrior, I have a dog. I have a dog. Therefore, I have a fox terrier.
   (*Answer:* Fallacy of affirming the consequent, F → D, D /∴F.
3. If Ray is 21, he is entitled to be served alcoholic beverages. Ray is 21. Therefore, he is entitled to be served alcoholic beverages.
   Answer: Modus ponens, R → S, R /∴S.

MODUS TOLLENS

A similarly important formal rule of inference is *modus tollens.* This form of argument consists in asserting an antecedent and consequent. We then find a denial of the consequent, and then deny the antecedent. This form of argument also figures heavily in testing scientific ideas. If a law or theory is true, there are no false instances. But if there are, then the law or theory is not true. If there are exceptions to a law, then the law is false.

We use modus tollens to affirm the antecedent, then the consequent. One then denies the consequent, followed by denial of the antecedent, as in

$$P \rightarrow Q$$
$$-Q \;/\therefore -P$$

Example:

If I have pneumonia, I'm sick.
I'm not sick.
∴ I don't have pneumonia.

We can write the formula vertically or horizontally, as in P → Q, −Q /∴−P. If Jones has diabetes, then he has a disease. He does not have a disease. Therefore, he does not have diabetes. Or, if I have a goat, I have an animal. I do not have an animal. So, I do not have a goat.

Or, in a more complex instance, if Ms. Kelly has diabetes, then she has an abnormal increase in blood glucose level. Ms. Kelly does not have an abnormal increase in blood glucose level. Therefore, Ms. Kelly does not have diabetes. Or, if Mr. King has pneumonia, then he has rusty sputum, temperature of 38.8C, respiratory rate of 45, and lethargy. He does not have rusty sputum and other symptoms. So, he does not have pneumonia.

We can, however, misuse modus tollens and commit a fallacy. Instead of denying the consequent, we can deny the antecedent. This is known as the fallacy of denying the antecedent. For example, if I have surgery, then I am a patient. I do not have surgery. Therefore, I am not a patient. Or if I have a cat, I have a pet. I do not have a cat. Therefore, I do not have a pet. Both are instances of fallacies, because even if I do not have surgery, I can still be a patient, and my not having a cat does not preclude my having a pet.

An example of the fallacy of denying the antecedent is: If Nightingale was killed in an airplane crash, then she is dead. Nightingale was not killed in an airplane crash. Therefore, she is not dead.

Other examples of modus ponens and modus tollens, as well as the fallacies of affirming the consequent and denying the antecedent, are as follows: If Jane takes antibiotics, then she will recover from pneumonia. Jane recovered. Therefore, she took antibiotics. This example commits the fallacy of affirming the consequent. She might have taken other measures or recovered without medication.

The difference between modus tollens and the fallacy of affirming the consequence is:

Modus Tollens	Fallacy of Affirming the Consequence
P → Q	P → Q
−Q /∴−P	Q /∴P

The difference between modus ponens and the fallacy of denying the antecedent is:

Modus Ponens	Fallacy of Denying the Antecedent
P → Q	P → Q
P /∴Q	−P /∴−Q

Exercises

Determine if the example is valid or invalid and why, and symbolize.

1. If Ms. H gains weight, her blood pressure will rise. She gains weight. Therefore, her blood pressure rises.
   Answer: Valid, modus ponens, G → R, G /∴R.

2. If Ms. H gains weight, her blood pressure rises. Her blood pressure rises. Therefore, she gains weight.
   Answer: Fallacy of affirming the consequent, $G \rightarrow R, R /\therefore G$. Invalid.
   Symbolize and check for validity:
3. If Nurse Brown gave Mr. Eliot digitalis, then she gave him a heart medication. She did not give him digitalis. What would follow? That she did not give him a heart medication? Not at all. What is the fallacy?
   Answer: Fallacy of denying the antecedent, $D \rightarrow H, -D /\therefore -H$. Invalid.
4. If Mr. T is on aminophylline, then he will have urinary frequency. He has urinary frequency. Therefore, he is on aminophylline.[26]
   Answer: Fallacy of affirming the consequent, $A \rightarrow U, U /\therefore A$.
   Using rules to date, cite the form of argument, symbolize and check for validity.
5. If Mr. C, a former drug addict, is not given treatment, he will regress and "shoot it up." If he shoots, he will be at risk for overdosing. Therefore, if he is not treated, he will be at risk for overdosing.
   Answer: Hypothetical syllogism, valid, $-T \rightarrow S, S \rightarrow O /\therefore -T \rightarrow O$.
6. Either Mr. S has a problem with peripheral pulses or lymph nodes. Mr. S does not have a problem with peripheral pulses. Therefore, he has a problem with lymph nodes.[27]
   Answer: $P \vee L, -P /L$, disjunctive syllogism valid.

SIMPLE AND COMPLEX DILEMMA

Two other forms of argument are *simple* and constructive dilemma. Nurses deal with dilemmas, and therefore, forms of argument dealing with dilemmas may be helpful. The formula of a simple dilemma reads:

$$
\begin{array}{ccc}
P & \vee & Q \\
P & \rightarrow & R \\
Q & \rightarrow & R \\
\hline
\multicolumn{3}{c}{\text{So, R.}}
\end{array}
\qquad \text{or} \qquad
\begin{array}{ccc}
A & \vee & M \\
A & \rightarrow & R \\
M & \rightarrow & R \\
\hline
\multicolumn{3}{c}{\text{So, R}}
\end{array}
$$

It is easy to see intuitively that simple dilemma is valid. "If one or the other of" P and Q "is true and moreover" if R "is true," when either P or Q is true, then you know that "R must be true."[28] Nurse Jones either gives Mr. Lee acetaminophen or morphine. If she gives him acetaminophen, then she will relieve his pain. If she gives him morphine, then she will relieve his pain. Therefore, she will relieve his pain.

A useful way to learn constructive dilemma is to use an example in nursing. If Nurse A gives morphine every 4 hours, the patient's pain is lessened, but the patient's rate of respiration is also undesirably decreased. We can symbolize this: M → P. And if Nurse A gives acetaminophen four times a day, then the rate of respiration is not undesirably decreased, but then there will be a moderate increase in pain. We can symbolize this: A → R. Either Nurse A gives morphine or acetaminophen. Therefore, either the patient's pain is lessened or the patient's respiration rate is not undesirably decreased. Constructive dilemma applied to our example reads:

$$(M \rightarrow P) \,\&\, (A \rightarrow R)$$

Where M = morphine; P = pain relief; A = acetaminophen; R = respiration not undesirably decreased.

$$M \vee A \;/\therefore P \vee R$$

In ordinary language, the above formula reads: If one gives morphine, then pain relief, and if one gives acetaminophen, then the rate of respiration is not undesirably decreased. Either one gives morphine or acetaminophen. Therefore, either the patient's pain is relieved or the patient's rate of respiration is not undesirably decreased.

SOME OTHER USEFUL RULES OF INFERENCE

Some other useful rules of inference for nursing are *simplification* and *addition.* Simplification entitles one to take a conjunction and assert one conjunct without the other. If a nurse cares for a patient with cardiac surgery, and if she "inspects suture line(s), observes for bleeding from body orifices, monitors vital signs . . .," then it is true that she does any one of these procedures. To symbolize, if I = inspects suture line(s), O = observes for bleeding . . ., we have I & O. I & O implies I. Simplification enables us to assert this formality; and this can be proved with a truth table. Moreover, simplification is an implication of conjunction.

Addition is to disjunction what simplification is to conjunction. With conjunction we may contract or eliminate. With addition, we may expand. If it is true that a nurse gives acetaminophen or codeine, then it is true that she gives one or the other, or both. All we are asserting in addition is that if it is true that she gives the one medication, then it is true that she gives that one or another. The formula applied to our example reads: $A \;/\therefore A \vee C$.

This seems to be a good occasion to repeat the point that validity in critical thinking means a conclusion follows from the premises. Validity does not mean soundness of the argument. Additional inductive criteria determine whether an argument, in addition to being valid, is also sound. To be a sound argument, both the premises and the conclusion, in addition to being structurally related, have to be shown to be true. The rules discussed above are rules of validity, not soundness.

SHORT-CUT METHOD

We cited the truth table method to prove formal arguments and we used the truth table to prove a disjunctive syllogism. Anyone encountering a problem with four or more symbols appreciates how long and cumbersome it is to do a truth table. With four or more symbols as in a constructive dilemma, a proof using truth tables involves 16 or more column. Fortunately, there is a short-cut method that helps cut down on the number of lines. This method generalizes on the main principles of the truth table.

Recall the definition of material implication. If the antecedent is true, the conclusion has to be true in a valid argument. If the antecedent is false, the conclusion may be either true or false in a valid argument. In the short-cut method, the procedure is to assign an F to the conclusion, and, out of consistency, we assign the same letter F to the same letter that appears in the premises. To start with our initial problem (A v C) & −A /∴ C, we assign an F to C in the conclusion. To be consistent, we also assign an F to C in the premises. We then do our best to show that the premises are true. If we assign true to −A, then we must assign false to A. Our problem now looks like this:

```
(A v C) & −A /∴ C.
 F   F     T     F
```

Anyone conversant with definitions of disjunction, conjunction, implication, and truth tables recognizes that for our left-hand parentheses, a disjunction with an F at either end implies an F. Our problem now looks like this:

```
(A v C) & −A /∴ C.
   F       T     F
```

Anyone conversant with conjunction recognizes that an F and a T implies an F. A conjunction, it may be recalled is true only if all of the conjuncts together are true; therefore our antecedent is false. A false antecedent implying a false conclusion is valid. If instead, we assign an F to −A, and a T to A, we will get the same result, a false antecedent. In all cases, the important principle to remember is T → F, which proves invalidity. If, when we assign an F to the conclusion, the antecedent is false, then the argument is valid. Let us take an earlier example, "If I have surgery, I'm a patient. I don't have surgery. Therefore, I'm not a patient." We said this commits the fallacy of denying the antecedent. Let us see if it does. The formula reads: (S → P) & −S /∴−P. We first assign an F to −P. Why? We are going through the essential task of the truth table that assigns an F to the conclusion. Next, we assign an F to any place in the premises in which −P appears. Instead, we have P, to which we assign T, the contradictory of −P. Next, we assign T to −S. This implies that we must assign F to S. Our problem now looks like this:

(S → P) & −S /∴ −P.
F   T   T   F

We know that an F, then a T implies a T; and a conjunction of Ts implies a T. So, when the above conclusion is false, the antecedent is true. A true antecedent followed by a false consequent makes an argument invalid.

This is an ingenious method, an indirect proof. Assign an F to the consequent. Next, do your best to show that the antecedent is, nevertheless, true whenever the consequent is false. If the antecedent is still false, whenever the consequent is false, the argument is valid. Sounds strange to some people, but that is the definition of material implication; and this is the procedure for testing arguments for their validity.

Let us use the short-cut method, finally, to prove that modus ponens is valid. It reads: P → Q & P /∴ Q. We assign an F to Q in the conclusion. We must do so in the premise as well. Next, we do our best to make the antecedent true. The problem now looks like this:

P → Q & P /∴ Q.
      F   F

Looking at the left side first, we must assign F to P, otherwise, we have an immediate T then F. But once we assign an F to the first use of P, we must, out of consistency, assign an F to the next use of P. Although an F then an F implies a true part of the antecedent, the next use of F to P shows that the antecedent is false. The problem now looks like this:

P → Q & P /∴ Q.
F   F   F   F

So modus ponens is a valid form of argument.

Exercises

Prove the following statements using the short-cut method.

1. A & C /∴ A.

F F T v F F
Answer: A & M /∴ A. Explanation: First assign F to A in the conclusion, then assign F to A in the first conjunct, out of consistency. Next, assign T or F to M. It does not matter, because an F and any other value still implies an F in a conjunction. So, if the consequent is F, and the antecedent is also F, the argument is valid.

2. S /∴ S v J.

F F F F
Answer: S /∴ S v J.

3. Symbolize and prove by the short-cut method. Nurse Rufus gave Mr. Willis acetylsalicylic Acid. Therefore, Nurse Rufus gave Mr. Willis acetylsalicylic acid or acetaminophen.

       F   F F F
   Answer: C /∴ C v A, valid.

NATURAL DEDUCTION

The most elegant and powerful value of symbolic logic is to be able to use rules of inference to generate other propositions and to prove or justify these propositions from their premises. First, let us put the Rules of Inference together.

Commonly Used Rules of Inference Applicable to Nursing

1. Modus Ponens: P → Q
P / ∴ Q
(P then Q. P. Therefore Q.)
2. Modus Tollens: P → Q
−Q /∴ −P
P then Q. Not Q. Therefore not P.)
3. Disjunctive Syllogism: P v Q
−P /∴ Q
4. Exclusion: −(P & Q)
P /∴ −Q
(Not both P and Q. P. Therefore not Q.)
5. Hypothetical Syllogism or Chain Argument:
P → Q
Q → R /∴ P → R
(P then Q. Q then R. Therefore P then R.)
6. Simple Dilemma
P v Q
P → R
Q → R /∴ R
(P or Q. P then R. Q then R. So R.)
7. Constructive Dilemma
(P → Q) & (R → S)
(P v R) /∴ (Q v S)
8. Simplification: P & Q /∴ P
(P and Q. Therefore P.)
9. Addition: P /∴ P v Q
(P. Therefore P or Q).

We can now put the rules to work using the forms or formulas of inference to generate new inferences. We start with this rather simplified word problem: Either Nurse Jones gets Mr. Lee, a patient with bed sores, out of bed, or she turns him every quarter hour. She does not get Mr. Lee out of bed. Therefore, she turns him every quarter hour. We symbolize this:

$O \vee T$ (Out of bed or turn)
$-O\ /\therefore\ T$ (Not out of bed, therefore, turn)

We can use either a truth table, a short cut, or one of the forms of inference to conclude T with certainty and justification. Which method shall we use? Let us try applying the rules of inference, or natural deduction, a wonderful and powerful method.

Given:

$O \vee T$ (O or T)
$-O$

How do we arrive at T? We consult the rules of inference. For this problem, we will not use modus ponens or modus tollens. We note, however, that the structure of this problem is identical to disjunctive syllogism, which is

$P \vee Q$
$P\ /\therefore\ Q$ (Rule 3)

Numbering our lines, we write the problem:

Line 1. $O \vee T$ Given
Line 2. $-O\ /\therefore\ T$ 1, 2, (Disjunctive syllogism)

On the left side after line 1, we write the first premise, and on the right of the first premise, we write the justification. In this case, $O \vee T$ is given. In line 2 we write the next premise, and follow this with the conclusion, T. On the right of the conclusion, T, we again write the justification, which in this case consists in referring to lines 1 and 2 along with the appropriate rule of inference, which in this case is disjunctive syllogism. We can now use the rules of inference to justify the passage from premises to conclusion.

Another example is: If Nurse Jones fails to put Mr. Lee's guard rail up, he is apt to fall out of bed. If he falls out of bed, he is apt to break a hip, suffer prolonged bed rest, and risk getting pneumonia. Therefore, if Nurse Jones fails to put Mr. Lee's guard rails up, he is at risk for getting pneumonia. We symbolize this example by: $-R$ = guard rails not up; B = falling out of bed; and P = risk getting pneumonia. Now we formulate the problem: $-R \rightarrow B$

$-R \rightarrow B$ (Not R, then B)
$B \rightarrow P$ (If B then P)
$\therefore -R \rightarrow P$ (Therefore, if not R, then P)

What form does this fit? Chain argument. We prove this:

1. $-R \rightarrow B$ Given
2. $B \rightarrow P$ Given
3. $\therefore -R \rightarrow P$ 1, 2 (Hypothetical syllogism)

We justify the conclusion P on the basis of 1 and 2, using hypothetical syllogism.

A slightly more complicated example is: If Mr. S is diagnosed as having Hodgkin's disease, he will receive MOPP (nitrogen mustard, vincristine (Oncovin), procarbazine, and prednisone) regimen. If Mr. S receives MOPP, he will get severe nausea. Therefore, if Mr. S has Hodgkin's disease, he will get severe nausea.[29] We then use the symbols: H = Mr. S's being diagnosed as having Hodgkin's; M = receiving MOPP; and N = getting severe nausea. We then set up the problem as follows:

1. $H \rightarrow M$
2. $M \rightarrow N / \therefore H \rightarrow N.$

How do we prove that $H \rightarrow N$ follows from premises 1 and 2? We do so by appealing to the relevant rule or form of inference.

1. $H \rightarrow M$ Given
2. $M \rightarrow N / \therefore H \rightarrow N$ 1, 2 (Hypothetical syllogism)

If prochlorperazine is administered before MOPP drugs, Mr. S's nausea will be relieved. Prochlorperazine is administered before MOPP drugs. Therefore, Mr. S's nausea is relieved.[30] We use the symbols: P = Prochlorperazine is administered before MOPP drugs and N = Mr. S's nausea will be relieved. We then symbolize the problem and prove the conclusion.

1. $P \rightarrow N$ P then N.
2. $P \rightarrow N$ 1, 2 (Modus ponens). P, therefore N.

N is justified by referring to steps 1 and 2, as applications of modus ponens.

If Nurse Quigly gave Mrs. Edison acetylsalicylic acid, then her leg joint pains were relieved. Ms. Quigly gave Ms. Edison acetylsalicylic acid and helped her move her legs. Therefore, Ms. Edison was relieved. We symbolize by looking at the italic letters for clues.

1. $A \rightarrow R$
2. $A \,\&\, M / \therefore R.$

Next we try to prove the conclusion. The question is: How do we get from the premises to the conclusion R? First, try doing it yourself. If you get stuck, here are steps 3 and 4: 3. A, 2 (Simplification). Why did we pick A? Because we want to derive or generate the all important letter R, the conclusion. We do so by using the premises along with Modus ponens. We are now ready for step 4: 4. R, 1, 3 (Modus ponens). In step 3, we eliminated M with the help of simplification to set up the application of Modus ponens. This may not seem like much, but by using two rules, we have shown that R must follow from the premises.

Here is another example. A team of physicians and nurses developed a new cardiac medication. If Nurse Rufus gave the new cardiac medication, M, to Mr. Willis, her patient, CM helped stabilize his condition. If Mr. Willis's condition was stabilized, then he experienced no further tachycardia episodes. Therefore, he experienced no further tachycardia episodes. We symbolize this by using our underlined letters for clues. It reads:

1. M	(Medication)
2. M → S	(If medication, then stability)
3. S → −E /∴ −E	(If stability, then no tachycardia episodes. Therefore, no episodes)

Now for the proof of −E from premises 1, 2, and 3. First, however, try to prove −E by applying the forms of inference. If you get stuck, here are steps 4 and 5:

4. S, 2, 1 Modus ponens and
5. −E 3, 4 Modus ponens

As we can "see" from deducing conclusions, we use established forms of reasoning as stepping stones or building blocks for reaching a definite and certain position, namely the conclusion.

Exercises

For practice in applying deductive forms, complete the deduction and cite the rule to justify the step.

1. 1. A → C
2. A /∴ C
3. ________
Answer: C, 1, 2, Modus ponens

2. 1. R → R v S
2. ________
Answer: R v S, 1, 2, Addition.

3. 1. R → W
2. W → U /∴ R → U
3. ________
Answer: R → U, 1, 2, Hypothetical syllogism.

4. 1. A → C
2. −C /∴ −A
3. ________
Answer: −A, 1, 2, Modus tollens.

5. 1. (S → J) & (R → B)
2. S v R/ ∴J v B
3. ________
Answer: J v B, 1, 2, Constructive dilemma.

6. 1. R v S
2. −R/ ∴S
3. ________
Answer: S, 1, 2, Disjunctive syllogism.

7. 1. M & N /∴ M
2. ________
Answer: M, 1, S, Simplification.

8. Symbolize and prove this word problem. Nurse Ronley says to L. White, MD that either Ms. Stowe, 28 years old, has signs and symptoms of appendicitis or diarrhea (A v D). If Ms. Stowe does not have an elevated blood count, then she does not have appendicitis (−C → −A). If there is an elevated blood count, then there is danger of peritonitis (C → P). There is no danger of peritonitis (−P). Therefore, Ms. Towe has diarrhea (D).

Answer: 1. A v D
2. −C → −A
3. C → P
4. −P /∴ D
5. −C 3, 4, Modus tollens.
6. −A 2, 5, Modus ponens.
7. D 1, 6, Disjunctive syllogism.

CONCLUSION

Deductive reasoning provides the outermost boundaries for distinguishing valid from invalid arguments. The relation between validity and invalidity and scientific truth and falsity may be put into concentric circles. An advantage of this graphic representation (Fig. 10–1) is that it shows that the outermost rational structure is provided through rules of deduction. If an argument is invalid, it is not worth pursuing further for the purpose of scientifically evaluating it as being either true or false. To take our simplest illustration, if A is bigger than B and B is bigger than C, then A cannot be smaller than C. So, what we gain by criteria of deductive reasoning is economy of effort in inquiry. An invalid argument is pointless to pursue further.

On the other hand, a valid argument is not necessarily a sound argument with true premises and a true conclusion. That is, again, a reason for putting the deductive circle outside. Once, validity is established, we proceed to find out if the content of a particular nursing statement is true. For example, the editors of a New State Board examination book assert

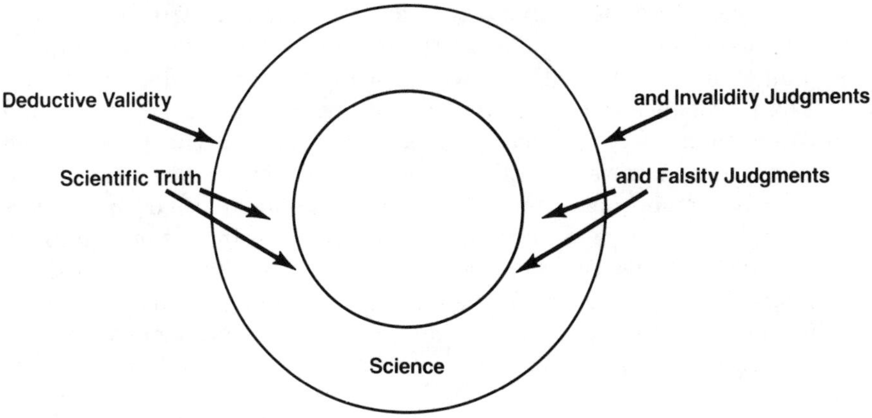

Figure 10-1. Deductive logic.

that "A Po_2 of 80 mmHg is normal"[31] for burn victims. Whether this is true depends on evidence, but the evidence will be external to the assertion. For a deductive argument, all that is required by way of evidence of proof is contained within the premises and rules of inference. In this respect, a deductive system, such as euclidean geometry or syllogistic or symbolic logic, is similar to the formal or structural rules of any game in that the rules specify the player's positions and allowable moves. For example, in baseball, "Out" means the batter has had three strikes. A batter may deny vehemently that the third strike was a pitch over home plate and between the batter's shoulder and knee. But for a batter to ask the umpire, "Give me a fourth strike" would be a contradiction of the rules of the game.

The rules of baseball, geometry, syllogism, symbolic logic, or chess do not, however, predict what will happen in the next game. Similarly, the rules of inference do not tell us how to predict the future, or how to treat or cure diseases, or how to give effective nursing care. Deductive rules of inference provide the rational boundaries and principles for the pursuit of inquiry. Canons of deductive reasoning provide the rational structures within which meaningful inquiry may be intelligently pursued.

Valid deductive arguments provide us with examples of certainty and provide a basis for training in certainty. To train students to understand uncertainty in arguments calls for training in certainty, as well as training in uncertainty, and training in the difference between certainty and uncertainty. Deductive reasoning helps us to achieve training in certainty.

The relation between syllogistic and symbolic deduction is that we use the system that is rationally helpful. For some problems, classical logic is helpful. For other problems, symbolic logic is a helpful guide to validity.

We use deduction to extract, extrapolate all that we can from a minimum set of premises, all of which are assumed to be true or prefaced with the hypothetical "if." These premises form the links of a chain, or stepping stones, to generate an ever growing web of valid connections.

Finally, deductive arguments have an intrinsic power, elegance and beauty of their own. Deductive arguments, such as the hypothetical syllogism, show how we may eliminate a middle term in the drive to draw deductively certain conclusions. Accordingly, we make use of the process of elimination to arrive at nursing judgments. The principle of simplification provides another way to eliminate terms on the way to establishing conclusions. Also, by such rules as addition, we may engage in hypothetical reconstruction, a veritable translation procedure, based on rules that provide adequate justification for our conclusions, conclusions that cannot rationally be disputed.

Deductive reasoning provides an indisputably powerful, reasoned touchstone, a model of the rational use of critical thinking, one that is applicable and significant to nursing judgments. The conclusions in some examples of deductive reasoning may be obvious, but it is elegant and conceptually powerful to use relevant rules of inference to justify the validity of nursing arguments by logical principles.

REFERENCES

1. Desharnais, A., et al. New State Board Examination (2nd ed.). East Norwalk, Conn.: Appleton-Century-Crofts and Fleschner Publishing Co., 1986, pp. 447, 459.
2. Ibid, p. 52.
3. Ibid, pp. 163, 178.
4. Ibid.
5. Mendelsohn, R., & Schwartz, L. Basic Logic. Englewood Cliffs, N.J.: Prentice-Hall, 1987, p. 122.
6. Desharnais, A., et al. New State Board Examination, p. 75.
7. Ibid, p. 34.
8. Ibid, p. 50.
9. Ibid, p. 161.
10. Ibid.
11. Mendelsohn, R., & Schwartz, L. Basic Logic, p. 206.
12. Ibid, p. 203.
13. Copi, I. Introduction to Logic (7th ed.). New York: Macmillan, 1986, pp. 279–283.
14. Ibid.
15. Ibid.
16. Charleston Community Memorial Hospital v. Dorrence Kenneth Darling, 33, Ill, 326, 211, NE 2nd 253, 1965.
17. Devereaux, A. Worksheets for Professor Devereaux's Logic Classes. New York: Unpublished manuscript, 1986, p. 138.
18. Desharnais, A., et al. New State Board Examination, p. 49.

19. Ibid, pp. 131, 146.
20. Ibid, p. 127.
21. Ibid, p. 161.
22. Ibid, p. 127.
23. Ibid.
24. Ibid, p. 134.
25. Ibid, p. 129.
26. Ibid, p. 25.
27. Ibid, p. 118, pp. 145, 147.
28. Mendelsohn, R., & Schwartz, L. Basic Logic, p. 203.
29. Desharnais, A., et al. New State Board Examination, p. 133.
30. Ibid.
31. Ibid, p. 148.

Chapter 11

Inductive Reasoning and Analogies

Study of this chapter enables the learner to:

1. Identify major issues in inductive and scientific reasoning that apply to nursing.
2. Recognize the difference between certainty and uncertainty.
3. Develop training in uncertainty.
4. Cope with uncertainty.
5. Justify reasoning procedures that help reach cogent conclusions.
6. Arrange and expedite critical thinking procedures to make sound nursing judgments.

INTRODUCTION

A nurse who uses critical thinking is concerned not only with validity, but also with making sound nursing judgments. Valid arguments are helpful to nurses, but nurses also need substantive truths to guide everyday nursing practices. Although deductive validity provides certainty, it applies to general forms of argument rather than to more particular substantive issues. Nurses depend on induction. Induction consists of actual evidence and arriving at both particular and general conclusions. But arguments based on induction can only be uncertain. Deduction gives us certainty but no actuality. Induction gives us actuality but no certainty. Nurses face the resulting dilemma of not knowing what will happen next in situations that sometimes involve life and death.

WHY MAKE INDUCTIONS?

Nurse Reilly tells Nurse Barshovsky, "I gave a new gastric ulcer medication to Ms. Wells, 58 years old, and she's better already." Ms. Barshovsky tells Ms. Reilly, "I used that medication last week with Mr. Monzey and Mrs. Peppys; and they, too, are showing astounding improvement," Ms. Reilly then says, "I bet that's a good medication to use on other gastric ulcer patients." Here, Ms. Reilly is drawing an inductive inference.

We frequently make inductive inferences. Nurse Sanders buys sneakers at the shoe store and says, "This is my third pair, and they're wonderful." She, too, is making an inductive inference. We buy groceries at stores that have the best deals. We make friends with people whom we believe we can count on and trust. We prepare for the winter. We train ourselves to make a living. On what basis do we trust our inductive conclusions? Our judgments are guided by past experiences along with the assumption that future events will be like the past. If a given pain reliever worked to relieve pain in the past, we use it again. A nurse reasons "If my sexually active client had used condoms, he might have avoided venereal disease." A physician reasons, "If I give Ms. Ellenburger, 66 years old, this cardiac medication, she will breathe easier."

These examples of daily inductive reasoning have several features in common. They show that (1) we seek certainty in our lives; (2) if we cannot have certainty, we seek high probability; and (3) if we cannot have high probabilities, we seek continuities and probabilities of some strength, therefore, we group or classify events; but with the avowed aim of having as much security, if not certainty, as we can derive from actual events. In patient care, we classify or group events, whether within ages and stages, or by diseases, alterations, dysfunctions, and nursing and medical diagnoses. We seek regularities, patterns, continuities, lawlike relations, or tendencies; and we do so to include, infer, or predict future particular events that affect us.

WHAT IS INDUCTION?

Aristotle (384–322 BC) remarks in *Book One* of his metaphysics that "All humans by nature desire to know. An indication of this is the delight we take in the senses; for even apart from their usefulness they are loved for themselves; and above all others the sense of sight."[1] In this remark, Aristotle helps us recognize how humans essentially come to know, notably through the senses, and inductively rather than through deductive inference from a given absolute. We look and see, hear and listen, touch and feel, smell and taste. Humans and nurses, in particular, learn in part, by experiencing what there is before them. Humans learn, in part, by perceiving. Deductive forms are schemata and are no substitute for a nurse's direct observation of a patient's condition. Most of what a nurse learns depends on her knowledge of facts about patients and their health and illnesses. These are gained inductively, perceptively, and learned through the other sense, such as hearing a cough or a heart sound. Nursing proceeds by describing; and description depends on a nurse's seeing, hearing, smelling, talking, and touching. A nurse looks for data. Nurses are taught to be alert and to confirm conjectures and impressions about a patient's condition.

Nurses make inductions from sense data. With the help of categories and generalizations in language, such as pain, anxiety alterations, dysfunctions, illness, disease, we form statements and arguments that are judged as true, false, valid and invalid, relevant, plausible or cogent, sound, and significant.

Inductive inference is drawn from experience. For example, John sees that this patient's color is blue. Therefore, John infers this patient's condition is one of cyanosis. Nurse Fitterly has found that acetylsalicylic acid has worked to relieve pain for many patients. Robert Johnson, a patient, has a minor neck ache. Therefore, Ms. Fitterly, believing that this medication will relieve Mr. Johnson's neck ache, gives him two tablets.

An inductive inference may conclude with a general or a particular statement, as these two examples illustrate. Nevertheless, in an inductive argument, the conclusion is uncertain. In a deductive argument, the focus of concern is on formal validity and invalidity; whereas in an inductive argument, attention is on the soundness or unsoundness of the constituent propositions that make up an argument.

DEDUCTIVE AND INDUCTIVE INFERENCE

In induction, we are guided by the search for true generalizations and true particulars. But among generalizations there are those that, in context, are not useful, such as "All nurses care for the whole patient." We need to have rational ways to evaluate which inductive inferences are useful from those that are useless. We find one source of help among deductions. Deductive forms help us decide which arguments are valid or invalid. We know from our study of deduction that if the premises are true and the conclusion is false, the argument is invalid. Even if the premises of an inductive argument are true, however, the conclusion is not necessarily true. If Nurse Roberts finds that in a given hospital, all nurses are women, and then concludes that all nurses in all hospitals in that city are women, that could lead to an invalid and an unsound argument. For if there is one male nurse, there would be an exception. The principle of modus tollens applies here:

$$P \rightarrow Q,\ -Q/\therefore -P.$$

One exception invalidates a generalization. (We added the subscript $_1$ to Q to refer to at least one counter-instance.) Although attention to deductive forms does not replace attention to induction, induction is largely aimless and unstructured without deductive criteria. Deductive arguments help us determine which arguments are valid or invalid. Deductive forms not only provide the certainty of their conclusions, they also provide criteria for evaluating inductive arguments. Immediately and obviously, if an inductive argument has true premises and a false conclusion, the argument is both invalid and unsound. An argument is sound if all its premises and its conclusions are true. An invalid argument, having true premises and a false conclusion, is unsound. For example, if all nurses in Hospital X are women, and Josie Jones is a nurse at Hospital X, then Josie Jones is a woman. This is a deductive argument. Now for an inductive argument. If all nurses observed to date at Hospital X are women and if Josie Jones is going to be a nurse in Hospital X, then Josie Jones is a woman. But in this case, one cannot be sure that Josie Jones is a woman.

Here is another example of an inductive argument with true premises and a possible false conclusion: Nurse Smith gave 50 patients acetaminophen last week and they all got over their headaches. Ms. Smith gave 75 patients acetaminophen the week before and they all felt better. The week before, Ms. Smith gave 71 patients acetaminophen, and always with the same result, all felt relieved. Ms. Smith, then, draws two conclusions: (1) that acetaminophen relieves all minor aches and (2) that she will give Mr. Gonzales acetaminophen on the basis of her past experiences. But what if Mr. Gonzales is allergic to acetaminophen? Ms. Smith's premises will be true, but her conclusions will be false.

SOME SIMILARITIES AND DIFFERENCES BETWEEN DEDUCTIVE AND INDUCTIVE ARGUMENTS

As inductive arguments draw on experience, and experience is never certain, such arguments are sometimes referred to as empirical arguments. Inductive or empirical arguments depend on experience for their truth value. In inductive or empirical arguments, the conclusion, unlike deductive arguments, is not included in the premises. In inductive arguments, the conclusion states more than we find in the premises. The premises of an inductive argument can never fully assure the truth of the conclusion. Just because acetaminophen helped relieve minor pain for a lot of patients in the past, it does not imply that acetaminophen will work for the next patient.

There are three ways an inductive argument can be unsound. First, if at least one of the premises, presumed true, turns out to be false. It used to be thought true, for example, that complete bed rest was indicated for postsurgical patients. It was reasoned that a 38-year-old postoperative cesarian patient should have complete bed rest. We now know this to be false. If an argument has a false premise and a false conclusion, it is valid but unsound.

Second, an inductive argument can be unsound if the premises used to be true, but conditions have now changed to make these same premises false. At one time, infants with low birth weights usually died. Today, most of them can be saved.

Third, an inductive argument may be unsound if the premises are all true to date, but then a new instance makes the conclusion false. If someone once believed that all nurses are women, the presence of a male nurse would show that such a belief was no longer true. At one time, swans in almost every continent were white. We can imagine an ornithologist collecting records on swan that were white, and doing so by adding or enumerating instances as follows:

Swan 1 is white
Swan 2 is white
Swan 3 is white
∴ All swan are white

This ornithologist, however, might have given us true premises and a false conclusion. For unkown to him, another ornithologist discovered a non-white swan. The moment that the first kidney transplant was achieved, generalizations regarding the inevitable fatality of renal end stage disease were invalidated. Similarly, generalizations regarding the impossibility of organ transplants were invalidated.

Another example of arguments with true premises and false conclusions, are surprises. Some health professionals assume that young patients will live. They have data to support their assumptions. We could formalize the reasoning process as follows:

> Mary, Henry, and Phillip were my patients last week and they were all young people. They recovered from minor surgery.
>
> Therefore, young people recover nicely from minor operations. Jane, 21 years old, is recovering nicely from a tonsillectomy. Therefore, Jane will continue to recover. But suddenly, Jane has a cardiac arrest and dies.

In inductive reasoning, therefore, even if the premises are true, we can never be sure of the conclusion.

SOME CONDITIONAL ARGUMENTS

Another type of an invalid inductive argument with true premises and a false conclusion is a conditional argument, also called a counter-factual argument. If I were Florence Nightingale, I would be a gifted nursing leader. I am not Florence Nightingale, therefore, I am not a gifted nursing leader. Both premises are true for some nurses; the conclusion may also be true. But the argument is invalid, as we could substitute the name of Clara Barton, Lydia Hall, or Hildegard Peplau, in the conclusion, making the conclusion false. Another fallacy committed in the foregoing argument, is the fallacy of denying the antecedent. Just because I am not Florence Nightingale (antecedent) does not mean that the person referred to in the conclusion is not a nursing leader.

Validity and invalidity have to do with the form into which to fit the facts. Any substitution for a valid deductive argument must have a true conclusion. But for an argument to be sound means it has a true conclusion and true premises. Inductive arguments, however, are judged primarily by the truth or falsity of their premises and conclusions.

The purpose and function of an inductive argument is also different from the purpose of a deductive argument. Deductive arguments are categorically valid or invalid. Althought inductive arguments are also valid or invalid, the main function of inductive arguments is to provide degrees of strength to arrive empirically at conclusions. In inductive arguments the strength of the conclusion in relation to the premises is a matter of degree. This is not to deny that an inductive argument may be invalid, as in an example of true premises followed by a false conclusion.

Because our aim in induction is to find out new things about the world, it is useful to assess inductive arguments as having conclusions that are supported by evidence that is inconclusive.

An invalid argument is one in which the conclusion does not follow from the premises. Every invalid argument has or could have at least one false statement, such as its conclusion. Because an argument with any false statement is unsound, every invalid argument is unsound. Accordingly, we have several levels of appraisal, including validity, soundness, relevance, and significance.

A VIEW OF DEDUCTION AND INDUCTION

Some nursing scholars identify deduction as proceeding from the general to the particular; and induction as moving from the particular to the general. Our view is that the main difference between deduction and induction is that in induction the conclusion is probable or contingent, whereas in deduction the conclusion of a valid argument is necessary and certain.

There is, however, an understandable inclination to draw inferences from *some* to *all* and to identify these with inductive inferences. For example, Pinnell and de Meneses write,

> With induction you gather pieces of unassociated information. Then you evaluate all the data that you have collected and arrive at a conclusion

> that can be supported by theoretical knowledge. For example, often a woman who experiences tiredness, nausea in the morning, emotional sensitivity and a late menses will conclude that she is pregnant, even before confirmation by a physician.[2]

If a sexually active client experiences tiredness, nausea, and delay of menstruation, she concludes that she is pregnant. Her argument is inductive whether started with symptoms or confirmed by generalization of pregnancy. From a general premise to a particular conclusion, the argument looks like this:

> All sexually active women with tiredness, morning nausea, and absence of menstruation, are pregnant.
> Mary is tired, has morning nausea, and missed her expected menstruation.
> ∴ Mary is pregnant.

The argument may be schematized in syllogistic form:

$$\begin{array}{l} T \text{ a } P \\ M \text{ a } T \\ \therefore M \text{ a } P \end{array}$$

This is a valid, deductive argument. We cannot conclude that Mary is pregnant without accepting as true the major premise that sexually active women who are tired, have morning nausea, and do not menstruate are pregnant. The author's argument is an enthymeme, an argument with a missing or suppressed premise. The suppressed premise is that sexually active women with tiredness, morning nausea, and absence of effective menstruation, are pregnant. If the connection between being tired, nausea, and pregnancy is established, then the above argument can be interpreted as deductive. To render this example as an inductive argument, we may express it as:

> Being tired, T, having morning nausea, MN, and missing menstruation, MM, are features or signs associated with being pregnant.
> Joan, Clara, Sue, and Isabelle have had T, MN, MM, and were pregnant. Mary has T, MN, and MM.
> ∴ Mary is probably pregnant.

Exercises

Show whether the following arguments are valid and sound.

1. If I were Ronald Reagan, I'd be an American. I'm not Ronald Reagan. Therefore, I'm not an American.
   Answer: Premises 1 and 2 are true; the conclusion could easily be false. Hence, the argument is invalid, and therefore also unsound.

2. If I were a face–neck burn patient, the most important thing would be to assess for changes in the circumferences of the neck. I am not a face–neck burn patient. Therefore, I should not be assessed for changes in the circumference of my neck.[3]
   Answer: Premises 1 and 2 are true and the conclusion is true, but if the second premise were true filled in by the name of a face–neck burn victim, and the conclusion remained as stated, it would be false, and therefore, invalid and unsound. More simply, this argument commits the fallacy of denying the antecedent.
3. If I were a face–neck burn patient, the most important thing would be to assess for changes in the circumference of the neck. And I am a face–neck burn patient. Therefore, I should be assessed for changes in the circumference of my neck.[4]
   Answer: This argument is valid and sound. The argument has or could have true premises and the conclusion is or could likewise be true.
4. Cite the missing premise. If a patient is immobile, elderly, and has a poor nutritional status, then the probability of (this patient developing) decubitus is 95 percent.
   Answer: Immobile, elderly, nutritionally inadequate patients have a 95 percent chance of developing decubitus.[5]
5. Is statement 4 deductive or inductive, and why?
   Answer: Inductive, because the outcome for a given patient is uncertain. It may be 95 percent more or less, but it is not certain to be 95 percent for the next patient.
6. Cite the missing premise. All nurses have high IQs. Therefore, this nurse has a high IQ.
   Answer: This is a nurse.[6]
7. Cite the missing premises for this conclusion. "This nurse has a high IQ.
   Answer: All nurses have a high IQ. This person is a nurse.
8. Are statements 6 and 7 deductive or inductive?
   Answer: Deductive, because the conclusion is implied completely by the premises.
9. Is this argument deductive or inductive? Most nurses have a high IQ. This is a nurse. Therefore, she has a high IQ.
   Answer: Inductive, as we cannot tell for sure from the premises whether the next nurse has a high IQ or not.

INDUCTIVE ARGUMENTS DO NOT ASSURE THEIR CONCLUSIONS

If Jones tastes the first sip of brand X coffee and infers subsequent cups of coffee to be like the first, he will be using an inductive enumerative argument. But the true premises of an inductive argument, which describe the first few tastes, cannot insure the truth of the conclusion, notably that the next sip of coffee will be like the previous sips.

According to B. Stevens,

> A typical inductive argument follows: Morphine is a narcotic and relieves pain. Codeine is a narcotic and relieves pain. Heroin is a narcotic and relieves pain. Therefore, all narcotics probably relieve pain.[7]

Stevens reminds the reader that *inductive arguments,* in contrast to *deductive arguments,* are

> based on probabilities rather than necessity. An inductive argument is based on cases known, and its probability factor can alway be changed by new and contrary cases.[8]

Stevens further reminds the reader that "this inductive argument is one that proves to be false, as there are some narcotics that do not relieve pain."[9] It takes only a single exception to "invalidate an inductive conclusion."[10] In an inductive argument, we cannot be sure that the conclusion is implied by the premises.

The force of modus tollens

$$P \rightarrow Q,$$
$$-Q \ / \therefore -P$$

is that an exception invalidates a generalization. To say that:

Nurse 1 is female;
Nurse 2 is female;
Nurse 3 is female;
Nurse 4 is female;

and conclude, therefore, that all nurses are female is only warranted or justified, in relation to the evidence. One exception invalidates a generalization. Two to four percent of nurses are male.

FUNCTION OF INDUCTIVE ARGUMENT

In an inductive argument, we use the premises to attempt to show that the conclusion has a degree of strength. The conclusion of the coffee example that the next sip will be like the previous tastes, is *probably* true, but not necessarily or certainly true. Hence, inductive conclusions are never absolutely true.

We learn about the world in several ways. One is by looking at repeated patterns of occurrences. To give acetaminophen to 100 patients, because it worked on previous patients' headaches, makes use of an inductive argument. If we find no false instance in which acetaminophen failed to work, our confidence in it is reasonably strengthened. If we found that acetaminophen had solely beneficial effects and no adverse reactions, and on a wide variety of patients of various ages and stages of diseases, we could increasingly count on this effect to provide a pattern of repeatability, such as our faith that the wheels of our cars will keep turning.

Repeatability undoubtedly has inductive advantages. For the same nurses, physicians, and hospitals to provide the same support day in and day out over many years, provides stability, continuity, reliability, and predictability. If, for example, patient A takes treatment Z and recovers; and B takes Z and recovers, and if we give it to patient C, who is similar in relevant respects to A and B, then we can predict that patient C will recover. Nurse A sees patients with AIDS come into the hospital repeatedly until they die. A reasonable inductive conclusion is that this disease is likely to be fatal to its victims.

EXCEPTIONS TO INDUCTION BY ENUMERATION

The appeal to induction by enumeration of instances and repeatability, in particular, is a way to draw inductive inferences. But repeatability has its drawback, as deftly cited in B. Russell's celebrated example of the chicken.[11] Everyday it is fed at a certain time. As it grows into a hen, it expects the same meal at the same time. Then one day, instead of receiving the same meal at the same time, it is beheaded and eaten. The more often people go to bed at night and get up in the morning, the more convinced they become that what has happened in the past will continue to reoccur. But one day, the repeatable event of one's life stops. We cannot use the idea of repeatability to insure the certainty of repeatability.

The growth of human knowledge depends on being open to new experiences, exceptions, and improved explanations. For centuries, people believed the earth was flat. Experience led people to that conclusion, until some people took seriously their observations of the disappearance of ships' sails as they moved away from shore. Moreover, no ship ever fell off or gave evidence of a flat earth. Moreover, when a ship approached the shore, the first visible part was the masthead, the top of the ship.

Until 1929, laboratory workers regarded mold on culture plates, as impurities to be discarded. Arthur Fleming observed that the mold prevented the growth of bacteria on the plate, and thus discovered the active agent of penicillin.[12] The intelligent, alert nurse looks for exceptions and differences rather than just similarities or likenesses. Some differences in patient symptoms call for nursing judgments.

FORMING HYPOTHESES, CONJECTURES, SPECULATIONS, AND BOLD GUESSES

Enumeration is generally a slow and not very sure method of aiming at sound inductive conclusions. It is fraught with questions, exceptions, and counter-examples. How many Scandinavians do we have to study to determine that they have a high cholesterol level due to a high dairy consumption? What is a high cholesterol level and what counts as a high dairy consumption? In using induction by enumeration, dealing with exceptions, qualifications, and counter-examples adds difficulties to an otherwise useful method of arriving at inductive conclusions.

One alternative to an endless addition of examples is to guess, speculate, or form hypotheses to account for some event. The hypothesis approach starts with a conjecture to explain a given phenomena. Some 19th Century lung specialists wondered about the correlation between chimney sweeps and lung disease. Instead of enumerating how many sweeps were afflicted, these specialists began with an initial assumption that exposure to tars and soot were causal factors in lung disease. Some great scientists, such as Darwin, Pasteur, and Freud, rather than laboriously counting instances of correlations between two phenomena, drew bold hypotheses to explain events.

Most of us are not as gifted as these theorists. Some researchers consequently engage in induction by enumeration. People have learned a great many valuable things by enumerating instance upon instance, ranging from early human observations of the effect of lunar tides on navigational safety, to presidential poll taking, and to correlations involving bladder cancer in laboratory animals and the use of saccharine. Nevertheless, there are other methods of drawing inductive inferences that are less painful and time consuming. One of these methods is the formation of an hypothesis. Another commonly used method, also compatible with forming hypotheses, is the use of argument by analogy.

ARGUMENT BY ANALOGY

We arrive at inductive conclusions by drawing analogies or comparisons between like phenomena. To say one argument is an argument by analogy is to say one argument is like another. An analogy is a likeness. Likenesses, similarities, comparisons, and analogies are near synonyms. If we know that one twin's last name is Esposito, we can correctly infer that the second twin, likewise is named Esposito. But we cannot be sure that the second Esposito is not married to a Mr. Green. Two women who are twins, but with different last names, present a disanalogy. Here, the similarity ends.

The principle that one thing, condition, or patient is like another, is an important inductive principle in nursing. This is the principle of similarity. If we know that patient Jones has a colostomy similar to some other person's, we may draw analogies concerning the nursing care of Jones and other patients, which is more helpful than if Jones was one of a kind, a unique patient with a brand new diagnosis.

A more serious objection to relying solely on enumeration rather than appealing to analogy is that in research, an appropriate analogy, such as experiments using chimpanzees or rats, may be most useful. Animal research may provide as much transferable data as thousands of enumerations tried only on humans. The enumeration test is generally too simple and too unrewarding. Animal research assumes analogies between ourselves and other animals.

An example of an analogy is the symbolic meaning attached to Florence Nightingale by nurses. Florence Nightingale was identified as the "lady with a lamp." The lamp sheds light on the darkness, just as Nightingale shed light on nursing practice as a way to combat the death and illness among wounded and sick soldiers. If a neurologist tells a cancer patient, "You have a time bomb," he is comparing the threat to life of this disease to the military metaphor of a detonating device that will go off at some unknown time. Cancer, also, is compared to the growth of cells invading healthy tissue, another military metaphor.

Exercises

1. The journal *Nursing Research* makes use of analogies. In a recent editorial, F.S. Downes refers to "Food For Thought."[13] What thoughts come to your mind when someone uses this analogy?
   Answer: The Editor then tells the reader that "nursing investigation is trying to uncover" a "wealth of information."[14] Therefore, information is one form of food for thought.
2. What analogy is conveyed by a "wealth of information?"
   Answer: Riches, abundance
3. When a stock market broker uses terms, such as *bullish, bearish,* and *belly up,* what analogies come to mind?
   Answer: Bulls are assertive. Bears are cautious. "Belly up" refers to a corporation going bankrupt or more exactly ceasing to exist as a corporate body.
4. Translate the following analogies.
   a. The pilot aborted Flight 701.
   Answer: The pilot terminated Flight 701 on route.
   b. Joe Collins nursed his martini.
   Answer: Collins drank slowly.
   c. Nurses are experiencing burn-out.
   Answer: Nurses are feeling used up. They are leaving the field after long service in the face of job frustration, low pay, poor rewards, and overwork.

HOW TO EVALUATE ANALOGIES

How do we evaluate analogies? Some are obviously better than others. But no analogy is perfect. If it were, it would be an identity or equation. If one thing A is another B, then we could give the converse and say B is A. But if A is like B, a cup and a saucer, in that both are porcelain, that does not mean that they are identical. Analogies range from near perfect to inappropriate. Some analogies may be trivial in comparison. Other analogies, metaphors, or word pictures, used for comparisons, may break down in application.[15] Analogies are inexact matters of degree.

We may identify several criteria for judging analogies.[16] First, is the number of instances of one thing being like another. If a brand of acetylsalicylic acid has proved effective over a large set of instances, the greater is the probability that the next tablet will have the same effect. A second criterion consists in testing how many diverse types of problems an item, such as acetylsalicylic acid, has affected positively. In evaluating a pain reliever, we consider the variety of aches in which a pain reliever has been effective. A third criterion is the relevance of the reasons cited in the premises to the conclusion. Judging the effectiveness of a pain reliever depends on relevant similarities between large number of users and on relevant similarities between diverse types of users.

An example may clarify these criteria for judging analogies. A home mortgage assessor strengthens his assessment of a home by producing the independent assessments of three comparable homes. If a home in question has twelve rooms, a two-car garage, four acres, and a pond, the reasons for accepting an assessor's value placed on that home is strengthened if three comparable homes have similar qualities.

We may formulate these criteria into a principle of similarity as follows: The greater the number of relevant and significant respects in which one thing can be compared with another, the greater is the likelihood of a further analogy between the two. This principle applies to pain relievers, patients, diseases, and to our assessment of health professionals. If an argument is weak, a way to show it is to construct a counter-analogy. Nurse A says Mr. L, 80 years old, is not responding to treatment for pneumonia with conventional antibiotics. Nurse B tells Nurse A about Mr. R, 82 years old, who responded, but only after the first week. Then the number of differences between Mr. L and Mr. R will affect the strength of the analogy between the two cases.

Exercises

Evaluate the strength or weakness of the following arguments by analogy. Try to use the criteria of numbers, diversity, and relevance.

1. Nurse Smith did well in her academic course work. She is yet to do her clinicals.

2. This bridge has withstood the effect of twelve-ton trucks, Atlantic ocean storms, millions of cars and trailers. This bridge will stand in the next three years.
3. Identify the analogy in these statements.
   a. Every cigarette is a nail in one's coffin.
   Answer: Every cigarette hastens one's death.
   b. The heart is a clock.
   Answer: Comparing the heart to a time piece for its rhythmic sound and for its regularity.
   c. The patient lost his fight for life.
   Answer: The patient died. This metaphor compares life to an armed struggle.

REFUTATION BY LOGICAL ANALOGY

We can refute an argument by showing that it fits into a deductive invalid form, where the premises are true and the conclusion is false; or where some other formal fallacy is committed. If the nurse does not supervise Patient B in his daily self-administration of insulin, then Patient B does not control his diabetes. His diabetes is not under control. Therefore, the nurse is not supervising his daily self-administration of insulin. This commits the fallacy of affirming the consequent. The nurse could be supervising, because, although Patient B takes the prescribed amount of insulin, he could be cheating on his diet or he could have an infection.

A refutation by logical analogy consists in providing an equally fallacious argument prefaced with, "You might as well argue that." For example, If Bias, the basketball player, took cocaine, then he died. He died. Therefore, he took cocaine. The conclusion in either case may be true, but it does not follow from the premises.

Exercises

Determine if the following inductive arguments are valid or invalid, sound or unsound, and show why.

1. If L got over the measles, then L is well. L is well. So, L got over the measles.
   Answer: Fallacy of affirming the consequent, $P \rightarrow Q, Q / \therefore P$.
2. If Drew took acetaminophen, then he got over his headache. Drew did not take acetaminophen. So, he didn't get over his headache.
   Answer: Fallacy of denying the antecedent, $P \rightarrow Q, -P / \therefore -Q$.
3. If millions of cancer victims took Laetrile and died, and if no cancer victim who took Laetrile ever recovered, then Laetrile is (a) useful, (b) useless, (c) worth considering, and (d) undecidable.
   Answer: (b) because of maximal positive correlation and the absence of negative correlation.

4. On Mr. T's third postoperative day after a cholecystectomy, T calls for the nurse and tells her "I feel my stitches popping up." What are some analogies to Mr. T's feeling?
Answer: Buttons coming off a suit.
5. A jaundiced patient says of her body image, "I feel like a summer squash." To a nurse, what problem does this patient communicate by using this analogy?
Answer: Abnormality in skin color or texture.

CONCLUSION

We achieve inductive support for inductive conclusions by demonstrating that we have the maximal number of positive, relevant, and significant analogies and a minimal number of negative analogies or dissimilarities. An inductive argument by analogy takes this form and is illustrated with this example:[17]

> Patients A, B, C, D, E and F all have fatigue, cough, chest pain, weight loss, rusty sputum and fever, r, s, t, u, v and w.
> Patients A, B, C, D and E all have positive sputum test for Mycobacterium tuberculosis, x.
>
> Therefore, Patient F probably also has a positive sputum test for Mycobacterium tuberculosis, x.

REFERENCES

1. McKeon, R. Introduction to Aristotle. New York: Modern Library, Random House, 1947, p. 238.
2. Pinnell, N., & de Meneses, M. The Nursing Process, Theory, Application and Related Processes. East Norwalk, Conn.: Appleton-Century-Crofts, 1986, p. 24.
3. Desharnais, A., et al. New State Board Examination (2nd ed.). East Norwalk, Conn.: Appleton-Fleschner, 1986, pp. 134, 148.
4. Ibid.
5. Tanner, C. Factors Influencing the Diagnostic Process, in Carnevali, D., et al. (Eds.), Diagnostic Reasoning in Nursing. Philadelphia: J.B. Lippincott, 1984, p. 63.
6. Schwerger, J., & Huey, R. Perspectives in Organizational Design, in Schwerger, J. (Ed.), Handbook for Front Line Nurse Managers. Bethany, Conn.: Fleschner, 1986, p. 13.
7. Stevens, B. Nursing Theory, Analysis, Application, Evaluation, (2nd ed.). Boston: Little, Brown, 1984, p. 63.
8. Ibid.
9. Ibid.
10. Ibid.
11. Russell, B. The Problems of Philosophy. New York: Oxford University Press, 1959, p. 63.

12. Copi, I. Introduction To Logic, (7th ed.). New York: Macmillan, 1986, pp. 418–419.
13. Downes, F. Food For Thought. *Nursing Research,* 1986; 35(3):131, May/June.
14. Ibid.
15. Scheffler, I. The Language of Education. Glencoe, Ill.: Thomas Publishers, 1960, p. 48.
16. Copi, I. Introduction To Logic, pp. 411–414.
17. Ibid, p. 406.

Chapter 12

Cause–Effect Relationships

The aims of this chapter include the following:

1. Enable the learner to understand and to work with cause–effect relationships that apply to nursing practice.
2. Encourage the learner to ask fundamental "Why?" questions about causes and effects that apply to nurse–patient relationships.
3. Promote the learner's skills and abilities in seeking explanations for the causes of nurse-related health care problems.
4. Explain causal patterns in terms of necessary and sufficient conditions.
5. Impart to the learner the idea that cause–effect patterns are uncertain.

INTRODUCTION

Nursing intervention and the nursing process assume the importance of cause–effect relationships. The search for the causes of ill health, and of both good and bad effects in human life, preoccupies workers in the sciences and health professions alike. We seek the causes of health-related events to find out what accounts for a health problem and to intervene with a health-related agent that may alleviate the problem.

To want to survive individually and collectively is to want to seek relevant knowledge of how to survive. We seek knowledge by inquiring, methodically asking, and trying to answer pertinent questions. To inquire is to look for the causes of events. The causes that health professionals seek are the control of conditions that contribute to health, disease, illness, and recovery.

WHY LOOK FOR CAUSES?

When an airplane crashes or when a bridge collapses, we look for the cause or causes. Likewise, the death of a patient calls for an autopsy to determine the cause of death. The presumable goal in seeking for the causes of an event in nursing is to develop criteria and guidelines for bringing about good effects. M. Gordon succinctly makes the point about the role of causality in nursing.

> We experience every day the fact that our actions do indeed change things. By inductive reasoning from experience, we attribute cause to action.[1]

CAUSES AS NECESSARY AND SUFFICIENT CONDITIONS

An assumption in the study of events leading to health and ill health is that health-related events do not occur without a cause. To understand cause–effect relationships calls for us to distinguish between the necessary and sufficient conditions of events. A necessary condition for an event is one in whose absence the event could not occur. A necessary condition for human life is the presence of adequate amounts of safe drinking water or equivalent fluids. But water is not enough. We cannot live without sufficient food, clothing, and shelter. These conditions are necessary conditions for life.

A sufficient condition is one in whose presence a given event must occur. Without life support systems, heart stoppage is a sufficient condition of death. *Cause* may refer either to a necessary or sufficient condition. Ideally, *cause* refers to both necessary and sufficient conditions. To find the cause of a disease or of a patient's death is to find condition(s) without which the effect could not occur and to find the condition(s) by which the event, such as a disease or a patient's death, must occur. To say that rain causes the pavement to be wet means that rain is a sufficient condition of the pavement being wet. A street sprinkler watering the pavement is another sufficient condition of a pavement being wet.[2]

SOME MEANINGS AND CRITERIA OF CAUSAL STATEMENTS

A cause has the logical character of being a universal statement, an *all type* statement; thus serving as a conceptual umbrella for conclusions about particular patients, diseases, or events. Part of the value of saying that X is the cause of Y is that all succeeding instances of X will probably be followed by Y. If X stands for immobile, elderly patients with poor nutrition, and Y stands for them developing decubitus ulcers, then we recognize that where X occurs, Y is apt to follow. If the cause is known, then the causal conditions can be prevented.

A function of cause in nursing and health care is also to forewarn a health professional that a health care intervention, such as surgery, implies health care problems for postsurgical patients, such as hemorrhagic shock, atelectasis, thrombophlebitis, wound infection, and urinary retention.[3] By recognizing these possible effects, we use causal factors to intervene against the occurrence of these postsurgical effects.

"WHY" QUESTIONS

From ancient times to the present, some people have wanted to know the causes of events. Why do stars and planets move in orbits? Why is there gravitation? Why does life occur in some places and not others? Why does the heart function? Why do certain patients with the same signs and symptoms recover at different rates, or not at all? Why are nurses undervalued? To answer these and other *Why* questions calls for adequate causal explanations.

To fulfill the conditions of a satisfactory explanation means we have reasons to rule out alternative explanations. For some problems, an explanation may be relatively easy to give. Why did Mary Rolinson, 26 years old, recover from her appendectomy? Because she was in good health; an expert operated on her. Her parents were wealthy. There were no complications after surgery and the round the clock nursing care was excellent. But for some patients and for some conditions, explanations are more complicated and are often unsatisfactory. Why did Rufus Jones, 18 years old, in H 206, arrest? Why do some people get certain cancers? Why was acquired immune deficiency syndrome undetected for so long? Why is Alzheimer's disease still largely a mystery? and Why do people age, break down, and die when they do?

An effort to answer these and other *Why* questions continues. If an ordinary event is not satisfactorily explained, one way to deal with it is to look for criteria to evaluate any explanation, and then apply these criteria to the case at hand.

An example of an explanation is: Why is this object red? Answer: It is a rose and all roses are red. Schematically, this type of explanation, developed by C. Hempel, a philosopher of science, looks like this:

T P_1 All red roses are red.
T P_2 This object is a rose.
T $\therefore C_1$ This object is red.[4]

Students of syllogistic logic will notice this to be a first figure AAA argument, one with two universal, affirmative premises and a universal, affirmative conclusion. The conclusion, the statement to be explained is called the *explanandum;* and the premises or reasons that account for the conclusion are called the *explanans.* For an explanation to be both valid and sound means that the premises and conclusion must be true.

For the simplified example, the explanation may be demonstrated to be true. But for some complex health care examples, we may not have sufficient evidence to establish the truth of the conclusion. But we can use the model of explanation to evaluate explanations that are offered in health care. One way to evaluate causal explanations is to reformulate them as if–then statements, and apply established if–then criteria to explanations.

CAUSATION AS A FORM OF IF–THEN REASONING

In nursing, as in other fields, statements of cause–effect relationships may be expressed as a form of if–then reasoning. The *if* refers to the antecedent, and the *then* refers to the conclusion of a causal sequence. M. Gordon writes,

> If jaundice, then abnormality in skin color; if abnormality in skin color, then change in outward appearance; if change in outward appearance, then feelings of being different; if feelings of being different, then negative perception of body or self, and if feelings of being different, then decreased family and social contacts.[5]

Readers of the deductive chapters (8, 9 and 10) will recognize this as a Chain argument of a sorites form, an argument with more than two premises.

Another example of if–then reasoning is provided by C. Tanner, who writes,

> If the patient is immobile, then there is a chance for decubitus ulcer formation. If the patient is immobile, and if the patient is elderly, and if the patient's nutritional status is poor, then the probability of decubitus is 95%.[6]

Immobility and poor nutritional status together may provide some causal conditions of a decubitus ulcer. But, unless the two conditions of immobility and poor nutrition in conjunction invariably result in this ulcer, we cannot say that we have found the complete cause of a decubitus ulcer.

Tanner examines this nursing student's generalization: If a patient lives in a mobile home, then the patient has a low income. If the patient has a low income, then she or he would get poor health care and inadequate help with special dietary needs.[7] If a patient lives in a mobile home and has a high income, then this causal statement is refuted.

ASSESSING CAUSAL STATEMENTS: USE OF COUNTER-FACTUAL CONDITIONAL JUDGMENTS IN NURSING

One way to assess a causal if–then statement in nursing is to consider subjunctive or counter-factual conditionals. A counter-factual conditional is contrary to fact. For example, "If Florence Nightingale had never existed, nursing would be worse off." We know as a matter of fact that she existed. So the antecedent is false. But we are asked to assume what would have happened to nursing if Nightingale had never existed.

One informal logician writes that:

> Counterfactuals are, in fact, extremely important both in science and in ordinary life. If is often important to make claims about what would have happened or would happen if conditions were different from what they are. In science and in ordinary life, we usually distinguish between counterfactuals, thinking that some are true or plausible and others are false or implausible.[8]

Some nursing examples are: (1) If nursing had moved into the academic mainstream early in this century, it would now be a well-established scientific discipline as is medicine. (2) If nursing had remained an apprenticeship-type training in hospitals, it would now be a well-established occupation in health care delivery. (3) If nursing education and practice moved to the same scientific level as medicine, it would attract great numbers of applicants. (4) If nursing had become independent of medicine and science 40 years ago, it would now be at the center of the health professions and attract large numbers of applicants.

We can argue that some counter-factual judgments, such as 1 and 3, are plausible, whereas 2 and 4 are likely to be false and even implausible, given the state of science and technology that surrounds modern nursing.

Although these examples of judgments may be debatable, the evaluation of counter-factual judgments in nursing may be quite useful. Even though the antecedent is known to be false, if we assume *ex hypothesi* that the antecedent is true and then examine the consequent in relation to the assumed antecedent, we can then determine whether a given counter-factual judgment is true, false, plausible, or implausible. We can then test judgments, such as "If Nurse Anderson had turned the patient every half hour, he would not have gotten a decubitus ulcer." and "If the gallbladder patient was not 60 pounds overweight and was not a heavy smoker, then he would not have gotten atelectasis." By assuming the truth of the antecedent, we can test whether nursing judgments, such as these, are true, false, probable, plausible, or implausible. We can translate counter-factual judgments into cause–effect relationships, using this form: (A) If X had not occurred, Y would not have occurred. (B) Assume the truth of X and test to determine if X is followed by Y, as follows: (C) X was a necessary or sufficient condition for Y. (D) Therefore, X is a causal factor in the occurrence of Y.

Exercises

Reformulate the following sentences into cause–effect statements.

1. Where there is thunder, there is lightning.
   Answer: Thunder causes lightning.
2. A stitch in time saves nine.
   Answer: Prevention pays off.
3. Irritability, tremulousness, cold and clammy skin and diaphoresis are signs and symptoms of hypoglycemia.[9]
   Answer: These signs and symptoms are indicative of a patient having little sugar.
4. A patient's immobility, old age, and poor nutritional status results in 95 percent chance of decubitius.[10]
   Answer: A patient's immobility, old age, and poor nutrition contribute to an overwhelming probability of decubitus.
5. Patients in mobile homes are poor.[11]
   Answer: Mobile homes are a causal factor in explaining poverty among patients.

Are these statements true or false? Where would we look for evidence?

6. The use of marijuana leads to heroin addiction.
   Proposed answer: Relevant medical journal.
7. Saccharine causes cancer of the bladder.
8. Cigarette smoking causes lung cancer.
9. Oral contraceptives cause fatal blood clots.
10. Vitamin C increases one's resistance to colds.[12]
11. Buckling up with a seat belt causes saving of lives.
12. Crime on television causes violence.
13. Heavy drinking causes high blood pressure.[13]
14. Church attendance causes fewer crimes.
15. Jaundice causes yellow skin and low self-esteem.
16. Teaching patients preoperatively causes 50 percent anxiety reduction.[14]

Identify the types of causal statements used and reformulate it into one that can be evaluated.

17. If Chad Green were living today with child leukemia and had chemotherapy in place of Laetrile, he would survive.
    Proposed answer: Counter-factual conditional. If there is a boy like Chad Green with respect to age and leukemia, and if he is treated with chemotherapy, then the probability is that he will survive.

The assumed truth of the antecedent places the burden on the evidence to be secured for the conclusion also being true as a condition for the counter-factual to be judged as true.

MILL'S METHODS FOR ESTABLISHING CAUSAL CONNECTIONS

J. S. Mill, a notable philosopher, lived 1806 to 1873. Several of his methods of ascertaining a causal connection are useful applications to c → e (cause–effect) relations in nursing. Suppose several nurses ate in the hospital cafeteria: Nurse A ate grapefruit, chicken, peach pie, and developed stomach cramps and diarrhea. Nurse B ate grapefruit, steak, salad, peach pie, and developed stomach cramps and diarrhea. Nurse C ate fruit cup, fish, salad, peach pie, and developed stomach cramps and diarrhea. Symbolized, we have:

A. grapefruit, chicken, peach pie—diarrhea.
B. grapefruit, steak, salad, peach pie—diarrhea.
C. fruit cup, fish, salad, peach pie—diarrhea.[15]

To use Mill's method of agreement, we assume that there is one cause of stomach cramps and diarrhea. A presumptive cause of cramps and diarrhea for Nurses A, B, and C is not grapefruit, chicken, steak, salad, fruit cup, or fish, but the peach pie.[16] The formula for the method of agreement is that if c is present (peach pie) followed by e being present (stomach cramps and diarrhea), then c is the cause of e.

Next, let us consider this argument: Nurse D ate chicken pie (cp), salad (s), ice cream (ic), and developed diarrhea (d). Nurse E ate chicken pie, salad, ate no ice cream, and was free of diarrhea. Nurse F ate no pie, ate no ice cream, and was also free of diarrhea. Again, the assumption is that the cause is one of the foods eaten. Using the method of difference, however, we reason that a factor absent in the antecedent and absent in the effect cannot be the cause. Therefore, by the process of elimination, ice cream is the cause of the diarrhea. In abbreviated form, we have:

D. cp, s, ic → d
E. cp, s, − ic → − d
F. −cp, s, −ic → −d

These are called the methods of agreement and difference. These examples show that the methods of agreement and difference are useful ways of identifying causal factors even in complex events.

A still more precise method is Mill's method of concomitant variation. Consider: Nurse G ate one hamburger (h), developed cramps and diarrhea and a temperature of 101F. Nurse H ate two hamburgers and developed stomach cramps and diarrhea (d) with 102F fever (t). Nurse I ate three hamburgers, developed stomach cramps and diarrhea with 103F fever. Here we are not concerned with the presence or absence of the effect when the cause is present, but with the degree in which both the cause and the effect are present. In abbreviated form:

G.	1h → d and t (temp)	101F
H.	2h → d and t	102F
I.	3h → d and t	103F

Mill's three methods state that if antecedent factors are present in conjunction with the consequent; or if, when the antecedent is absent, the consequent is absent; or if the antecedent is present in varying degrees, followed by the consequent in varying degrees, then the antecedent is regarded as the cause of the consequent. In the presence of c_1 and e_1 the amount or degree of c_1 is correlated with e_1, with c_1 as the causal factor of e_1.

Mill's methods work to correlate phenomena in the natural and social sciences. They do, however, assume a definite set of antecedent causal factors and correlate gross phenomena. Mill's methods are helpful in attempting to determine if poverty or broken homes are a more important cause of juvenile delinquency; or to determine if smokers are at higher risk for lung cancer; or if the use of seatbelts reduces the number of automobile fatalities. In the nineteenth century, studies applying Mill's methods showed that chimney sweeps in England contracted lung diseases at a higher rate than the rest of the population. In nursing, scholars, such as N. Woods, have applied Mill's methods to diagnostic reasoning.[17]

Despite some notable uses and successes, there are limits to Mill's methods. The cause of an event among a given set of antecedents and consequents may be overlooked. A patient's clues may not include the relevant and significant causal factors. Moreover, the items in the antecedent–consequent correlation may be too general to be useful.

Exercises

Which of Mill's methods would you cite for the following?

1. Patients A, B, and C smoke two packs a day. Patient D smokes one pack. A, B, and C cough 34 to 37 times per day. D coughs 12 times a day.
   Answer: Concomitant variation. Cough causally correlated with amount of smoking.
2. Bob, Harry, Bill, and Henry smoke, sing, and cough. Mike does not smoke and he does not cough, but he sings. What causes their cough?
   Answer: Smoking, method of difference.
3. Mr. K had a permanent pacemaker inserted and a day later, the nurse noticed a bulging around "the area." The effect of post-

operative bulging is generally not caused by impending infection, subcutaneous bleeding, or accumulated serosanguineous drainage, but rather is an expected outcome of the insertion of permanent pacemakers.[18]
Answer: Combined methods of agreement and difference.

4. Mr. K has a heart block with a ventricular rate of 40. The physician orders a bolus of atropine sulfate 1 mg intravenously (IV push). This is expected to result not in decreased respiratory secretions, in dilating the coronary arteries, or in reduced artery pressure, but in an increase in heart rate.[19] The finding that atropine causes an increase in the heart rate is explained by which of Mill's methods?
Answer: Method of agreement.
5. As a side effect, Isuprel causes Mr. K's heart to start "pounding in his chest."
Answer: Combined methods of agreement and difference.

THREE INTERPRETATIONS OF CAUSE–EFFECT RELATIONS APPLICABLE TO NURSING

We make several assumptions when looking for causes of health-related events. One assumption is that every event must have a cause. One view of cause–effect relations is that "Every event has a cause;" and this statement is certain and necessarily true. We call this the natural necessity view.[20] According to this statement, there cannot be an uncaused event. Every disease must have a cause. The only question, then, is to find it. This view has been held by such diverse thinkers as Thomas Aquinas (1225–1274) and John Locke (1632–1704).

Another philosopher, David Hume (1711–1776), challenged the natural necessity view; and he did so with a powerful argument. Hume held that the only way we know anything about the world is through sense impressions in experience. Every idea is traceable to sense impressions. According to Hume, to infer a cause means it has to constitute a plausible part of our experience; there are "no ideas without sense impressions." The notion that every event has a cause is an idea, but what impressions do we have of this idea? We have the "habit of expecting" that if we take a kettle of water and put sufficient flame under it, the water will boil. But how do we know that the water will boil? Because when a sufficient flame was placed under a kettle of water in the past, we noticed that the water boiled shortly afterward. But we have no sense impression of one event causing another. According to Hume's argument, the idea of causality is nothing more than a *constant conjunction* of two events in the past going together in our minds. We form an association, therefore, of the two events as if they were inseparably linked in the world. But even out of a past tense "constant conjunction" of events that we think are connected, being connected in our minds, we cannot (knowingly) say that one is the cause of the cause of the other in the real world. We then expect or form the "habit of expecting" or of supposing that the first is the cause of the second.

In the past, we have seen the spirochete followed by syphilis, the pneumococcus followed by pneumonia, and streptococcus and staphylococcus followed by infections. If we notice these pathogens, we conclude that they cause these effects.

One of Hume's points is that although constant conjunctions occur, we cannot be sure that the next spirochete, pneumococcus, streptococcus, or staphylococcus will be followed by their respective infections. Another point in Hume's argument is that although we have experienced events in the world, we have never experienced the cause of an event. We surmise or infer a causal link between the two phenomena.

Hume's account leaves room for surprises, and most important, it protects against drawing false inductive conclusions, because in his analysis, we can never know whether every event has a cause. We have, at most, a statistical regularity view of past events; and we project a future event on the basis of the past.

This view helps us to identify causal factors as probable rather than certain or necessary. M. Gordon expresses a position similar to the Humean view in nursing:

> Causal relationships in the health professions are recognized as plausible, not ultimate, necessary or sufficient causes. Thus, . . . etiological factors are thought of as probable causes.[22]

Gordon's view, however, attributes reality to the cause–effect link, whereas Hume questions the idea that there are causes that are known.

An assumption we make in inferring that the future will resemble the past is called the *Principle of the Uniformity of Nature* (PUN).[23] To have predictive laws, which exemplify causal connections stated in a valid deduction, requires the inclusion of the principle of the uniformity of nature in a hypotheticodeductive explanatory scheme. The hypotheticodeductive scheme, using the principle of the uniformity of nature, looks like this:

> Those uniformities that we believe to constitute laws of nature, that have occurred regularly in the past will continue to occur regularly in the future.
> This uniformity (or causal law) has occurred regularly in the past.
> Therefore, this uniformity (or causal law) will occur regularly in the future.[24]

To get the desired conclusion depends on the assumption that the principle of the uniformity of nature is true. But using Hume's analysis, (no ideas without impressions to justify those ideas), there is no justification for the assumption that nature is uniform or that events are connected causally. There may be evidence for the principle of the uniformity of nature. But all the evidence is not sufficient to justify holding this principle as one that is necessarily true. Laws, theories, and explanations are summaries of past regularities rather than future predictions.

The Aquinas–Locke view of *natural necessity* has the advantage of enabling us to assign a truth value in front of the *causal principle* and to the principle of the uniformity of nature, in conjunction with other statements. The difference between the natural necessity view and the *statistical regularity* (Humean) view are schematized by:

The natural necessity view:

> True—Principle of the uniformity of nature. The uniformities that have occurred in the past will occur in the future.
> True—This uniformity has occurred in the past (e.g., acetylsalicylic acid has been safely given and has relieved minor pain).
> True—Therefore, this uniformity will occur in the future.

Using Hume's statistical regularity analysis, we cannot assign a truth value to the major premise or top line of this argument. Even if we assigned a truth value to the second premise, specifying that this uniformity has occurred in the past, we do not have a valid basis for the conclusion. On Hume's analysis, we are left without a conclusion.

A third view, first held by I. Kant (1724–1804) and recently by L. Wittgenstein is that causal laws and the principle of the uniformity of nature are neither true nor false, but are proposals, rules, "inference tickets," leading assumptions, recipes, or regulative principles that justify and guide us in making causal inductions. The principle of the uniformity of nature, which underlies the causal principle, is justified not because it is true or certain, or empirically true, but because adopting this principle pays off in practical results. The causal principle and the principle of the uniformity of nature work and are highly useful to nursing and to all other pursuits of causal relationships. As a physician once said to a patient, "the only remedy is an operation. Whether it works one can't tell. One knows . . . however, that without it, there is no hope."[25] Whether the causal principle or the principle of the uniformity of nature is true is unknown. But if there are predictive causal laws in nature, the principle of the uniformity of nature is assumed as a guiding principle. On this third view, however, we recognize that there is no way to prove that it is true.

The three views of causal connections are: (1) The natural necessity view, (2) the statistical regularity view, and (3) the regulative principle view, which like a map, guides the investigator.

As Gordon writes, "some philosophers argue that the concept of causality should be abandoned; others that it is so implicit in human thinking that it cannot be discarded."[26] Humeans reject causality; Lockeans find it impossible for the world to be without causality; and Kantians find it "implicit in human thinking."

An appropriate synthesis of these three views of cause–effect relations, natural necessity, statistical regularity, and pragmatic justification, strengthens inductive arguments in nursing. The first of these views emphasizes deductive validity and ideal truth. The second emphasizes inductive soundness and substantial, empirical truth; and the third emphasizes the pragmatic justification for making use of the earlier views of cause–effect relationships. But proving the causal principle is like trying to prove that a distant star exists that is forever humanly inaccessible. We believe that this star exists, but only believe this on indirect evidence, through its effects on other stars and planets. Believing in this star seems to give coherence to the rest of the universe. But in the absence of decisive tests, what are we to believe?

A useful distinction to make is between the *task* or *try* and *success* or *achievement* uses of cause in health care. If a cause of a health problem is well established, then we refer to the *success sense,* as in the "conquest" of such diseases as polio. If we are still looking for the cause of a dreaded disease, such as acquired immune deficiency syndrome, then we refer to the task or try sense of causality.

CAUSALITY IN NURSING

What difference do these interpretations of causality make in nursing? And what criteria are relevant to choice? If nurses are committed to the kind of scientific rigor associated with Mill's principles, then the nurse will prefer Hume's view to the natural necessity view. Nurses concerned with an analysis of causality will also appreciate the importance of seeking pragmatic justification to assess both the principle of the uniformity of nature and the causal principle.

Nurses who work with the nursing process and with diagnosis are apt to appreciate the conceptual link between diagnosis and causality. Without assuming causality, there could be no diagnosis, either nursing or medical. To diagnose is to infer a causal factor or a probable causal factor of a health problem. The principle of the uniformity of nature and the causal principle work; they have worked, and the assumption is that they will continue to work. We have no other justification. We accept, therefore, the statement that "Every disease has a cause." But how do we justify accepting this premise in the future? What status do we confer on a cause–effect link? Is an identified cause certain, probable, or only a plausible guess or conjecture, until a better conjecture comes along? Only by accepting the principle of the uniformity of nature as true do we have the basis for the deductive validity and soundness required to conclude that a given causal relation is true. There is, accordingly, a minimal sense in which we accept the natural necessity view of causality; and that is as an assumption that we hope is true.

SOME CAUSAL FALLACIES

The assertion that X causes Y may be fallacious. One fallacy is *false cause,* sometimes known as *post hoc ergo propter hoc.*[27] Here, we assert that just because one event precedes another, the first is the cause of the second. To say that "Nurse A gave care to Mr. B just before he died and that, therefore, she is the cause of his death," is an example of false cause. Or to assert that "Nurse C practiced touch therapy on Ms. L and she recovered. Therefore, Nurse C has healing powers," is another example of false cause.

One version of false cause is to confuse a correlation with a cause. The fact that children have spots and fever does not mean that the spots are a cause of the fever. Both spots and fever are said to be caused by the measles virus.[28]

Exercises

Evaluate the following causal statements as either dubious, plausible, probable, certain and/or useful.

1. Saccharine causes bladder cancer in laboratory animals and, therefore, in humans.
   Answer: Uncertain, plausible, but a useful guideline.
2. Vitamin C increases one's resistance to colds.
   Answer: Uncertain and probable, but also a useful guideline in nursing as health education.
3. Drum beating causes rain to fall.
   Answer: False cause fallacy.
4. Laetrile causes cancer to be cured.
   Answer: False cause fallacy.[29]
5. A bolus of atropine sulfate causes an increased heart rate.[30]
   Answer: Probable.
6. Decreased oxygen to the brain causes syncope (or fainting).[31]
   Answer: Probable.
7. After a permanent demand pacemaker is surgically inserted in a patient's chest wall, nursing care of the patient is to do range of motion exercises with the arm of the affected side, which otherwise causes frozen shoulder syndrome.[32]
   Answer: Probable.
8. Of the roughly 30 agents known to cause cancer in humans, all of them cause cancer in laboratory rats—in high doses.[33]
   Answer: Probable. Questions arise, however, such as: Do agents

known to cause cancer in laboratory rats also cause cancer in humans? And do agents known to not cause cancer in rats also not cause cancer in humans? Is the amount of the dose the critical factor in developing cancer?

9. If Jones had not smoked two packs a day for 30 years, he would not have gotten lung cancer.
Answer: Counter-factual judgment. By assuming the truth of the antecedent, we test whether the consequent is likely to follow from the premise. Given several other conditions, such as a high family lung cancer history, this judgment can be translated into a judgment of the patient's smoking being a probable cause.

10. If this cancer patient had not been exposed to asbestos for 25 years, then he would not have developed asbestosis.
Answer: Translate counter-factual into causal statement: asbestos–asbestosis. Assuming research design, the antecedent is a probable cause of the patient's disease.

CONCLUSION

The intricate nature of certainty, uncertainty, and pragmatic views of cause–effect relationships is a yet undecided issue in induction. For practical nursing purposes, the following statement may be useful: Nursing depends on the continuing search for the causes of, as well as responses to, health problems. To help rationally decide between these views, and to clarify related issues of induction relevant to nursing calls for attention to the nature of evidence and probability.

REFERENCES

1. Gordon, M. Nursing Diagnosis, Process and Application. New York: McGraw-Hill, 1982, p. 103.
2. Hospers, J. An Introduction to Philosophical Analysis (2nd ed.). Englewood-Cliffs, N.J.: Prentice Hall, 1967, p. 291.
3. Gordon, M. Nursing Diagnosis, Process and Application, pp. 103–104, 165.
4. Hempel, C., & Oppenheim, P. The Logic of Explanation, in Feigl, H., & Brodbeck, M. (Eds.), Readings in the Philosophy of Science. New York: Appleton-Century-Crofts, 1953, pp. 319–352.
5. Gordon, M. Nursing Diagnosis, Process and Application, p. 179.
6. Tanner, C. Factors Influencing Diagnostic Process, in Carnevali, D., et al. (Eds.), Diagnostic Reasoning in Nursing. Philadelphia: J.B. Lippincott, 1984, p. 63.
7. Tanner, C. Factors Influencing Diagnostic Process, p. 65.
8. Govier, T. A Practical Study of Argument. Belmont. Belmont, Calif.: Wadsworth, 1985, p. 207.
9. Tanner, C. Factors Influencing the Diagnostic Process, p. 63.

10. Ibid.
11. Ibid.
12. Giere, R. Understanding Scientific Reasoning (2nd ed.). New York: Holt, Rinehart, Winston, 1984, p. 190.
13. Ibid, p. 268.
14. Tanner, C. Factors Influencing the Diagnostic Process, p. 63.
15. Barker, S. Elements of Logic (4th ed.). New York: McGraw-Hill, 1986, p. 257.
16. Ibid.
17. Woods, N. Methods for Studying Diagnostic Reasoning in Nursing, in Carnevali, D., et al. (Eds.), Diagnostic Reasoning in Nursing. Philadelphia: J.B. Lippincott, 1984, p. 197.
18. Desharnais, A., et al. New State Board Examination (2nd Ed.). Norwalk, Conn.: Fleschner Publishing, 1986, p. 120.
19. Ibid, pp. 119, 137.
20. Toulmin, S. Philosophy of Science, London: Hutchinson University Press, 1960, pp. 91–103.
21. Hospers, J. An Introduction to Philosophical Analysis, pp. 207, 250–257.
22. Gordon, M. Nursing Diagnosis, Process and Application, p. 47.
23. Hospers, J., An Introduction to Philosophical Analysis, 3rd edition, Englewood Cliffs, N.J., Prentice Hall, 1988, p. 191.
24. Ibid.
25. Ibid, p. 191.
26. Gordon, M. Nursing Diagnosis, Process and Application, p. 37.
27. Copi, I. Introduction to Logic (7th ed.). New York: Macmillan, 1986, p. 101.
28. Giere, R. Understanding Scientific Reasoning, p. 187.
29. Ibid, p. 313.
30. Desharnais, A., et al. New State Board Examination, pp. 119, 137.
31. Ibid.
32. Ibid.
33. Giere, R. Understanding Scientific Reasoning, p. 283.

Chapter 13

Evidence and Probability

Study of this chapter enables the learner to:

1. Make nursing judgments proportional to the degree of evidence for them.
2. Evaluate the degree of evidence and probability for cause–effect judgments in nursing.
3. Distinguish evidence in nursing from related terms, such as verification, falsification, and testing.
4. Recognize how degrees of evidence affect the credibility of nursing judgments.
5. Recognize the role of probability and uncertainty in nursing.
6. Distinguish three theories of probability and apply them to nursing judgments.
7. Apply Bayes' theorem to nursing judgments.
8. Expose major inductive fallacies.

INTRODUCTION

Nursing judgments and conclusions are more apt to be trusted when backed by appropriate evidence than when judgments lack evidential standards. Mr. M's ankles show signs of edema. He smokes one half of a pack of cigarettes daily. He eats at a fast food restaurant across the street. His meals consist of hamburgers, fried chicken, fried fish, cole slaw, french fried potatoes, and pastries. He tells the nurse, "I ask them to salt the fries."[1] How does the nurse confirm her hypothesis that the patient is retaining fluid? C. Tanner gives these indications. She tells Mr. M:

> . . . perhaps the reason you've put on so much weight and have trouble breathing is from fluid retention.[2]

Tanner cites the reasoning process, the "stringing together of concepts: edema, shortness of breath, weight gain, fluid retention, increased sodium intake."[3] Edema of the ankles provides partial confirmation of fluid retention. Confirmation is one type of evidence or backing for a nursing judgment. Other evidence that needs evaluation is the patient's increase in weight, change in medications, and activity.

Evidence is not certain proof, but a matter of degree. Evidence involves an assessment of probabilities, an evaluation of what the chances are that A rather than B is the cause of X.

MEANING OF SOME KEY TERMS IN RELATION TO EVIDENCE

A statement has meaning if it can be verified analytically or empirically. To say "all diabetics are noncompliant" or that "All acetylsalicylic acid tablets are harmless" requires that complete evidence that each and every diabetic is indeed noncompliant and that each and every acetylsalicylic acid tablet is harmless. One exception invalidates a generalization. How would we ever know that the next diabetic would also be noncompliant? This statement could never be completely verified, because there are always more diabetic patients to follow. Suppose the statement "All acetylsalicylic acid tablets are harmless" has been true in the past. But the truth of this statement in the past does not guarantee its truth for future tablets. The statement, therefore, that "all acetylsalicylic acid tablets are harmless" is not fully verifiable.

To offset the vagueness of verifiability, two further terms are distinguished. One is confirmability. A statement, law, or theory may be confirmed repeatedly through accretion of evidence. To confirm a statement is to increase the likelihood of that statement being true. To falsify a statement is to show a counter-instance. If I say that "All acetylsalicylic acid tablets are harmless," and find an instance of a fatality as a direct consequence of taking such tablets, then I have falsified the above generalization.

A further term clarifies the process of verifying a statement, namely that the statement is testable in the *here and now.* The *operationalist criterion,* as this is called, holds that a scientific statement is meaningful if a method or a set of steps or operations or a recipe can be specified showing how the statement is true.[4] Statements about a patient's pallor, blood count, temperature, respiration, and blood pressure are testable rather than merely verifiable or confirmable. The criteria of verifiability, confirmability, falsifiability, and testing rule out statements that have no evidence.

A fundamental principle of critical thinking in nursing is that every statement is given appropriate cognitive backing in the form of sound evidential reasons.

THE NATURE OF EVIDENCE

A purpose in emphasizing three aspects of evidence, verification, confirmation, falsification or testing, is to look for appropriate backing for different kinds of statements. If Mr. Jones is to have restored motion in an injured shoulder, he will need a range of motion exercises or surgery. Why? Because a frozen shoulder syndrome may be more difficult to treat than the original condition. Smith needs postoperative prostatectomy treatment. Why? To avoid or minimize the postoperative complications of a prostatectomy. Evidential backing is: X needs Y treatment. Why? Because he has just had Z and Y is needed to help X's recovery; and nurses are qualified to give Y treatment.

Qualified judgments that depend on data in the form of relevant evidence take the place of intuitions or feelings. One way to measure evidence is to assess the probability or likelihood that an event will occur on the basis of past occasions.

THREE THEORIES OF PROBABILITY

Because certainty is unobtainable in the world, we settle for the next best thing—maximal probability or the strongest likelihood of the occurrence of an event. Probability refers to the chance that one event out of a finite number of possible events will occur. We use a numerator over a denominator to designate the chances of the event occurring. If 9,000 out of 10,000 quadruple bypass operations have survived for a 5-year period, then a cardiac surgeon may tell the next candidate that he or she has nine out of ten chances of surviving a 5-year period. There are problems with this formulation. We do not always know the denominator. A desperately ill patient with a fatal disease, such as acquired immune deficiency syndrome (AIDS), may or may not be willing to accept an experimental medication with possibly lethal side effects without knowing the denominator.

The chance of turning up a king of hearts in a deck of 52 cards is 1/52. The chance of a coin turning heads on the next flip is 1/2. If 250 people died in a bubonic plague out of 1,000, then the next patient's chance of dying in those circumstances is 1/4. In each of these cases, one knows the denominator, the total number of instances. We are, furthermore, given the numerator. We then calculate the chance of the occurrence of positive and negative events. To compute a probability of the foregoing kind is known as the *a priori theory*. The a priori theory of probability is ideal and is clearly suitable when there are equal chances for the occurrence of an event. This occurs in lotteries, coin tosses, dice throws, and chances of knowing the next card. But as almost everyone knows, the chance that most health care events occur is seldom, if ever, exactly equal. This difficulty with the a priori theory leads us to an alternative theory of probability.

An alternative theory, the *relative frequency* view, holds that we need further specification of the denominator before we can compute the probability of the occurrence of an event. "Of 1,000 25-year-old women, if 971" survive "at least one additional year, the number .971 is assigned as the probability coefficient . . ."[5]

The relative frequency theory, being empirical, is useful in statistical studies, whereas the a priori, classical theory, formulates the basic ground rules of probability theory. The a priori theory of probability assumes that all possibilities are equal. They are when the quantity of the denominator is determined, as in tossed coins, cards, or dice.

A third view of probability is the *subjective* or *common sense view.* Here we say, "This is probable . . ." The usual meaning of this statement is: "I think this is likely to occur" or "I would bank on it." To say, "This is probable" expresses a person's degree of trust or credibility in that judgment. An example in the third sense is that of a nurse who says, "It's likely that Mr. Smith will die tonight." Or a nurse says, "I think the new medication will lower Mr. Jones's blood pressure. He'll do better now."

APPLICATIONS OF PROBABILITY THEORY TO NURSING

A central point about all three theories of probability is that they reflect the uncertainty we acknowledge in arriving at a health care decision. If the chance of an event occurring is 100 percent, we assign a 1 in the numerator over a 1 in the denominator to that event. For example, everyone dies is a 1/1.

According to C. Seaman and P. Verhonick,

> . . . the theory of probability deals with the possibility of events occurring by chance.[6]

These authors distinguish three theories as they apply to nursing:

> 1), A subjective determination of fair odds; 2), relative frequencies expected to occur in a series of events; and 3), an equally likely set of events mathematically calculated.[7]

We all make decisions that affect aspects of our lives. We give probability assignments to our decisions in the hope or assumption of maximizing benefits and minimizing harm to ourselves and others we care for. We may be mistaken, but we go by probabilities in a subjective or common sense way. The chances of an AIDS patient recovering from repeated infections are currently 0; and the chances of his or her dying is 1; which means that on the basis of known AIDS patients dying, it is highly probably that an AIDS patient with recurrent infections will die. We may formulate this example as a subjective or common sense probability : "It's highly unlikely that a treatment to reverse AIDS can be developed for a patient currently suffering from AIDS." Seaman and Verhonick write that

> Much of nursing practice depends upon subjectively experienced, anticipated probabilities . . . the decision to give one type of nursing care may be based upon the nurse's present experience and knowledge of the probability that the patient will experience benefit from this type of nursing care.[8]

They go on to say that "diagnosis and therapy" depend heavily on "subjective internal mental processes."[9] The attempt to formalize "these probabilities in order to make more accurate diagnoses" leads us to the other theories of probability, the empirical relative frequency theory and the a priori mathematical theory previously discussed.

Tanner points out that

> . . . the use of probability statements is commonplace in medicine. On informed consents for medical procedures, . . . many states require that the probability of complications be explicitly stated, e.g. the chance of developing a blood clot after an arteriogram is 5%.[10]

Probabilities are also stated as the conditions of the patient's age and physical status. Tanner claims that the systematic observations of large numbers of people are a necessary empirical basis for precise statements of probabilities. Effective clinical decision making in both diagnosis and prognosis depends "at least on the informal assignment of probabilities to clinical data."[11] Ignoring probabilistic relations "between cues and client states leads . . . to errors in diagnosis."[12] Tanner gives this example. Nursing students learn that signs and symptoms of hypoglycemia, related to short-acting insulin, include change in behavior,

> . . . irritability, tremulousness, cold and clammy skin and diaphoresis. They also learn that the causes of hypoglycemic reaction are delayed or omitted meals; excessive exercise, or insulin overdosage . . The diagnosis is confirmed through accumulation of data and informally revising the probability of the hypothesis with each datum.[13]

A blood sugar test, however, is "the only cue that might bear a positive relationship to hypoglycemia of sufficient magnitude that no other data would be needed."[14] A blood sugar sample provides a sufficient condition of hypoglycemia.

Tanner points out that "probabilistic relationships between cues and diagnosis increases the thoroughness of data collection and improves diagnostic accuracy."[15] In general, nurse practitioners need to collect more data as the basis for increased probabilistic relationships between cues and diagnosis.

Although differences exist among subjective, relative frequency, and a priori theories of probability, a point of overlap is that there are probabilities in place of certainties in all theories. In citing these examples in nursing, we recognize that the effort is to approach the a priori theory of probability, but to settle for the frequency theory, and when the other theories are not accessible, to use the subjective theory. The a priori view provides an unachievable ideal of probability, an ideal model of a statistically sound basis for predictions. The relative frequency view provides an account of how some nursing problems are actually solvable. Here we deal with the actual data and criteria of statistical sampling. The subjective view indicates how guardedly we give our word or authority to our inductive assertions.

BAYES' THEOREM IN NURSING

A problem with all three theories of probability is that they leave us with a "superabundance of hypotheses"[16] in the denominator, the lower number in the fraction. This leaves probability too open-ended and "hopelessly inclusive."[17] We need a ruling out device to prune down on the wealth of possibilities. The probability calculus can be useful at this point.

Diagnoses involve various judgments. One is that the patient has certain diseases. To consider prior probabilities or likelihoods, giving them special weight rather than counting them as equally possible, appeals to Bayes' theorem. This is formally rendered:

$$P(D/C) = \frac{P(C/D)\ P(D)^{18}}{P(C)}$$

P(D/C) is the posterior probability, and refers to "the patient's chances or probability of having the disease D, given symptom C; P(C/D) is the likelihood of a patient's exhibiting C, given that he or she has D; P(D) is the prior probability that the patient has D; and P(C) is the probability that the patient will exhibit C whether or not he has D."[19] For our purposes, the gist of Bayes' theorem is that a health professional is aware of some diseases being more likely with some patients than others. A health professional's orientation or initial predisposition to regard a patient's having a disease, "is directly proportional to the incidence of that disease in the population he serves."[20]

> If the flu bug is on the rampage, and the patient has fever and chills, the prior probability that your patient has the flu is quite high, although of course, it could conceivably turn out to be tuberculosis or malaria.[21]

Applying Bayes' theorem consists in giving a patient's prior conditions a probability rating, and in not regarding "every disease as equally probable."[22] Another way to state Bayes' theorem is to start with the simplest, most common hypothesis. We then proceed to test for increasingly complex hypotheses as simpler hypotheses are eliminated.

Exercises

1. How would we estimate the chances of black and non-black youngsters getting Tay-Sachs disease in a rural southern community?
   An answer: We compare rural and nonrural regions, the percentage of blacks and non-blacks, and the frequency of Tay-Sachs disease among both groups.
2. If Nurse A says, "Mr. J, an AIDS patient, will most probably die of AIDS within a few years," which theory of probability is she using?
   Answer: She is using primarily the a priori theory, which at this point of uncertainty assigns a 100 percent death rate to all AIDS patients.
3. Betty, an 8-year-old child, comes into the pediatric nurse practitioner's office with spots all over her body, and a fever. The nurse asks "What illnesses have there been in her school?" Betty's mother says, "The teacher told me that two children had the chicken pox." What presumptive or initial diagnosis is the pediatric nurse practitioner likely to make on the basis of the available data?
   Answer: Chicken pox.
4. Which probability theorem helps the pediatric nurse practitioner decide what Betty has?
   Answer: Bayes' theorem.
5. What does Bayes' theorem state for nursing diagnosis?
   Answer: Among diseases presented, assign special weight or prior probability to those diseases that are currently present in one's environment.

EXPECTATIONS AND UNUSUAL SURPRISES

A strength of Bayes' theorem is to start with an expected disease. A difficulty with Bayes' theorem, however, is that it ignores unlikely and rare diseases. In health and disease, there are good and bad surprises. A point about induction is to be aware of surprises and thereby to cope with them.

The more frequently repeated an event F is, the more likely it is that the event F will not continue. A clock, car, train, plane, ship, washing machine, pacemaker, or human body wears down. A diagnosis that rules in the obvious disease by appealing to prior probability may lose precious time in which to rule out the rare, less commonplace disease. Reluctance to consider the rare and uncommonplace can also lead to erroneous judgments.

The problem for nurses is to decide when to invoke Bayes' theorem and when to consider less likely possibilities. A suggested principle is to hope for the expected, but not rule out unexpected surprises or rare conditions.

INDUCTIVE FALLACIES

Five inductive fallacies are apt to occur. The first is *hasty generalization.* Take one, two, or a few instances in which X's and Y's, and infer that, therefore, all X's are Y's. An experimental drug may work on a patient for a short time, but that does not prove that such a drug works for that patient or for all patients all the time. Hasty generalization consist in making a universal inference on the basis of a limited sample.

Suppose Physician Yan, an intern, meets Nurse Ying, a supervisor at Q hospital. Ying turns out to be an ardent feminist, who insists that women should have equal courtship rights, such as proposing marriage to men. Yan, a traditional man, is shocked and reports to his fellow interns that all the nurses at Q hospital are ardent feminists. Ying will then have committed the hasty generalization fallacy.[23] Or for example, if one old patient smells badly, we cannot validly infer that all old patients smell badly. Sexist, racist, religious, or ethnic stereotyping also generalizes about people of a particular sex, race, sect, or ethnic group on the basis of a small sample.

A second inductive fallacy is *forgetful induction.* This fallacy may occur in a statistical sampling, where there is a thorough sampling of one region or part of a study only to completely ignore or forget another. Forgetful induction consists in neglecting relevant empirical evidence. In Hospital R an interviewer finds that there are 500 employees. The interviewer visits the eye clinic and finds that out of 50 employees in that department, 20 percent are over age 62. If the interviewer infers that, therefore, 20 percent of all 500 hospital employees are over age 62, the interviewer commits the forgetful induction fallacy.

A third fallacy is to treat a conclusion as certain when the evidence runs against it. We prefer not to accept a distasteful conclusion, such as the impending death of a beloved relative. This fallacy is known as *slothful induction,* and consists in the refusal to allow any evidence to be considered that refutes our preferred conclusion. Slothful induction is a way to insulate ourself against rational criticism.[24]

An aspect of critical thinking consists in exposing and challenging dogmas, and to question ideas. An antidote to slothful induction is the right to inquire, no matter where the inquiry leads. A nurse, physician, or patient who refuses to question a particular treatment or diagnosis just because it coincides with deeply ingrained habits, whether by a specialist in the disease or a nonspecialist, is committing the fallacy of slothful induction.

A fourth mistake in reasoning is to infer that if a regular sequence occurs, such as a toss of the coin, showing heads in five throws, that the next flip of the coin must result in a tail. This is known as the *Monte Carlo fallacy.* Obstetrical nurses assisting in the deliveries of an unbroken sequence of male babies incorrectly infer that the next birth must be that of a female. An intensive care unit nurse has worked for five consecutive days without the occurrence of a patient's death. On the fifth day of practice, Nurse Jones says, "Someone will surely die today." Her argument commits the Monte Carlo fallacy.

A fifth fallacy, known as the *false cause fallacy,* occurs if a speaker assumes that because two events have occurred in temporal sequence, the first is the cause of the second. Nurse A sees a patient, Ms. L, who had taken Laetrile. Ms. L is in remission of cancer. If Nurse A concludes that Laetrile caused the cancer remission, she or he commits the fallacy of false cause.

Exercises

Identify the fallacy and explain why it is a fallacy.

1. Nurse Jones sees Amie O'Reilly, 16 years old, sweet, pug-nosed, happy disposition, fresh from Ireland, making the best of her diagnosis. Ms. Jones concludes that all young Irish women are sweet, pug-nosed, and happy.
   Answer: Fallacy of hasty generalization.
2. Ms. Jackson, 45 years old, a mastectomy patient, has not see her husband in 6 days. He promised to see her within 2 weeks of her surgery. On the basis of probability, she concludes that her husband is more likely to see her the next day.
   Answer: Monte Carlo fallacy. It does not follow that he is more likely to see her on the seventh day as he did not see her the first 6 days.
3. A nurse investigator is studying the effects of therapeutic touch. TT, on tension headache pain, and concludes that TT causes headache pain reduction after 4 hours.
   Answer: Fallacy of false cause. The readers, however, are invited to study E. Keller's and V. Bzdek's article on this subject to deter-

mine for themselves if the evidence rationally shows that TT causes headache pain reduction after 4 hours.[25]

4. Massage causes relief of tension.
   Answer: Fallacy of false cause. Unless we can show that a prior event is a necessary and sufficient condition for a later event, we have not succeeded in establishing a causal conclusion.[26]
5. Suppose a study shows that among baccalaureate nurses in a big city, those who are married, aged 45 to 60, 24 percent experience a burn out. The investigator concludes that 24 percent of American middle-aged nurses experience burn out.
   Answer: Fallacy of forgetful induction.

LAWS, CAUSAL EXPLANATIONS, AND PREDICTIONS DISTINGUISHED FROM PROPHECY IN NURSING

A strength of appealing to rigorous standards of logic and science is that we seek the best explanation for events, one that provides the best chance for prediction rather than prophecy. A prophecy is vague, open-ended. If we go to a fortune-teller, we are told our future in such general terms that hardly anything can ever count to refute a given prophecy. A fortune-teller says to Jones, a young person, "I see a lot of traveling to far-away places in your hand." If Jones is a nearby town farmer, and has never traveled; and does not travel for ten years after the fortune-teller's prophecy and Jones sees the fortune-teller, what does the fortune-teller say to Jones? "You have to wait awhile, and then you'll travel far." Supposing there is a war and Jones joins the armed forces and is sent overseas. Has the fortune-teller's prophecy been vindicated? Inasmuch as Jones finally traveled, the prophecy is fulfilled; but there is a salient feature still lacking in a prophecy. It lacks a method for duplicating the initial success of this fortune-teller's prophecy. Looking into Jones's hand and inferring that Jones will travel far is a vague generalization; one that has no causal connection to the lines in his hand. We could tag the fortune-teller with the false cause fallacy.

Moreover, a prophecy is so vague that it has no ruling out devices. A key aspect of critical thinking consists in being open-minded; but a state of open-mindedness is self-critical and welcomes the rational criticism of other inquirers. To be open-minded and self-critical is to know what to include and exclude among candidates for serious conclusions and judgments.

A virtue of nurses appealing to science to justify their judgments is that they do not conclude with prophecies that are too vague, and are never alllowed to be refuted. To offset this difficulty, they seek predictions that are precise anticipations of future events, and that are open to rational refutation or falsification. In science, truth and falsity are never far away from statements that are to be evaluated. The use of true and false to evaluate judgments helps to explain the role of testing, confirmation, falsification, and verification.

Another reason to prefer prediction over prophecy is that prediction occurs in the context of scientific laws and causal explanations within a coherent, structural fabric of interlocking relations. An important value of science consists in its traditions and methods, as well as the accumulated impact of its results. This includes the lessons learned from the working procedures of scientists. It is not that scientists individually are open-minded. It is that the degree of credibility of scientific work depends on acceptable evidence that is open to any investigator to consider. Multiple checks and balances prevent relevant and significant questions from being ignored or silenced. Science and also critical thinking implies scrutiny, investigation, inquiry, rigorous cross-examination as a prelude to rational acceptance.

THE VALUE OF CRITICAL THINKING AND SCIENCE IN NURSING

A value of the role of science in nursing consists in demonstrated respect for evidence. Three attributes in conjunction highlight the scientific approach to human problems. The first is publicness, exposure to public scrutiny and examination of ideas and hypotheses. Scientific inquiry is a glass bowl, not a sealed vault, nor a private antechamber. A second closely related feature of a scientific approach to inquiry is openness to rational reconsideration from any quarter. No matter how fixed or incontrovertible a conclusion seems to be, there is always room for doubt, qualification, and refinement. Questions are never closed to new investigations. A third related feature of a scientific approach is that science is self-correctable through methods of testability. What counts in science is results, not hopes, wishes, fantasies, or intentions. Individual expression of sincerity in the minds of nurse practitioners are laudable, but what counts are scientifically established results.

The upshot for nursing is that the improvement of nursing practice and theory depends on incorporating publicness and openness, and in implementing self-corrective procedures in the evaluation of nursing theory, process, and practice. In short, nursing depends on the incorporation of critical thinking and scientific approaches to nursing problems.

Exercises

In your answers to these questions, try to use criteria of critical thinking and cite fallacies wherever appropriate.

1. What is nursing?
2. Give an example of a nursing prophecy and a nursing prediction? What differences are between these?

3. What is the role of publicness, openness to rational reconsideration, and self-corrective feedback in nursing? Use these considerations critically to evaluate holism, touch therapy, and nonscientific approaches to nursing.

CONCLUSION

In this chapter and in previous chapters of this book, distinctions between ideas and hypotheses and methods of testing have been drawn. An idea or hypothesis in nursing is not self-certifying or self-evident. The best ideas and theories still call for independent testing.

In Anglo-Saxon justice there is a principle that no person can be a judge in his or her own case. We look to third parties to decide cases. So, too, in a physical or nursing theory, no matter how bold or imaginative, it requires appropriate verification. For that purpose, there is no substitute for the "tried and true methods" of both deductive and inductive logic. These are tried and true because they work.

The unfathomable depths of inquiry about the universe and human nature present mysteries, puzzles, dilemmas vastly transcending the power of a single mind to grasp. To help fill the void, the lacuna of ignorance and bafflement, comes the increasingly effective mosaic of scientific inquirers. They respect established canons of reasoning as the basis for the rational settlement of disputes.

The methods of proof or verification and examination are distinguished from ideas, hypotheses, wishes, hopes, fantasies, and desires. Imagination belongs perhaps closer to ideas than to proof; and through imagination the arts enter in the human search for the minimization of suffering. A purpose for distinguishing ideas from methods of proof is to applaud the free flow of ideas and hypotheses, to apply tolerance to ideas of all kinds, origins and, outcomes. But another purpose for distinguishing ideas from methods of proof is to be tough on what produces results. Critical thinking, therefore, enters in two ways, in helping to create ideas and in testing them. We collectively search for rational standards to examine the ideas that come before us. The hardest part is testing them. The temptation may be to make our ideas come out true without testing them. But that is precisely what critical thinking enjoins us not to do. Critical thinking beckons that we examine the ideas that come before us.

Several assumptions operate in the use of critical thinking in nursing. One is that the truth matters, finding it and stating it. We regard this as a firmly entrenched principle, the principle of integrity. A second assumption of critical thinking in nursing is the principle that we use truth to do good. One form of goodness is caring. A third assumption is that we shape our work and our social institutions to achieve truth and goodness. We use methods appropriate to those ends and aspirations.

REFERENCES

1. Tanner, C. Diagnostic Problem Solving Strategies, in Carnevali, D., et al. (Eds.), Diagnostic Reasoning in Nursing. Philadelphia: J.B. Lippincott, 1984, pp. 90–95.
2. Ibid, p. 95.
3. Ibid.
4. Bridgman, P. The Logic of Modern Physics. Cambridge, Mass.: Harvard University Press, 1948.
5. Copi, I. Introduction to Logic (7th ed.). New York: Macmillan, 1986, p. 531.
6. Seaman, C., & Verhonick, P.J. Research Methods for Undergraduate Students in Nursing. New York: Appleton-Century-Crofts, 1982, p. 136.
7. Ibid.
8. Ibid, p. 137.
9. Ibid.
10. Tanner, C. Factors Influencing the Diagnostic Process, in Carnevali, D., et al. (Eds.), Diagnostic Reasoning in Nursing, p. 63.
11. Ibid.
12. Ibid.
13. Ibid, pp. 63–64.
14. Ibid, p. 64.
15. Ibid.
16. Salmon, W. The Foundations of Scientific Inference. Pittsburgh: University of Pittsburgh Press, 1967, pp. 115–116.
17. Ibid.
18. Schaffner, K. Logic of Discovery and Diagnosis in Medicine. Berkeley, Calif.: University of California Press, 1985, p. 7.
19. Ibid.
20. Clauser, K. Approaching the Logic of Diagnosis, in Schaffner, K. (Ed.), Logic of Discovery and Diagnosis in Medicine, p. 39.
21. Ibid.
22. Ibid.
23. Barker, S. Elements of Logic (4th ed.). New York: McGraw Hill, 1985, p. 245.
24. Ibid, p. 246.
25. Keller, E., & Bzdek, V. Effects of Therapeutic Touch on Tension Headache Pain. *Nursing Research* 1986; 35(2):101–103, March/April.
26. Kurland, H. Treatment of Headache with Auto Acupressure. *Current Psychiatric Therapies* 17(21):271–274.

Glossary

Analytic. A statement whose truth is demonstrated by inspecting its parts without reference to external verification, e.g., "A tall nurse is a nurse."

Antecedent. The premise or premises of an argument; the "if" part of an "if–then" logical relationship.

A Priori. A statement whose truth is independent of experience, e.g., "A nurse is a health professional."

Chain Argument. An argument with two premises, including a middle term that is eliminated in the conclusion. $P \rightarrow Q, Q \rightarrow R / \therefore P \rightarrow R$

Conclusion. A claim one argues for supported by reasons.

Conditional. An "If–then" argument consisting of a premise and a conclusion.

Contradictory. Two statements that have opposite truth values. If one is true, the other is false, and vice versa.

Contrary. Two statements that may both be false but that may not both be true, e.g., "Nurse A is highly qualified. Nurse A is unqualified."

Controversial Issue. A debatable issue morally, politically, esthetically, ideologically, e.g., "Abortion is murder. Abortion is a woman's right."

Counter-factual–Subjunctive Conditional. A conditional cast in the subjunctive mood with a false antecedent, e.g., "If he had gone to the hospital sooner, he would have survived."

Decision Making with Certainty, Uncertainty, or Risk. Decision making with certainty depends upon definite knowledge of the state of the world. When nothing is known about the state of the world, a decision is made with uncertainty. When knowledge is incomplete, probable, or statistical, decisions are made with risk.

Denying the Antecedent. Formal fallacy of using an antecedent consequent relation in which the denial of the consequent entitles one to deny the antecedent, but not to first deny the antecedent followed by denying the consequent, e.g., "If a nurse were here, someone would help the patient. The nurse wasn't here. So, no one helped the patient."

Dilemma. A problem all of whose solutions are unsatisfactory.

Disjunction. The use of "or" either inclusively or exclusively. If "or" is used exclusively, then one or both disjuncts P or Q may be true, e.g., a nurse has an option of giving acetaminophen or codeine, meaning one or the other or both. In the exclusive use of "or," if one disjunct is true, the other is false, e.g., "A nurse chooses to give acetaminophen or acetylsaclicylic acid, meaning one or the other, but not both."

Division Fallacy. Informal fallacy of arguing that because a characteristic applies to a group, class, or collection, therefore, that characteristic belongs to the members of that group, e.g., "Hospital S is good. So, every health professional who works there is good."

Double Negative. The negation of a negation, which formally implies a positive, e.g., $- - P = P$.

Empirical. A statement based on experience.

Enthymeme. An argument with a premise or a conclusion missing or assumed; e.g., "All nurses are hardworking. Ms. Anderson is hardworking. Missing premise. Ms. Anderson is a nurse."

Evidence. Relevant factual reasons for an empirical conclusion.

Exclusion. A formal principle that denies that a conjunction of two propositions is true. The formula is: $-(P \& Q),\ P /\therefore -Q$.

Existential Fallacy. The presence of exclusively universal premises followed by a particular conclusion.

Fallacy. A mistake in an argument or in the critical thinking process that makes an argument invalid.

Fallacy of Appeal to Force. Informal fallacy in which one argues that because one has power, one is right.

Fallacy of Appeal to Ignorance. Informal fallacy in which one argues that because the opposite of a given proposition has not been proved, the initial proposition is true; e.g., "It's never been proved that smoking causes cancer. Therefore, smoking doesn't cause cancer."

Fallacy of Appeal to Irrelevant Authority. Taking the word of someone who does not have relevant authority.

Fallacy of Begging the Question. Assuming as true what is to be proved, e.g., "Touch therapy is true. Ask any believer."

Fallacy of Black or White Thinking. Either–or fallacy of supposing that two contraries exhaust all alternatives, e.g., "Live free or die" (New Hampshire license plate slogan).

Hasty Generalization. Inductive fallacy in which one leaps from a few particular instances to a universal statement, e.g., "Some nurses are women. Therefore, all nurses are women."

If–Then. One or more sentences in which the antecedent, a set of reasons, is followed by a conclusion.

Illicit Major. Fallacy in which the predicate is distributed in the conclusion but not in the premise.

Illicit Minor. Fallacy in which the subject is distributed in the conclusion but not in the premise.

Implication. A formal relation between two or more propositions, one of which follows from the other(s). An implication may also refer to a suggestion or command, e.g., "The patient is not breathing, may imply: Get some help."

Inclusive Use of "Or". Interpretation of a disjunction, which holds that one or both disjuncts are true, e.g., "All our nurses in Hospital Z are women or men."

Inference. Taking one proposition as given and guessing that another proposition follows, e.g., "I see a person in green pajamas in Hospital R. Therefore, that person is a patient."

Induction. Logical process of arriving at a substantive conclusion that is uncertain and probable, and depends on verification that is external, e.g., "Nurses observed in this hospital are women. Therefore, it is probable that all nurses in this hospital are women."

Justification. A set of reasons that establishes a conclusion.

Major Term. The predicate of a conclusion in a categorical syllogism.

Material Implication. A formal relation between two or more propositions between an antecedent and a consequent that requires that if the antecedent is true, the consequent cannot be false for an argument to be valid. If, however, the antecedent is false, the argument is valid, whether the consequent is true or false. In $P \rightarrow Q$, if P is true, Q must be true. If P is false, Q may be true or false, and the argument will still be valid.

Metaphor. An analogy using a word picture.

Middle Term. The term used in each of the premises along with the minor and major terms, but not used in the conclusion of a valid argument.

Minor Term. The subject of the conclusion in a categorical syllogism.

Modus Ponens. The assertion of an antecedent–consequent relation, P then Q. If this relation P, then Q is followed by the assertion of the antecedent P, then one is entitled to assert the consequent Q; e.g., "If physicians marry smart nurses, they will both be happy. Joe, a physician, married Helen, a smart nurse.. Therefore, they are both happy."

Modus Tollens. The assertion of an antecedent–consequent relationship, $P \rightarrow Q$, followed by denial of the consequent, $-Q$. This implies denial of the antecedent, $-P$.

Natural Deduction. An argument with premises and conclusion as given, followed by a demonstration of the premises implying the conclusion, with justifying reasons drawn from appropriate rules of inference.

Necessary Condition. A causal factor without which a conclusion of an inductive argument does not follow.

Negation. The denial of a proposition.

Non Sequitur. Does not follow from the premises.

Nursing. The diagnosis and treatment of human responses to actual or potential health problems.

Nursing Diagnosis. The effort to name a perceived difficulty or need as the basis for understanding its meaning to institute treatment and resolution.

Nursing Process. A systematic, sequential approach to assessment of the patient's situation involving data collection and diagnosis, planning, treatment, and evaluation. The plan includes joint patient/family and nurse participation and implementation of all phases of the process.

Nursing Theory. Concepts, principles, and processes basic to nursing actions. Nursing theory is drawn from nursing research and from other sciences on the basis of their explanatory value to nursing diagnosis and treatment.

Operationalist Criterion. Judging the truth of a theory by the procedures for testing it.

Paradigm Case Argument. An argument that makes use of a standard example of a principle to illustrate the principle; e.g., "If people have rights, they have health care rights to give informed consent, a right that black people were denied in the Tuskeegee syphilis study."

Performative. A term or set of terms that when uttered simultaneously makes something happen, e.g. "I now pronounce you man and wife."

Premise. Antecedent of an argument that helps to justify the conclusion.

Principle of Coherence. Criterion of inclusiveness in characterizing a system or theory of thought.

Principle of Consistency. To assert the same values throughout a system of values without contradictions.

Principle of Integrity. Assumption that people engaged in inquiry seek to find, identify, and communicate the truth.

Scientific Method. A codified sequence of steps used in the formulation, testing, evaluation and reporting of scientific ideas.

Square of Opposition. A formal relation between universal affirmative (A), universal negative (E), particular affirmative (I), and particular negative (O) propositions, showing the implications of contraries, contradictories, and subcontraries, e.g., "If an A proposition is true, then an O proposition is false."

Sufficient Condition. A causal condition by which an event must occur, e.g., "If it rains, the garden will be wet."

Truth Table. A formal procedure for assigning true and false values in an argument, which enables one to prove that an argument is valid or invalid.

Umbrella Statement. A general value statement that by inclusion of particular values provides justification for the particular values.

Vague. A term without clear boundaries for determining meaning, e.g., bald, big, small, alive, rich, game, cold, hot.

Valid Argument. A formal criterion for evaluating an argument in which the premises imply a conclusion. The criterion is the impermissibility of premises that are all true followed by a false conclusion.

Index

Italicized page numbers followed by italicized letters indicate tables (*t*) and figures (*f*).

Italicized page numbers followed by italicized letters indicate tables (*t*) and figures (*f*).

Italicized page numbers followed by italicized letters indicate tables (*t*) and figures (*f*).